End-of-Life Care for Children and Adults With Intellectual and Developmental Disabilities

End-of-Life Care for Children and Adults With Intellectual and Developmental Disabilities

Edited by
Sandra L. Friedman, MD, MPH
and
David T. Helm, PhD

Foreword by Allen C. Crocker, MD

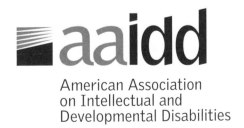

aaidd

American Association
on Intellectual and
Developmental Disabilities

Published by
American Association on Intellectual and Developmental Disabilities
501 3rd Street, NW, Suite 200
Washington, DC 20001-2760

Printed in the United States of America

Library of Congress Cataloging-in-Publication Data

End-of-life care for children and adults with intellectual and developmental
disabilities / edited by Sandra L. Friedman and David T. Helm.
    p. ; cm.
  Includes bibliographical references and index.
  ISBN 978-1-935304-07-4
  1. Terminal care. 2. People with mental disabilities—Care. 3. Developmentally
disabled—Care. I. Friedman, Sandra L. II. Helm, David T. III. American Association
on Intellectual and Developmental Disabilities.
  [DNLM: 1. Mentally Disabled Persons. 2. Terminal Care—ethics. 3. Adult.
4. Bioethical Issues. 5. Child. WB 310 E553 2010]
  R726.8.E5323 2010
    362.17'5—dc22   2010003479

In loving memory of my father, Dr. William W. Friedman, and my sister, Joan Friedman, whose lives ended far too soon. They continue to provide me with inspiration.

SLF

To my parents—my father, Dr. John D. Helm, Jr., who showed me how to provide a dignified and supported end of life for my mother, Grace H. Helm.

DTH

Contents

Foreword

ALLEN C. CROCKER

This book is a thorough and thoughtful compilation on the phenomena connected with end of life in the setting of intellectual and developmental disabilities (IDD). The editors have chosen well, and all of the authors are to be commended for their energy and sensitivity. The phenomenology of aging as it affects persons with IDD is humanistically described (almost in family terms), and the effects of aging on caretakers is also considered. As an addition to notes on the culture of aging well, we now added the anticipation of dying well, and a good death is reflected upon here. These considerations are earnestly described.

There is a fellowship of sorts to approaching death, and in this book it receives a notable respect. I have a special sympathy for this given my own sunset position. This book on dying is solemn but not dispirited. Palliative care and its strategies are warmly presented. Hospice emerges with special richness.

To make up this introduction, an excerpt of varying length is presented from each chapter in direct quotation. Taken together they capture key messages from the text and portray the depth of material covered. The call for stewardship is clear; this book will help.

1

The merging of the social consequences of an increasingly more defined bioethical stance toward patients' rights both in research and in clinical work, the recognition of the consequences of the medicalization of the dying process, and the increased influence of the disability rights movement have resulted in a more humanistic and respectful process in end-of-life care.

How to anticipate upcoming needs of patients and how to secure resources to assist them are crucial for successful planning at the end of life. Providers and families can maximize end-of-life care that is compassionate and competent, dignified, and respectful. Although the end of life is inevitable for all individuals, it is becoming increasingly possible that children and adults with IDD can participate in constructing their own end-of-life scenario to obtain a "good death," or at least one that is as good as a well-planned ending can be.

2

Against a backdrop of increased community inclusion, decisions about health care and end-of-life care have moved center stage for people with IDD, their families, disability

ix

self-advocacy organizations, hospitals, hospices, disability service providers, bioethicists, attorneys, and legislators.

The average life expectancy of people with IDD is currently nearly that of the general population's, and, like the general population, they confront aging and end-of-life issues.

In addition to social policies, four social movements have influenced the attitudes of the general population and those of people with IDD and their families about health and end-of-life decision making: the hospice movement; the civil rights movement; the movement for consumers' rights in health care; and the self-advocacy movement among people with IDD, mental illnesses, and physical disabilities.

People with disabilities are often excluded (more often described as "shielded") from confrontation with life's difficult discussions and experiences, such as illness, aging, loss and dying. They have often been excluded from family funerals, conversations about a roommate's or parent's illness, visiting someone in the hospital, and other normal grief experiences. Families and professionals have explained their exclusion of people with IDD as an effort to spare their feelings, to avoid upsetting them, to prevent them for upsetting other people, or to avoid confusing them in the belief that "they would understand anyway." As a result, exclusion with IDD may be unprepared to participate in discussions about their health care and end-of-life options.

There is no doubt that palliative care choices such as hospices are increasingly utilized by both the general public and for the population of people with disabilities. Families may access hospice care. However, while the general public is increasingly aware of the hospice options, health care professionals do not necessarily consider people with IDD and their families for hospice information or care.

3

People with IDD, similar to the population in general, are living longer due to advances in health care at all phases of life. In 1996, according to a study in California, the difference in projected life expectancy for people with IDD was only 10 years less on average than that of the rest of the population.

Patient preference refers to the right of an individual to make decisions about personal health care treatment. The issue of autonomy and the self-determination of people with IDD is a much discussed topic in health care for people with disabilities. Quality of life varies from person to person, and it may be perceived differently by patients and their health care providers, especially when the patient has IDD. Contextual issues relate to family and provider influences on patient decision making and financial, religious, cultural, confidentiality, resource allocation, legal, research, or conflict of interest issues.

In his book by the same name, Ira Byock, a physician, coins the term "dying well" to describe a process that includes life as well as death, rather than using the popular term "good death," which seems to focus on the end result and gives us little information about the process itself and is therefore of limited value. The concept of "dying well" can be applied to children and adults with IDD and their families. The author notes that this process is very individualized, and the actual specifics for a given person, child or adult, result from that person's unique characteristics. This is consistent with the principle of autonomy, which requires that we respect individuals' unique beliefs and preferences.

4

It is important to note that these medical issues need to be considered in the context of an individual child's medical stability, quality of life, and goals of care. These issues often change with time, and therefore ongoing medical review and communication between the health care team and family with regards to treatment and management decisions are crucial. There are times in which it is appropriate to choose aggressive medical management, times when it is ethically appropriate to choose different options of care, and times when aggressive procedures and treatments may not be recommended.

While the neurological condition associated with cerebral palsy or static encephalopathy may not be progressive, the changes in the neuromuscular and orthopedic systems may progress over time. Significant increase in muscle tone may contribute to discomfort and pain, as well as difficulties with seating, positioning, and providing daily care. To address these issues, muscle relaxants, such as Valium and Baclofen, have been used orally or per gastrostomy tube (G-tube). Medication may also be administered intrathecally, such as with a Baclofen pump. At times, injections of Botox or Phenol are administered, followed by serial casting. In situations in which there is severe impairment, surgical interventions to improve motor function are used, such as selective dorsal root rhizotomy.

There are no easy ways to address all of these issues, and families often approach decisions about the type, intensity, and duration of treatments quite differently. It is always important for accurate information to be presented to families on a proactive and ongoing basis, with opportunities for families to express their values, wishes, and concerns. Respect for the life of a child and for a family's hopes are always important. There are times, however, when our knowledge, expertise, and skills cannot stop the inevitability of death. It is at those times that we must continue to support the comfort and dignity of the patient, and remember that he or she is part of a larger social and family network that also requires our support.

5

Previously, physicians routinely informed mothers of infants with significant IDD that their babies would die within the first 6 months of life. As a result, many people have come to believe that adults with IDD have already long outlived their life expectancies. Consequently, they might believe that it is reasonable to ignore any medical issue that adults with IDD encounter.

However, many of those dire predictions of physicians in the mid-20th century have proven to be erroneous. Indeed, many of the individuals predicted to die within the first 6 months of life are still alive today, some now in their late 90s. In addition, more physicians now advocate for aggressive interventions for reversible, life-threatening conditions in infants with severe developmental and medical problems resulting in an even further increase in life expectancy for individuals with IDD. It is often reported that the only issues that significantly affected life expectancy are mobility and feeding method. It was noted that mobility needed to be quite severely impaired in order to have an effect on life expectancy. In that study, individuals who were independent in feeding orally and able to roll over or sit up on their own had life expectancies within approximately 10 years of those of the general population.

6

Fear over development of respiratory depression is one of the greatest barriers to the use of opioids, including at end of life. This is an unwarranted fear, as opioid-induced respiratory depression is unlikely with a low starting does, appropriate and standard dosing and titration, and adjustment for renal or hepatic impairment in individuals with altered mental status or compromised breathing. An exception can occur if there is a sudden change in the ability to clear opioids or a reduction in pain stimulation. The association of opioid use with end-of-life care can result in an assumption that opioids either hasten death or indicate that someone is dying when he or she is not. When used appropriately and for stated goals, opioids do not hasten death but can assure comfort throughout life.

7

Nutrition for people facing end-of-life care may provide many challenges for the patient, caregiver, and medical team. The provision of nutrition not only offers sustenance with potential comfort and sensory pleasure; it may also cause discomfort at the end of life. In the best of circumstances, the patient, caregiver, and medical team can face these challenges together and come to a consensus on the nutritional support method. For some people with IDD, however, communication may not always be optimal. During these times, the caregiver and the medical team must make decisions based on the presumed wishes and the best interest of the patient in terms of nutritional support versus burden/discomfort in end-of-life care.

8

A hospitalized patient may have an order written by his or her physician for Do Not Resuscitate (DNR). This order typically means the person will not receive cardiopulmonary resuscitation (CPR) in the event his or her heart stops. A physician writes this order based on the wishes of the decision maker(s) and taking into consideration the medical condition of the patient. This is usually used when someone has a condition in which death is imminent or there is little likelihood of surviving CPR. The individual therefore will not receive artificial means to promote breathing or resumption of his or her heartbeat. A person may have a DNR order yet continue to receive treatment for acute illnesses, such as pneumonia, urinary tract infections, fractures, and other acute conditions. Generally, a DNR order assumes that a patient will not be intubated—with a tube placed in is trachea to which oxygen and artificial respiratory support is delivered—or be on a ventilator or other mechanical means of breathing.

9

In general, cognitively competent persons now have a well-established right to make his or her own decisions about health care that includes both informed consent for hospitalization, transfer, treatments, procedures, and surgeries they want to have—including

CPR—and informed refusal of those they do not, including DNR. By extension, persons with IDD have the same right, though it must be exercised by a surrogate decision maker, usually in the case of children his or her parent(s), who is presumed to be responsible for determining either what their child or ward would want if they could choose for themselves (substituted judgment) or what would be best for them (best interests).

10

There are an increasing number of conditions that, while previously considered "lethal," are currently treated "successfully" insofar as they lengthen the life span of these affected individuals. Second, there are an increasing number of conditions that require long-term treatments or therapies, changing them from "acute" to "chronic" conditions. Finally, there are an increasing number of treatment options that extend life with variable "costs" and "benefits."

Devices that support life include mechanical ventilators as well as systems to deliver oxygen other than ventilators, devices to assist circulation for extended periods, devices to clean the body of toxins, and devices to deliver nutritional support. Each one of these treatment interventions, which substitute for major organ systems of the human body, requires significant clinical and technical expertise to initiate, but some require considerably less expertise to maintain. This discrepancy in required expertise between initiation and maintenance of treatment interventions has caused decisions around the foregoing or withdrawing of such supports to be an ethically contentious arena of health care in which families and clinicians may disagree.

11

Many people hold that nutrition and hydration are special—that even if other life supports can be withdrawn, nutrition and hydration still should be provided. It is suggested that basic care is required for all human beings even if they are beyond benefit from medical treatments.

In 1982, a baby born in Indiana with Down syndrome and a cardiac septal defect was left to die on the basis of his parents' decision not to provide treatment.

Regardless of the interpretation of that case, it stimulated considerable public debate and led to the Reagan administration's development of legislation calling for regulations called the "Baby Doe Regulations." After several false starts, a set of regulations was promulgated that requires every state receiving federal funds of activities to protect against child abuse to have in place regulations conforming with federal standards. Under these standards no infant can be allowed to die by the forgoing of life support.

12

An attempt was made between 1992 and 1993 to bring some standardization to the diagnosis and prognosis of persistent vegetative state (PVS). The basic elements of treatment for PVS involve comprehensive supportive care. Nutrition and hydration typically require placement of a feeding tube. Although some nutrition may be swallowed orally by some individuals, it is not usually sufficient to maintain body weight and function. The choice of a nutritional product for chronic maintenance requires careful consideration of the individual's long-term metabolic needs. Periodic monitoring of body weight and laboratory tests to monitor metabolic levels, such as serum albumin levels, provides a measure of nutritional balance. Elimination usually requires assistance using stool softeners or other agents to promote regularity.

Measures to prevent infections are appropriate, and prompt treatment is essential to avoid septicemia and other complications. Skin care is critically important. Bedsores can develop quickly due to the immobility that is typically present and can become secondarily infected.

13

The chapter will begin with an examination of the concept of devaluation, because people with IDD are typically seen as devalued and are treated accordingly. This examination will include the socially devalued roles into which many people with IDD have been cast and the consequence of perception in this devaluation process. It will then explore the themes of dignity, social role valorization, and humanness in order to perceive and understand people with IDD differently and more positively. It will continue by briefly touching upon the barriers that stand in the way of people with IDD in the area of medical and end-of-life care. Finally, it will focus on the dignity-conserving care model and discuss its appropriateness as a strategy to minimize devaluation and to promote best practice in caring for people with IDD who are in fact at the end of their lives.

14

Hundreds of definitions of culture seek to explain a known but at times elusive concept that encompasses and forms everyone's life. Culture provides the lens through which we view, interpret, and find meaning in the world in which we live. Culture structures perceptions, shapes behaviors, and defines our sense of reality. Culture defines health and well-being. It also defines and determines the manner in which we recognize and cope with illness and disability. Culture frames attitudes and beliefs about death and determines mourning rituals. It is not uncommon that under stress, a person relies on aspects of culture that have long been neglected or thought of as unimportant. The cultural beliefs and practices of families, and the communities in which they live, are assets and a great source of strength to a person with IDD throughout life and at the time of death.

15

One of the familiar spiritual symbols from Eastern traditions is the Chinese character for "crisis," consisting of characters for both "challenge" and "opportunity." Professionals, families, friends, and caregivers who work with people with IDD simply cannot deal with end-of-life issues and experiences without encountering profound spiritual feelings, questions, and opportunities. The challenges come from the ways that IDD relates to our own understandings of spirituality; our own conceptions of how people with IDD deal with grief and loss; and the ways that issues of grief, loss, and death pervade our systems of care even without being named and addressed. This chapter will thus first provide a framework for understanding spirituality and IDD, and the ways that end-of-life issues raise both universal and unique spiritual questions in the world of IDD.

16

Along with the trend toward increased longevity, there have been significant strides in normalizing the lives of individuals with IDD. Many of them now live within the community in group homes, with family members, in special assisted-living facilities, or even on their own. They have, as other people do, created and sustained attachments to a variety of persons—family members, fellow residents and consumers, staff members, coworkers, members of their faith communities, and other friends.

One of the prices of such attachments is that individuals with IDD experience loss just like everyone else. They are now likely to outlive their parents. Loss inherently is a part of communal living as staff members and other residents relocate or die. In fact, individuals with IDD may experience significant secondary losses that may complicate grief. The death of a parent or caregiver, for example, may necessitate a change in residence leading to a range of losses that might include friends, neighbors, and employment.

17

Rituals around healthcare and end of life are often significant and hold great meaning to the person with whom we are planning. Rituals can bring comfort, solace, and a sense of familiarity and consistency; they deserve the attention of planners and must be addressed in planning.

18

Results of a retrospective study of parents whose children died in the intensive care unit revealed that more than half of the parents reported that they had little control during their child's final days. Moreover, one-fourth of the parents reported that if they had another chance, they would have acted differently. Furthermore, it was the physician (90% of the time) who initiated discussion about withdrawal of life support, although nearly half of the parents had considered it before the conversation was ever formally raised.

19

The decision to transition to end-of-life care should be based on a realistic prognosis for a cure; knowledge of the preferences of the people with disabilities or if those preferences are not known, preferences of the family, close friends, or direct care staff; and a balance of the benefits and burdens to the people with disabilities.

When individuals with disabilities are diagnosed with a terminal condition, there should not be an automatic assumption that treatment will be refused. As with anyone with a terminal condition, the benefits and burdens should be weighed.

20

Hospice is a philosophy-driven system of care that is focused on noncurative services provided in the last 6 months of life. Hospice provides continuous palliative and supportive services to dying people and their families, through physical, psychological, social, and spiritual care given in the home or in freestanding centers. Hospice reimbursement requires physician certification and explicit redirection of care from curative to palliative treatment.

Preface

Doreen Croser, Executive Director of the American Association on Intellectual and Developmental Disabilities, first mentioned the idea of writing a book on the subject of end-of-life care for people with intellectual and developmental disabilities (IDD) a few years ago. This conversation occurred after the public debate regarding Terri Schiavo, who did not have a developmental disability per se, but rather an acquired etiology for her persistent vegetative state. Because of that case, more public attention was being given to end-of-life issues, particularly withdrawal of support. Much controversy and confusion continues to exist regarding the medical and ethical issues surrounding the end of life for all people, not just those with disabilities. This book was born from the desire to provide clarification and insight to some of these compelling issues.

Book Organization

There have been many publications on the subject of end-of-life care although few, if any, that take the subject of people with IDD from broad social, political, medical, ethical, and practical perspectives. People with IDD have similar issues related to death and dying to those in the general population. However, they also have many unique challenges that must be considered and addressed in order to provide comprehensive, humanistic, and high-quality care at end of life.

The subjects covered in this book are written by individuals with expertise in their respective professional fields. Some of the information may be considered controversial, and some of the chapters touch upon similar information, which was expected when putting together this group of authors and selected topics. The chapters were written to be read within the context of the other chapters, or to stand alone and be read individually, if so desired. Each author brings his or her own vantage point to this complex subject. In many instances, there is no "right" or "wrong" way to approach a particular issue, but rather the need to individualize care as part of a process that includes ongoing communication among the patient, if possible, his or her surrogates, other stakeholders, and the medical team. However, certain fundamental ethical tenets underlie the process of making decisions and providing care. At the center of these discussions is the importance for respect, dignity, and the needs of the person with whom, or for whom, decisions are being made. Hopefully, the topics presented will provide a broad perspective, leading to more conversations about how to best address these issues and make important decisions.

The first section provides historical and foundational materials to end-of-life care for children and adults with IDD. Although the scope of the book does not allow a complete history in this area, these chapters accentuate the salient issues that affect the current state of practice and care. The authors chose critical events in the historical and social context that they believe would be informative and, at times, provocative. From this section, the reader will better understand and appreciate how policies impact practices at the end of life in the areas of medicine, law, and ethics.

The second section provides information regarding medical conditions that may be associated with a lower life expectancy, as well as common conditions encountered at the end of life. Frameworks of care are provided, particularly with emphasis on challenges in decision making when caring for adults and children with IDD. Chronic and acute management of various medical and nutritional issues are presented. In this section the reader is provided with a health-related overview in order to obtain an appreciation for the complexity of issues involved in caring for this population.

End-of-life care, particularly for vulnerable populations, is inherently controversial. There are many ways to approach the same problem, with social, religious, and emotional elements influencing people's viewpoints. The third section of the book discusses many of these controversies and also provides some guidelines for making decisions that are thoughtful, respectful, and ethical. The reader will be presented with the complexities of these issues and will understand the importance of involving all relevant stakeholders when making decisions.

The fourth part of this book more directly addresses the social, emotional, and spiritual needs of the patients, their families, and caregivers. The authors provide practical frameworks to approach these topics that are often overlooked but are critical to providing comprehensive and compassionate care. The familial, religious, and cultural contexts are important considerations when supporting the broad needs at end of life. The reader will gain a better understanding of the perspective of people with IDD when these individuals are confronted with issues related to death and dying.

The fifth section of the book provides information about how to support children, adults, and their families in planning for the end of life. Community services and resources, written material and curricula, and practical management tools are referenced. The reader will understand the scope of resources available to families and providers to which they may refer to and use when caring for people with IDD at the end of life.

TERMINOLOGY

We would like to provide a word about terminology and language. Throughout the book, "person-first" language was used (e.g., children with disabilities rather than disabled children). We combined intellectual and developmental disabilities into one term, IDD. More strictly defined, a person with an intellectual disability demonstrates significant limitations in the areas of intellectual functioning and adaptive behavior and skills, and they often require more community supports. A person with a developmental disability may present with impairments in a number of developmental and related domains, such as in the areas of cognitive, sensory, neurological, emotional, and behavioral abilities and functioning.

In this book, "end of life" is used as a noun, referring to a state before dying. "End-of-life" is used as an adjective, when describing a particular state or situation (e.g., end-of-life care, end-of-life decisions).

ACKNOWLEDGMENTS

We wish to acknowledge a number of people who kindly and generously contributed their time and expertise to the writing of this book. We thank Doreen Croser for her encouragement and foresight. We also thank the people on the editorial board of the American Association on Intellectual and Developmental Disabilities (AAIDD) who wisely provided the initial input on our proposed content. We are most grateful for the generous support and confidence provided by the editorial staff of AAIDD, particularly Bruce Appelgren and Anu Prabhla. While each of the chapters were read, reviewed, and edited by both of us, we had a group of peer reviewers—also experts in their respective fields who read and provided invaluable feedback for each of the chapters. These peer reviewers included Jay Berry, Sharon Cermak, Allen Crocker, Beverley Gilligan, Laurie Glader, Janet Hirsch, David Hoff, Angela Howell-Moneta, Kerim Munir, Wendy Nehring, Priscilla Osborne, Stephanie Porter, Patricia Rissmiller, and Ludwik Szymanski.

A special thanks to Allen Crocker, for his thoughtful and forever wise words. We are most grateful to all of our contributing authors, who each took upon his or her chapter with genuine interest and passion for the subject about which they wrote. And last, but certainly not least, we are most appreciative to our families—Terry, Jon, and Zach Patinkin, and Janet Hirsch, Alex, and Daniel Helm—for their continued love and support.

Sandra L. Friedman and David T. Helm

PART I

Historical Perspective

CHAPTER 1

Constructing a "Good Death"

Historical and Social Frameworks

DAVID T. HELM AND SANDRA L. FRIEDMAN

The end of life is inevitable. The ability to control and participate in one's own life-ending scenario is not. Longer lives, heightened awareness of impending death, and various planning strategies permit us to construct an all-things-being-equal plan for controlling our own "good death" scenario. That vision is certainly culturally prescribed and varies greatly from individual to individual or from family to family. It is, however, centrally connected to a sense of justice and fairness and to an ethically and competently administered and facilitated sequence. In hospice and palliative care settings, the definition of a "good death" refers to a process wherein the dying, their loved ones, and health care workers mutually accept the approaching death and share end-of-life decisions (Conway, 2007; McNamara, 1998). The goal of the chapters that follow is to help facilitate a process in which individuals with intellectual and developmental disabilities (IDD), their families, and loved ones can join with health care providers to reach that end. Unfortunately, the imagined as compared to the experienced end of life are often far removed.

The face of death has changed over the years. Death is rarely the family or community event it once was. The process of dying is now more often mediated by a bevy of health care providers, hospital administrators or regulators of some ilk, insurance overseers, and a host of other unrelated parties (Kellehear, 2007). This chapter looks at the connection between the individual's social construction of a good death and the realities and responsibilities of those whose job it is to ensure that the individual's or family's wishes for end-of-life care are carried out with compassion, competence, and dignity to the best of everyone's abilities.

It is well known that gains have been made in the areas of life expectancy, social and community inclusion, and participation in everyday activities for individuals with IDD. However, we have not yet realized all that can be done to improve the lives of people with disabilities, which includes end-of-life care. The end-of-life experiences and options for people with IDD should, and now more frequently do, mirror those of their peers without disabilities. Participation in the planning of one's own death or end-of-life care needs to be carefully reviewed and orchestrated such that whatever the image may be, the "good death" or "best way to die" can be thoughtful and carried out with dignity and caring for both the individuals and their families. Attention to the differing notions or constructions of what that may mean will vary across cultural contexts, but with planning, a "good death" can be realized. In the general population, this is occurring with increased frequency as more people demand control over their end-of-life decision making and care. It is only recently that individuals with IDD and their families started to demand those rights and procure those assurances. The process of recognizing that these rights also include individuals who have traditionally been excluded from equal rights or who have been devalued has been long and has often been fought in the courts and through legislation.

Death in this and other industrialized countries has become medicalized in most circumstances, with over 80% of individuals in the general population dying in hospital or institutional care (Klinenberg, 2001; Office of National Statistics, 2004). By comparison, it used to be that the death of an individual occurred within one's home, was embraced by one's community, and was a relatively short process supported by friends and neighbors. The epidemiological transition that has been occurring over the course of the century—that is, the transition from acute illnesses to chronic or degenerative illnesses as the primary cause of death and the consequently longer, more drawn-out dying process—has resulted in longer hospitalizations and institutional care. This propensity of a slow decline has naturally required an increase in medical treatments with the concurrent medicalization of the dying process. The resulting care, including management of pain and complex medical treatments, has too often prevented dying patients from being able to participate in, let alone control, their end-of-life care. The implementation of more palliative care processes has created the opportunity to rehumanize the process that had become dehumanized and detached from the family. Asserting control over one's own death, to some degree, or one's end-of-life care is becoming a new reality for many.

Death in earlier times was more normalized, visible, and part of everyday life. Modern medicine associated with caring for the dying, typically within a hospital setting, has made death and dying a hidden phenomenon, one controlled by experts and those often not related to the individuals or their culture. Death and the regulations surrounding the process are, at least partially, removed from the emotional and spiritual realm and focus more on the procedural. However, that being said, regulations do not necessarily foreclose the possibility of including the individual and their family from the process or planning for the end of life and operationalizing goals of care that take into account the individual's and family's wishes and cultural beliefs. These processes have been particularly difficult to realize if the individual has IDD or is removed from the setting of his or her family and is residing in an institutional setting. Historically these difficulties stem from a number of social and political ambiguities, including a lack of ethical clarity, the reliance on the growing influence of medical expertise to solve all problems, and the longstanding social devaluation of individuals with severe IDD. Some of these changing historical and sociological trends have had a profound impact on the current social, emotional, medical, and cultural landscapes that contribute to creating a "good death."

BIOETHICAL FOUNDATIONS

For centuries medical personnel have taken seriously the basic tenets of the Hippocratic oath, including the promise to do no harm as well as other guidelines that forswear euthanasia, the seduction of patients, or the divulging of patients' secrets. However, it is only since the 1960s that bioethics, the study of ethical issues pertaining to the biological sciences and health care, emerged as a distinct field and began to capture the public's concern. This has had a strong impact on both research and clinical practice, which have a history replete with instances where vulnerable populations, including individuals with IDD, were treated in ways that would now be considered blatantly unethical.

Since its beginning in 1847, the American Medical Association (AMA) required its members to subscribe to its Code of Ethics. This code primarily pertained to medical etiquette rather than to what we might now consider to be bioethics. The genesis of much of our current foundation for ethical decision making stems from the Nuremberg Trials and the resultant Nuremberg Code (1948). These trials brought to light the extent to which human rights can be violated when left unchecked (Yan & Munir, 2004). The policies and practices that occurred in Germany and elsewhere at that time reflected a belief in eugenics. Some of these policies were also unfortunately enacted in the United States, although to a lesser extent (Lifton, 1986). The atrocities that occurred in Europe are now well known and widely reported as they came to light during the Nuremberg Trials. The decision of those trials formed the basis of the Nuremberg Code. The Code particularly highlighted that subjects must give informed consent with full understanding of potential risks and benefits before they participate in any research. For our purposes, it is of issue to note that this informed consent must come from the participants themselves, thus putting children or individuals with IDD at some continued risk.

The trials had received some publicity in the United States, but their immediate impact on medical practice in the United States was minimal (Rothman, 1991). As new technologies were developed and as health care costs continued to rise through the 1960s, new ethical questions began to be raised regarding the use of life-support systems for persons in a coma, access to new procedures such as kidney dialysis, and the development of organ transplant waiting lists. The spark that ignited the public debate was an article written by Henry Beecher in the *New England Journal of Medicine* in 1966. Here he described 22 research studies published in peer-reviewed journals that had used ethically questionable methods. He then looked at 100 consecutive research studies published in medical journals and found that researchers in 12 of the studies had not told their subjects the risks involved in participating in the research or, in some cases, that they were even involved in an experiment (Beecher, 1966; Weitz, 2001). Beecher's work not only captured the attention of the professional and medical world but also awoke the public's concern. The result of this revelation was the 1966 publication by the U.S. Public Health Service of a new and revamped guideline for protecting human subjects in medical research. The 1960s are often proclaimed as the birth of the bioethics movement (Fox, 1974; Rothman, 1991). Yet the 1970s would reveal that these ethical dilemmas had not disappeared.

The revelations discovered and made public in the Willowbrook hepatitis study, the Tuskegee syphilis study, and the Karen Quinlan case all stimulated more regulations and guidelines for medical practice. The Willowbrook hepatitis study reported on experiments on children with IDD who were either intentionally infected with hepatitis or knowingly not treated when diagnosed in order to study the natural course of the disease. The research began in 1956 and continued up until 1972. It was successfully argued that the children were not properly informed (if at all) nor did their parents voluntarily provide consent for their children to participate (Ramsey, 1970). The debate and public outcry halted the research shortly thereafter. Similarly, the Tuskegee syphilis study, which began as early as 1932, was discovered to be ongoing as late as 1972. It was revealed that 399 poor and mostly illiterate African-American men who were infected with late-stage syphilis were left untreated in order to carry out medical research about the effects of the infection even though penicillin, discovered in the 1940s, was known to be an effective treatment. The study exposed medical research practices that preyed upon the disenfranchised, the uneducated, and others who were fundamentally powerless in society: namely, minority populations, including those who had IDD (Jones, 1993). The resulting legacy continues today with many African-American communities not trusting public health workers and the "medical-industrial complex" in general.

In 1975, a few years after both studies, the case of Karen Ann Quinlan garnered much public attention. At the age of 21, Quinlan had fallen into a coma after ingesting a combination of drugs. She suffered extensive brain damage, and medical experts believed there was no chance of her regaining mental or physical functioning. The debate centered on the right to die and her parents' request that she be removed from all life-sustaining machines. After a yearlong court battle, she was removed from the ventilator, although she remained alive for an additional 10 years as staff continued to provide her with artificial nutrition and hydration as well as antibiotics for acute infections. This case was widely debated in the public and raised the issue of the right to die. For the first time, it also posed problems related to too much, rather than too little, access to medical technology (Weitz, 2001). The legal system was now entering the health care decision-making process in full force.

In the 1980s and 1990s, new ethical dilemmas regarding the control of medical technology, or the rights to gain access to it, were confronted. How far can or should medical interventions go to disrupt or change the natural human process in life and death decisions? Reproductive technology came to the forefront when the "test-tube baby" hit the front pages of the news. Questions arose regarding who should have the ability to control human conception, what the parameters for human engineering would be, and how the future of medical technology was to be controlled. The issue of in vitro fertilization posed the initial ethical dilemma regarding modern medicine's active role in human development outside of the traditional or natural processes. These debates continue in today's world with issues raised from the human genome project, cloning technologies, and prenatal testing protocols.

The result of these public revelations of morally debatable, and often reprehensible, events has been the development of ethics committees, institutional review boards, and professional standards. The impact on research, medical education, and clinical practice has been substantial, if at times controversial (Annas, 1991; Hafferty & Franks, 1994, Zussman, 1992). The public interest must be protected and researchers and clinicians are required to live up to reviewable standards and codes of ethical behavior. It is this background that sets the foundation for clinical behaviors relating to the clinical practice at the end of life.

Medicalization of Death

As the population began to rely more heavily on medical interventions to ease pain, as the dominance of the biomedical model grew along with technology, and as dying became a more drawn-out experience, death became medicalized (Illich, 1976). We often now talk about the medicalization of society—the slow transformation of all human conditions into treatable disorders (Conrad, 2007). That is, conditions, circumstances, and behaviors have become defined and are treated as medical problems. This trend has been written about for years (Balard & Elston, 2005; Lock, 2001), and some have called it "one of the most potent transformations of the last half century in the West" (Clarke, Shim, Mamo, Fosket, & Fishman, 2003, p. 161). Many social factors have contributed to this trend and have set the context in which this transformation has flourished, including the increased faith in science to solve problems and possibly the decreased faith in religion to do the same. Similarly, technological progress and general humanitarian trends in Western civilization have promoted medical intervention. Thus, as opposed to individual medical or health care personnel attempting to control new conditions or circumstances, there have been a number of social trends pushing medicine to do so. Although many social scientists at least imply a critical overtone toward excessive involvement or too much control from medicine, some have called for collaboration between patient and doctor, differentiating between medicalization and medical dominance (Broom & Westward, 1996). Others argue that we are now in a demedicalization trend, moving toward holistic treatments and complementary and alternative medicine (CAM), and some prefer the term "biomedicalization," which brings stronger connotations of technological and scientific findings and procedures (Clarke et al., 2003). Conrad argues that the influences of the ongoing trend of medicalization can be summarized as the coming together of biotechnology (pharmaceutical advancements and genetics), consumer demands and preferences, and managed care (Conrad, 2007, 2009).

Each component of these social trends has increased the demand for medical intervention to enhance human comfort and thus prolong a good life. It is clear that biotechnology, often in the form of pharmaceutical advancements, is seen everywhere, in all phases of life from birth to death. Drugs are viewed as the cure-all, the least invasive medical treatment used to prevent problems (e.g., lowering cholesterol and risk for heart attack) and solve problems (e.g., depression, hyperactivity). This appeal has been taken directly to the consumer since the U.S. Food and Drug Administration passed the Modernization Act in 1997, allowing for wider and more direct promotion of products, most evident on television. Patients have demanded more access to drugs, and the pharmaceutical companies have taken hold of that demand to satisfy the outcry and, at times, to create new markets (Conrad & Potter, 2004; Koerner, 2002). This consumer demand has strengthened the medicalization movement in all facets of health and illness, including end-of-life care.

Consumers themselves have demanded medical intervention and treatment not only for "classic" medical maladies such as heart disease and cancer but also for the "correction" of human variation through selective surgery (Sullivan, 2001) and medication for mood disorders or personality variations of all kinds (Barsky & Boros, 1995; Shaw & Woodward, 2004). Thus, medical treatment of human problems has become the rule rather than the exception.

It is beyond the scope of this chapter to fully discuss these social trends and resulting influences on medicalization; however, a third element that must be discussed is the oversight of this pharmaceutical explosion and consumer demand by managed care systems. The delivery of health care in the United States is clearly dominated by managed care organizations with various bureaucratic gatekeepers actively involved throughout the process. This is a complex relationship that both encourages and limits medicalization (Conrad, 2009). Thus, for instance, managed care may reduce coverage for psychotherapy for individuals with mental and emotional problems (Shore & Beigal, 1996) but may be more open to paying for psychiatric medications (Goode, 2002). These social forces come together to begin to transform human differences into pathological conditions, all with a medical remedy or intervention. Unfortunately, "the great danger here is that transforming all differences into pathology diminishes our tolerance for and appreciation of the diversity of human life" (Conrad, 2007, p. 148).

The results of medicalization have generally been positive, with new hope generated for cure, treatment, and care of a host of human maladies. Similarly, "blame," or acceptance of responsibility for an individual's condition, is mitigated when a medical diagnosis is attached: one is typically not held accountable for one's behavior or actions if it is deemed to be caused by a medical condition beyond the control of the individual. We must remember, however, that the positive aspects of the trend toward medicalization of behaviors or conditions may also be accompanied by social risk, negative outcomes, and pockets of resistance. That is, medicine can now often be seen as the definer of what is "normal," and thus medicalization creates an insidious stigma for those who are deemed different. This has generated resistance to a number of facets of the medicalization of life, especially in disability communities or elsewhere where differences can be and are celebrated. The disability rights movement is particularly wary of too much adherence to and acceptance of the medical model as opposed to celebration of human differences and variations.

DISABILITY RIGHTS MOVEMENT

As an extension of the civil rights movement, the disability rights movement has been increasingly active and growing for decades (Batavia & Schriner, 2001; Fleischer & Zamers, 2001; Shapiro, 1993, 1994) as the voices of individuals with disabilities, their family members, and supporters have been addressing classic rights for access to employment, housing, education, and community inclusion in general. The success of this movement is well known and includes many legislative advances, epitomized by the American with Disabilities Act (ADA) in 1990 and the American with Disabilities Act Amendments Act of 2008 (ADA-AA). The rights of individuals with IDD have been advancing in all facets of social life, including in the relationships between individuals and the medical world and the attitudes within the medical world.

Throughout history, medical views on individuals with IDD have not been altogether favorable, nor have medical attitudes been particularly welcoming (see chapters in this volume by Botsford & King, and Levy & van Stone). Individuals who are different, or who have conditions that create functional limitations or shortened life expectancies, have often been looked at as inferior and substandard. Only a brief reminder of the eugenics movements will bring this to light all too quickly (Pfeiffer, 1994). Those ideological stances have been successfully defeated for the most part, although remnants of that era reappear from time to time. The lasting social or attitudinal remnant that is often unintentionally sustained by the medicalization movement is that individuals with disabilities are still devalued in all sorts of obvious and covert ways (see chapter by Lutfiyya & Schwartz). This, then, can play a role in the end-of-life care expected by or given to individuals with IDD.

Individuals with disabilities routinely look warily toward the broad social view that focuses on the narrower medical realm that designates them as sick, a realm that often assumes or forces them to take on the sick role when in fact they are not ill. The lack of distinction between a medical model and a disability model can be traced to the root of social discrimination and exclusion and can thus play a role in end-of-life care and related social expectations as well as policy (Turnbull & Stowe, 2001). That is, when a medical definition or norm becomes the basis of what society regards as normal for bodily functions, intellectual capacity, articulation, or possibly hearing, for example, then those who do not meet such standards are deemed less worthy and possibly stigmatized as "subhuman." The deaf community certainly has stood up to such characterizations, as have many in the disability rights movement (Conrad, 2007; Fleischer & Zamers, 2001). It is the notion of the medical sense of "normal" that can confront or compromise the end-of-life care provided individuals with IDD.

In the broader social and policy arena, such organizations as ADAPT (Johnson & Shaw, 2001) and Not Dead Yet (http://www.notdeadyet.org/docs/about.html) have been particularly vocal in dissent and resistance to the right-to-die movement that had been epitomized in the Dr. Kevorkian and, later, the Teri Schiavo situations. Both organizations call for more public discussion about who controls end-of-life scenarios and how policy and public opinion will play a role in individual choices surrounding this issue. Professional caregivers play critical roles in working with and assisting individuals to make these difficult yet important decisions.

A backdrop to increasing end-of-life care options for individuals with IDD is the broader patient rights movement. Within this movement there is a segment of the patient population that gained momentum from Kubler-Ross's (1969) publication of *On Death and Dying*, which called attention to the dehumanizing aspects of modern medical treatment for the dying, including any individual who had been given a terminal diagnosis, which is typically accompanied by chronic or degenerative conditions where life expectancies are severely limited and death is imminent. In this case, ethical dilemmas of control and caring within the circumstances of the individual's end-of-life care become paramount. The relationship between care providers and consumers "is fraught with ethical issues relating to power" (Friedman, Helm, & Marrone, 1999, p. 349). It is how this power is utilized that makes end-of-life care comforting or not.

Role relationships between providers and patients have a long history in sociological literature beginning in the 1950s and continuing today (Anderson & Helm, 1979; Love, Mainour, Talvet, & Hager, 2000; Parsons, 1951; Szasz & Hollander, 1957), and who is in the best position to make decisions in life-and-death situations has likewise been a topic for study and debate (Hackler & Hiller, 1990; Nursey, Rohde, & Farmer, 1990). The relationship challenge, however, still lies in being able to provide the best and most comprehensive care to an individual with IDD while working closely with the family and other caregivers

(Friedman, Helm, & Marrone, 1999). The disability rights movement, as do all similar political movements, essentially boils down to respecting all individuals equally, thus providing them with person-centered and culturally competent care that fosters their autonomy and independence and therefore their right to make their own decisions.

Conclusions

The merging of the social consequences of an increasingly more defined bioethical stance toward patients' rights both in research and in clinical work, the recognition of the consequences of the medicalization of the dying process, and the increased influence of the disability rights movement have resulted in a more humanistic and respectful process in end-of-life care. These historical and social trends create the backdrop on which this book focuses.

The remaining chapters of the book provide information on children and adults with IDD and some of the risks they face that may bring on premature death. How to anticipate upcoming needs of patients and how to secure resources to assist them is crucial for successful planning at the end of life. Providers and families can maximize end-of-life care that is compassionate and competent, dignified and respectful. Although the end of life is inevitable for all individuals, it is becoming increasingly possible that children and adults with IDD can participate in constructing their own end-of-life scenario to obtain a "good death," or at least one that is as good as a well-planned ending can be.

References

Anderson, W. T., & Helm, D. T. (1979). The patient-physician encounter: A process of reality negotiation. In E. G. Jaco (Ed.), *Patients, physicians and illness* (3rd ed., pp. 259–271). New York: Free Press.

Annas, G. J. (1991, May–June). Ethics committees: From ethical comfort to ethical cover. *Hastings Center Report, 21*, 18–21.

Balard, K., & Elston, M. A. (2005). Medicalization: A multi-dimensional concept. *Social Theory and Health, 3*, 228–241.

Barsky, A. J., & Borus, J. F. (1995). Somatization and medicalization in the era of managed care. *Journal of the American Medical Association, 274*, 1931–1934.

Batavia, A. I., & Schriner, K. (2001). The Americans With Disabilities Act as engine of social change. *Policy Studies Journal, 29*, 690–702.

Beecher, H. K. (1966). Ethics and clinical research. *New England Journal of Medicine, 274*, 1354–1360.

Broom, D. H., & Woodward, R. V. (1996). Medicalization reconsidered: Toward a collaborative approach to care. *Sociology of Health and Illness, 18*, 357–378.

Clarke, A. E., Shim, J. K., Mamo, L., Fosket, J. R., & Fishman, J. R. (2003). Biomedicalization: Technoscientific transformations of health, illness and U.S. biomedicine. *American Sociological Review, 68*, 161–194.

Conrad, P. (2007). *The medicalization of society: On the transformation of human conditions into treatable disorders*. Baltimore: John Hopkins University Press.

Conrad, P. (2009). The shifting engines of medicalization. In P. Conrad (Ed.), *The sociology of health & illness: Critical perspectives* (8th ed., pp. 480–492). New York: Worth.

Conrad, P., & Potter, D. (2004). Human growth hormone and the temptations of biomedical enhancement. *Sociology of Health & Illness, 26*, 184–215.

Conway, S. (2007). The changing face of death: Implications for public health. *Critical Public Health, 17*(3), 195–202.

Fleischer, D. Z., & Zames, F. (2000). *Disability rights movement: From charity to confrontation.* Philadelphia: Temple University Press.

Fox, R. C. (1974). Ethical and existential developments in contemporaneous American medicine: Their implications for culture and society. *MillBank Memorial Fund Quarterly, 52,* 445–483.

Friedman, S. L., Helm, D. T., & Marrone, J. (1999). Caring, control, and clinicians' influence: Ethical dilemmas in developmental disabilities. *Ethics & Behavior, 9*(4), 349–364.

Goode, E. (2002, November 6). Psychotherapy shows a rise over decade, but time falls. *New York Times,* p. A21.

Hackler, J. C., & Hiller, F. C. (1990). Family consent to orders not to resuscitate. *Journal of the American Medical Association, 264,* 1281.

Hafferty, F. W., & Franks, R. (1994). The hidden curriculum, ethics teaching, and the structure of medical education. *Academic Medicine, 69,* 861–867.

Illich, I. (1976). *Medical nemesis.* New York: Pantheon.

Johnson, M., & Shaw, B. (Eds.). (2001). *To ride the public's busses: The fight that built a movement.* Louisville, KY: Advocado Press.

Jones, J. (1993). *Bad blood: The Tuskegee Syphilis Experiment* (Rev. ed.). New York: Free Press.

Kellehear, A. (2007). The end of death in late modernity: An emerging public health challenge. *Critical Public Health, 17,* 71–79.

Klinenberg, E. (2001). Dying alone: The social production of urban isolation. *Ethnography, 2*(4), 501–531.

Koerner, B. I. (2002). Disorders, made to order. *Mother Jones, 27,* 58–63.

Kubler-Ross, E. (1969). *On death and dying.* New York: Macmillan.

Lifton, R. (1986). *The Nazi doctors: Medical killing and the psychology of genocide.* New York: Basic Books.

Lock, M. (2001). Medicalization: Cultural concerns. In N. J. Smelser & P. B. Baltes (Eds.), *International encyclopedia of the social and behavioral sciences* (pp. 9534–9539). New York: Elsevier.

Love, M. M., Mainour, A. F., Talvet, J. C., & Hager, G. L. (2000). Continuity of care and the physician-patient relationship. *Journal of Family Practice, 49,* 998–1004.

McNamara, B. (1998). A good enough death? In A. Peterson & C. Waddell (Eds.), *Health matters: A sociology of illness prevention and care* (pp. 169–184). Buckingham: Open University Press.

Not Dead Yet. (n.d.). Retrieved March 27, 2009, from http://www.notdeadyet.org/docs/about.html

Nursey, A. D., Rohde, J. R., & Farmer, R. D. (1990). A study of doctors' and parents' attitudes to people with mental handicaps. *Journal of Mental Deficiency, 34,* 143–155.

Office of National Statistics. (2004). *Mortality statistics* (Series DH1, No. 37). London: Author.

Parsons, T. (1951). *The social system.* New York: Free Press.

Pfeiffer, D. (1994). Eugenics and disability discrimination. *Disability & Society, 9,* 481–499.

Ramsey, P. (1970). *The patient as person.* New Haven, CT: Yale University Press.

Rothman, D. (1991). *Strangers at the bedside: A history of how law and bioethics transformed medical decision-making.* New York: Basic.

Shapiro J. P. (1993). *No pity: People with disabilities forging a new civil rights movement.* New York: Times Books.

Shapiro, J. P. (1994). Disability policy and the media: A stealth civil rights movement bypasses the press and defies conventional wisdom. *Policy Studies Journal 22,* 123–32.

Shaw, I., & Woodward, L. (2004). The medicalization of unhappiness?: The management of mental distress in primary care. In I. Shaw & K. Kauppinen (Eds.), *Constructions of health and illness: European perspectives.* Aldershot, UK: Ashgate Press.

Shore, M. F. & Beigel, A. (1996). The challenges posed by managed behavioral health care. *New England Journal of Medicine 334,* 116–18.

Sullivan, D. A. (2001). *Cosmetic surgery: The cutting edge of commercial medicine in America.* New Brunswick, NJ: Rutgers University Press.

Szasz, T., & Hollander, M. (1956). A contribution to the philosophy of medicine: The basic models of doctor-patient relationships. *Journal of the American Medical Association, 97,* 585–592.

Weitz, R. (2001). *The sociology of health, illness and health care.* Belmont, CA: Wadsworth.

Yan, E. G., & Munir, K. M. (2004). Regulatory and ethical principles in research involving children and individuals with developmental disabilities. *Ethics & Behavior, 14*(1), 31–40.

Zussman, R. (1992). *Intensive care: Medical ethics and the medical profession.* Chicago: University of Chicago Press.

Chapter 2

End-of-Life Policies and Practices

Anne L. Botsford and Angela King

Introduction

Against a backdrop of increased community inclusion,* decisions about health care and end-of-life care have moved center stage for people with intellectual and developmental disabilities (IDD), their families, disability self-advocacy organizations, hospitals, hospices, disability service providers, bioethicists, attorneys, and legislators. Professional books, articles, conferences, research papers, staff development trainings, national and statewide initiatives, coalitions, and commissions all testify to the myriad questions and discussions these issues have generated at many levels of society. To a great extent, the controversies and conflicts about this population's health, and end-of-life decision making in particular, are bound to the historical, legal, political, economic, bioethical, cultural, and ideological contexts that have always impacted people with IDD. While these contexts may be generally known, the purpose of briefly reviewing them here is to underscore

---

* In the last 25 years, people with IDD have increasingly received services in community-based settings. Of the 4.7 million people with IDD in the United States, 2.8 million live primarily with their families (Braddock, Hemp, & Rizzolo, 2008). Of the 536,476 people who were living in "out-of-home" residential services in 2006, 376,567 individuals (70%) were in settings of fewer than 6 persons, including public and private group homes, apartments, intermediate care facilities (ICFs), foster homes, and "supported living" arrangements in neighborhoods across the country (Braddock et al., 2008). Of the 11% (58, 493) of the people residing in facilities of more than 15 people, 21,031 persons lived in ICFs and 371,462 lived in group homes. Of the 19% (67,531) of the individuals who remained in large state or private institutions, 33,885 were in nursing homes. The remaining population resided in private and public institutions for "special populations" of people with ID and behavioral, psychiatric, or criminal histories (Rizzolo, Hemp, Braddock, & Pomeranz-Essley, 2004).

Individuals with IDD living and working in the community have greater opportunities to participate in the mainstream of life. More than half a million (542,127) people with IDD are currently employed in day work and another 116,797 are employed in supported and competitive employment (Braddock et al., 2008). Classrooms, recreational settings, transportation, and most public buildings have become more accessible to people with disabilities as the result of legislation. In addition, as the result of the demands of their families and self-advocacy organizations, lobbying, and litigation, there are more residential, educational, employment, transportation, and recreational opportunities for people with IDD and more support services—such as respite, personal assistance, and habilitation—that enable individuals to live better and more independently and that support family members in providing care for relatives with IDD at home.

both their separate and their cumulative relevance to current controversies about health care and end-of-life care decision making and people with IDD. One caveat is that, given the scope of the chapter, the review is not and cannot be comprehensive. Despite this limitation, the goal is to consider how the past may influence present practice and policies affecting people with IDD and end-of-life decision making.

CONTEXTS AND THEMES INFLUENCING HEALTH AND END-OF-LIFE DECISIONS

From as early as colonial times, the history of people with IDD in the United States confirms that then, as now, they most often lived with their families as part of the community (Scheerenberger, 1987). The average life expectancy for the general population was significantly shorter because childhood mortality was significantly higher, particularly for newborns and children with IDD, if they survived infancy. The general population also had less likelihood of surviving common, often fatal childhood diseases. (These circumstances continue to be the case in less developed countries.) At the beginning of the 20th century in the United States, the initial concern about a newborn was whether he or she would survive. In the case of an infant born with a disability, a second issue was whether or not to provide nutrition, hydration, and the limited neonatal care that was then available. Such decisions were considered "private," that is, only within the realm of parents' rights. Because of the medical, technological, and legal developments since then, these decisions have become more complex and the options available have become broader (Batshaw & Silber, 2004). Parents' historical right to make decisions about their infants and children continues to be a controversial issue in some health care and end-of-life debates; for example, to what extent do parents have a legal right to decide whether a potentially lifesaving medical intervention should be provided or withheld from a newborn or child? In addition, a key bioethical concern is that a tacit policy of "selective infanticide" inside the context of the newborn nursery could potentially morph into one of "selective genocide" outside the nursery. Since the introduction of immunizations, improved nutrition, public health, sanitation, and more advanced obstetrical and neonatal care during the 20th century, infant mortality has significantly decreased in the United States. Research that began in the 1950s, and continues today, has led to progressive identification of risk factors for IDD and to medical interventions and technology to reduce risks to newborns and children. Antibiotic, diagnostic, and surgical options have effectively increased the quality of life for many people with IDD. At the same time, some medical treatments and interventions have also been responsible for some disabilities, such as retinopathy of prematurity (ROP) in premature infants as the result of oxygen toxicity and disabilities in some infants whose mothers took thalidomide, a prescribed sedative.

The average life expectancy of people with IDD is currently nearly that of the general population's, and, like the general population, they confront aging and end-of-life issues (Janicki, Dalton, Henderson, & Davidson, 1999). Their likelihood of outliving their family caregivers is therefore likewise increased, as are their need for increased services and support (Braddock, Hemp, & Rizzolo, 2008). The development of additional health care options, increased longevity of a growing number of older people, and increased costs of care over longer periods of time present cost-containment, health care, and bioethical challenges. The fields of bioethics and medical ethics struggle to keep pace with additional technological and health care options, as well as with changing social attitudes about the issues of medical research, physician-assisted suicide (PAS), aging, dying, and quality of life. People with IDD and their families now share these concerns.

Residential education, influenced by European models, was a 19th century response to the needs of caring for people with IDD. This approach was intended to socialize people with IDD and to educate them for employment and maximum self-sufficiency when they returned to the community (Kanner, 1964). Such reformers established special schools, farms, and villages where children with IDD would be taught vocational skills, such as farming, as well as basic communication and self-care skills, including what would now be described as "activities of daily living." The goals of these programs reflected an inclusive ideology that people with IDD could have productive lives in the community.

Early reformers' aspirations were limited by a paucity of knowledge about the needs of people with diverse IDD and about effective methods of special education and rehabilitation. In addition, parents were generally reluctant to send a child with an IDD away from home unless the parents were unable to provide care, either because of their insufficient resources or the severity of the child's disability (Ferguson, 1994). As a result, children admitted to the schools were more likely to have severe disabilities, less family support, and more intensive needs than reformers had envisioned. Once the school deemed that the child's educational experience was complete, the child's parents and the communities frequently resisted the school's return of the child (Kanner, 1964). For children with IDD who survived to adulthood, there were limited community resources and opportunities. Despite the fact that residential schools produced segregation and that their educational effectiveness varied widely, they continued to be the educational model for children with IDD in the United States until 1975, when Public Law 94-142—now known as the Individuals With Disabilities Education Act (IDEA)—mandated that public school systems provide educational opportunities for children with disabilities. Once the neighborhood school became an educational option, many families were able to keep their children at home.

Institutionalization, which also developed in the United States in the mid-19th century, provided a notorious model of "care and treatment" of people with IDD. Contrasted with the earlier almshouses and poorhouses—which admitted the poor, old, sick, orphaned, alcoholic, mentally ill, epileptic, and the physically and intellectually disabled—developmental centers ensured social exclusion of people with IDD of all ages and diverse categories in separate institutions built specifically for them. The labels for categorizing people were broad and vague, and therefore even the developmental centers admitted people with a wide range of IDD, mentally illness, epilepsy, abandonment, and "incorrigibility." Because they were considered socially undesirable, they were stigmatized, ostracized, and dehumanized (Castellani, 2005).

The phrase "end of life" within the context of the era of institutionalization could aptly describe the existence of people confined to institutions where they were devalued and abandoned (Ferguson, 1994). Ferguson, for example, describes a recommended treatment called "rock therapy," in which inmates repetitiously moved rocks from one location to another for exercise and diversion (1994). The final testament to their insignificance in the eyes of society was reflected in the manner in which they were treated if they died within the institutions: Their graves outside the walls were marked only with numbers. The social policies that established and maintained this institutional nightmare continue to influence the concerns of people with IDD and their families about health care and end-of-life decisions. To many older individuals who lived through that era, it is still very relevant that the inhumane "treatment and care" they experienced was developed, funded, administered, and delivered by experts and "professionals"—physicians, social workers, psychologists, psychiatrists, nurses, therapists, attorneys, state and national legislators, and others. These providers and purported experts knew of and witnessed the effects of institutionalization on thousands of people with IDD, including infants and children with severe disabilities (Castellani, 2005). In fact, the institutionalization era should not be considered over as long as there are still thousands of people with IDD in developmental centers, nursing homes, and congregate residences for over seven people, as well as people on long waiting lists for appropriate housing to meet their needs (Castellani, 2005). Thus, while people may speak of the institutional era as past in the belief that "it's different now," this is far from the case. For the last 25 years, the shift from institutionalization to community-based services in terms of ideology, funding, services, and organization has been steady and progressive. The official beginning of deinstitutionalization for people with IDD was marked by the Willowbrook case, after which time New York State closed a few developmental centers and in 1987 committed to closing all of the developmental centers by 2000 (Castellani, 2005). A social movement for "normalization" paralleled the social policy of deinstitutionalization, and while the impetus and principles of these movements were different, they jointly influenced the new ideology, the redefinition of service organizations, and the new goals for community-based services (Scheerenberger, 1987; Wolfensberger, 1972).

In his history of the deinstitutionalization of people with mental illness, Koyanagi (2007) identified economic policy as a significant factor in the shift from institutionalization to community-based services. States' anticipation of cost savings from Medicaid reimbursement for nursing homes motivated the transfer of people from institutions for people with mental illness and IDD into institutions for older people—nursing homes—which were viewed at the time as "more normalized." Once the Home and Community Based (HCBS) Waiver program was authorized in 1981, states also took advantage of Medicaid reimbursement to finance a broad range of community services, including community housing, case management, medical care, transportation, respite, habilitation, family support, and supported employment.

The rapid rise of HCBS was the result of lobbying and litigation by people with IDD and their families to gain support for the development of individualized services. As of 2006, 57% of the 39.30 billion dollars in federal and state funding for people with IDD was for HCBS funding (Braddock et al., 2008). In the past few years, the Medicaid payment structure—allocated to person-centered planning and individualized supports—has financed services to people with disabilities in their family homes, their own homes, small group homes, and an array of other community-based residences throughout the country. Some of these opportunities have come as large state or private institutions downsized and closed, allowing people who have spent a lifetime in such settings to transition to smaller homes in the community. Meanwhile, cohorts of younger individuals with IDD have accessed services from home from the start. They and their families have higher expectations and a wider definition of "community-based care," and they have continued to push the system for a broader range of supports including transportation, recreation, education, residential arrangements, vocational opportunities, and, of course, health care.

Economic realities have assumed even greater importance in the last decade due to increases in health care costs, long-term care, and end-of-life care for both the general population and those with IDD. As a result, the expansion of Medicaid in particular has become a major concern for state and national budgeting. Managed care and de facto health care rationing are among the cost-saving and cost-cutting strategies implemented to reduce these costs.

Subsequent policies such as the Fair Housing Act Amendments in 1988, which provided housing protection in the community; the American Disabilities Act in 1990, which provided broad legal rights; and the Olmstead Decision, which mandated "the least restrictive environment" as the appropriate residential setting for people with IDD, have continued to expand the rights of people with IDD. In addition, rights to benefits such as SSD, SSI, Medicare, and Medicaid advanced the status of people with IDD. An amendment to the ADA in 2008 extended these rights and benefits to include people with a broader range of disabilities, such as cerebral palsy, multiple sclerosis, cancer, epilepsy, and diabetes—those who previously had been excluded by judicial interpretations of the ADA.

In addition to social policies, four social movements have influenced the attitudes of the general population and those of people with IDD and their families about health and end-of-life decision making: the hospice movement; the civil rights movement; the movement for consumers' rights in health care; and the self-advocacy movement among people with IDD, mental illnesses, and physical disabilities. The U.S. hospice movement dramatically raised the general public and health care professionals' awareness about the needs of terminally ill patients for better care, especially for pain management. From individual programs, to federally funded demonstration programs, to passage of the Medicare Hospice Benefit in 1986, the hospice movement effectively expanded the number of hospices and therefore the number of patients for whom hospice care was an option. In the 1960s and 1970s, the self-advocacy Independent Living Movement and consumers' rights movements grew out of the civil rights movement with broadly based demands for social justice and equality for poor people; women; African Americans; gay, bisexual, lesbian, and transgendered people (GBLT); and people with IDD, mental illness, and/or physical disability. By the 1970s, a number of self-advocacy groups coalesced into a disabilities rights movement organized around issues of individual rights and access to community health care. During this same period, the consumer rights movement in health care developed in which consumer advocates—including Ralph Nader, the American Association for Retired People, and others—challenged health care professionals, legislators, hospitals, and nursing homes to recognize patients' rights to information, education, choices, representation, and decision making about their own health care.

While the priorities and goals of these movements overlapped, disability advocates focused on housing, health care, employment, education, and transportation concerns because their options were fewer in all of these areas. For example, they focused on the long waiting lists for housing, poverty-level incomes, and the shortage of health care providers serving Medicaid patients. The Independent Living Movement espoused the core values of self-determination and autonomy in decision making in all aspects of one's life, from housing and health care to employment and end-of-life planning. Despite differences in priorities and politics, disability self-advocacy groups united on these values.

The roles of professionals in relation to people with IDD have changed with new political contexts and ideologies. In the current context of community-based services, one might assume that professionals are more knowledgeable, enlightened, and inclusive in our professional roles and thus think, "It's different now than it was then." However, some disability self-advocacy organizations are skeptical of the efforts of professional and provider organizations to establish and promulgate guidelines for end-of-life decision making *for* those with IDD rather than *with* them. A major concern expressed by Not Dead Yet (NDY), for example, is that the "end-of-life movement" could become the "euthanasia for the disabled" movement. In the following section, this concern is explored.

Issues in Practice With People With IDD and End-of-Life Decisions

Health care has presented a particularly difficult challenge to the full participation in the community of people with IDD. Transitioning from a system that focused on the "health and safety" of people with IDD to a system driven by "choice" for those with IDD has been neither easy nor smooth for individuals or service providers. States and providers are still struggling to define acceptable risks, to delegate health care tasks, and to support options for individuals with IDD in the community. A national survey of state developmental disability directors demonstrated a wide range of policies, or absence of policies, on end-of-life care options for people with IDD (Botsford & King, 2005).

Medical providers were not adequately prepared for an influx of people with IDD into community health care systems. Physicians, nurses, and other health care providers lacked knowledge about assessment, communication, and special health needs of individuals with IDD. In addition, other high profile medical and legal issues—health care rationing, PAS, surrogate health care decision making, Do-Not-Resuscitate orders (DNR), "futile care"—have emerged in the health care policy arena. These issues have significant implications for what is at stake not only for the general public but also particularly for people with IDD and their families.

Nothing About Us Without Us, John Charleton's book (1997) on disability oppression and empowerment, expresses the core values of self-determination and inclusion of people with IDD and their families in end-of-life coalitions and partnerships with public and private agencies, health care providers, hospices, disability services providers, ethics committees, and legislation that concern people with IDD. Disability self-advocacy organizations are adamant and articulate in their opposition to bioethicists, hospice organizations, physicians, and attorneys establishing guidelines for decisions that disability advocates claim are rightly their own to make.

For the last 20 years, health care organizations and organizations for aging people have exhorted the general population to complete "advance directives" by selecting health care proxies for medical situations in which they may be temporarily or permanently unable to make decisions or by completing a living will to document specific health care and end-of-life care preferences. The focus on end-of-life issues for people with IDD specifically emerged from a broad-based end-of-life movement concerned with an array of issues, including advance directives, PAS, DNRs, health care rationing, and informed consent. In view of the history of people with IDD, it is not surprising that self-advocacy organizations have expressed resistance to advance directives and guardianship on the grounds that prejudice against people with IDD could result in discrimination against them. Examples of such discrimination occur when a spouse or parent is pressured by a health care provider (a) to agree to forgo or withdraw treatment, (b) to urge agreement to a "futile care" policy, (c) to agree to written DNR orders, and (d) to withdraw treatment—including hydration and nutrition—based on a presumption that the value or quality of life of the person with a disability is insufferable (Johnson, 2003a, 2003b). Given society's difficulty grasping the possibility of life having both quality and disability, disability self-advocacy organizations have a realistic basis for these concerns.

In testimony before the U.S. Senate Committee on the Judiciary on the "Consequences of Legalized Assisted Suicide and Euthanasia," the president of NDY, Diane Coleman (also an attorney and the executive director of the Progress Center for Independent Living in Forest Park, Illinois) stated the "problem of physicians as gatekeepers" as follows:

> The disability rights movement has a long history of healthy skepticism toward medical professionals, and there's an established body of research demonstrating that physicians underrate the quality of life of people with disabilities compared with our own assessments. Our skepticism has grown into outright distrust in our profit-driven health care system. (Coleman, 2006)

Health care rationing, or "deciding who gets thrown out" of the cost equation in resource allocation, is an important issue for disability self-advocacy organizations, particularly because any "quality of life" standard that might be used to make decisions on the basis of quality of life lacks objective criteria. Still another concern is the potential conflict of interest for a state guardian who is appointed to represent a person receiving Medicaid, a program partially funded by states that, at the same time, is motivated to reduce Medicaid costs. In addition, "futile care" laws in some states allow physicians, generally in combination with a hospital ethics committee, to overrule both patient and surrogate and to make a decision to withhold or withdraw care on the grounds that treatment is "futile"—although definitions of "futile" are as ambiguous as the criteria for "quality of life."

The general population shares similar concerns about health care and end-of-life decisions, and it is reasonable to generalize the concerns of disability self-advocacy organizations about the impact of the health care system to older people and minority groups, whose health care disparities are well documented (Lillie-Blanton, 2008). In her article "Race, Religion and Informed Consent—Lessons from Social Science," Dayna Matthew writes, "Ironically, the solution to the discrimination felt by the excluded members of society may turn out to provide the remedy for the informed consent doctrine as a whole" (2008). This observation also applies to advance directives, health care proxies, and of end-of-life decision making. In a similar vein, Adrienne Asch writes, "At the end-of-life, facing decline and death, these 'disability issues' are issues for everyone—learning how to affirm and celebrate what gives life meaning and simultaneously acknowledge loss of capacity and eventually loss of life itself" (2005). Asch also points out that the participation of disability scholars and self-advocacy groups such as NDY and ADAPT is essential to reforming the end-of-life policies and practices within the ethics committees of both hospitals and hospices; to educating physicians, nurses, and social workers; and to mainstreaming dialogue about the allocation of national health resources generally (Asch, 2005).

Self-advocates and ethicists struggle to clarify the controversies created by increased health care options by questioning the rights of individuals and their families and, on occasion, by increasing media attention to the plight of a particular circumstance. What were once private decisions between health care providers, their patients, and patients' families have become public battlefields, pitting the conflicting opinions of the general public, courts, legislators, and sometimes *amicus curiae* against the private anguish of individuals and families. There are no easy answers as recent cases, such as Terri Schiavo's, have illustrated. In addition, broader social and legal controversies often shift the discussion of end-of-life care for people with IDD to the question of whether people with IDD have the rights and options for accessing the full range of health care choices. The issue is complicated further by the fact that surrogates for many individuals with significant cognitive disabilities make decisions for them. When family members serve as legal guardians, they may find themselves at odds with other surrogate decision makers, including court-appointed ad litem attorneys. Individual providers of services and caretakers, who have supported and known an individual for many years, may be discounted when distant relatives make a last minute appearance and implement decisions for a person they barely know. Guilt and disenfranchised grief often become an important part of the decision-making process, too, as family members struggle to make the best possible decisions. In the case of "unbefriended" individuals—people with no family support—the person's case may be assigned to a hospital ethics board that debates and, in some cases, decides the course of their health care. In short, the process of decision making varies from complex interpersonal, judicial, and legislative conflicts to quiet bedside discussions with no clear policy direction or precedents.

Prior to decisions about the end of life, there are often other health care decisions that must be made that may present barriers to people with IDD. Complex treatment options are often the beginning of decision-making processes that include the individual, their family members, service providers, and, on occasion, the legal system. Diagnostic testing, chemotherapy, surgical interventions, and other health care treatments require informed consent, which may not be possible to obtain from a person with significant cognitive or communication disabilities. If a person is assumed not to understand or have the ability to communicate their preferences, the person will likely be excluded from information, from considering options, from asking questions, and from the opportunity to express their opinions.

People with disabilities are often excluded (often described as "shielded") from confrontation with life's difficult discussions and experiences, such as illness, aging, loss, and dying. They have often been excluded from family funerals, conversations about a roommate' or parent's illness, visiting someone in the hospital, and other normal grief experiences. Families and professionals have explained their exclusion of people with IDD as an effort to spare their feelings, to avoid upsetting them, to prevent them from upsetting other people, or to avoid confusing them in the belief that "they wouldn't understand anyway." However, exclusion reduces a person's ability to participate in and cope with life. As a result of such exclusion, a person with IDD may be unprepared to participate in discussions about his or her health care and end-of-life options.

"Best practice" is not to exclude persons with IDD from discussions about an illness or imminent death, but to include, engage, educate, and inform them well in advance of a medical crisis (Kingsbury, 2005). For the general population and for people with IDD, health care planning and decision making are ongoing, rather than one-time, conversations, and decisions change over the course of one's life and health. Dialogue between people with IDD and their family members, other people with IDD, case managers, health care professionals, and long-term disability services providers can stimulate and inform the planning process, as well as engage the individual in talking about their health, health care choices, and how they might want to be cared for at the end of life.

There is no doubt that palliative care choices such as hospice are increasingly utilized by both the general public and the population of people with disabilities. Families may access hospice care. Through the HCBS Medicaid waiver system, family members may receive assistance with in-home support staff, respite, transportation, day programs, and other supports that are essential for the family to provide care. Caseworkers may assist in coordinating this care, suggesting hospice options, and ensuring that the family receives quality service. However, while the general public is increasingly aware of hospice options, health care professionals do not necessarily consider people with IDD and their families for hospice information or care.

For both the general public and for people with IDD and their families, it is most often the medical professional who is charged with referring the individual and the family to a hospice for palliative and end-of-life care. Depending on the medical professional's knowledge and perception both of people with IDD and of hospice care, hospice may or may not be suggested as a resource. As is the case with the general public, family members who expect a more aggressive, acute level of care are sometimes reluctant to select hospice care and may need education about hospice care as an option. In addition to educating physicians, outreach and coordination by hospice with aging services, public health services, and providers of disability services can increase awareness and education about hospice and related service options for people with IDD and their families.

Hospice care for people with IDD may encompass additional lifelong medical complications such as epilepsy, mobility limitations, secondary health problems, and mental health concerns such as Alzheimer's Disease in the case of Down syndrome (Coppus et al., 2006). Secondary medical problems pose additional caretaking and treatment considerations, which may be associated with health care and end-of-life decisions at an early age. Medical procedures and treatments, such as chemotherapy and invasive diagnostic tests, are decision-making traumas for people with IDD and their families, particularly people with severe cognitive limitations that may preclude clear expression of an understanding of the procedures or expression of their preferences and choices.

Almost all Medicaid-funded programs for people with IDD allow them to access hospice services within their settings, and while this is becoming more commonplace, there are still regional barriers to consistent access to and utilization of this care option. The essential concept of Medicaid HCBS waivers was that each state was allowed to develop programs and supports that best met the needs of the state. One of the critical variations in states' Medicaid waivers is the availability of nursing supports. The more that access to nursing supports is provided by the state's Medicaid waiver, the more likely it is that individuals are able to remain in their homes (with family members or in supported group residences) for care until the end of their life. Nursing care is a primary function of hospice services and nursing oversight is generally required for a terminally ill patient. To provide continuity of care, a nurse employed by a provider of disability services that has provided services to an individual for many years should be able to advise, advocate, and arrange for medical supports to enable the individual to transition to hospice care and to remain in his or her home.

Some states, such as Virginia and Indiana, have very limited nursing care available in their Medicaid waiver programs. As a result, individuals with greater needs for nursing care are transferred from their home to other settings such as nursing homes. Some states, such as Tennessee, provide extensive medical supports under the HCBS Waiver program, which allows the individual to die "at home," in their supported living residence. Without this nursing option under the state HCBS waiver program, providers may be forced to seek other residential options, often nursing homes, to provide the necessary nursing care, rather than to care for the individual within their own home.

Medical decisions often have negative, unintended consequences beyond health care. Ongoing medical interventions may require a change in a person's longtime living arrangement with important consequences for their daily life. In some states, such as Texas, direct support staff in Medicaid-funded group homes are not legally permitted to administer tube feedings. Consequently, if an individual receives a feeding tube as part of a medical intervention, the provider may be forced to move the person out of their long-term residence ("home") and into a nursing home where the feedings can be provided by licensed personnel. What appear to be simple medical decisions may have far-reaching consequences for an individual with IDD.

Many disability organizations serve an increasingly older and frailer population with IDD. The accessibility of homes is a major barrier for older people with IDD who want to continue to live in the community. Lack of accessible transportation and the expense of home modifications may require organizations to relocate individuals from one community residence to another residence or even to a nursing home. Residential moves and dislocations may separate individuals from long-term roommates, staff, and family. This loss of social networks therefore may adversely impact their quality of life at the end of life.

PROFESSIONAL EDUCATION

The growing body of research, journal articles, and professional training materials testify to increased professional awareness about the importance of end-of-life decision making and end-of-life care for people with IDD and their families. Recognition of the training needs of hospital and hospice nurses, physicians, social workers, attorneys, and people with IDD and their families has increased in the last decade. More educational curricula and materials have been developed for these purposes (Barbara, Pitch, & Howell, 1989;

Behrman & Field, 2003; Beifus & Yanok, 1993; Hedger & Smith, 1993; Kauffman, 2005; Kennedy, Sed, & Sterns, 2000; Kingsbury, 2004, 2005; Watchman, n.d.).

In addition, professional organizations have initiated consumer education, professional education curricula, staff development, and consultation services to address gaps in professional education for medical, hospital, hospice, nursing, clergy, and social work professions. In a recent study of palliative care in the UK, for example, hospice staff in London were found to lack training, skills, and experience for providing palliative care for people with IDD (Tuffrey-Wijne, McEnhill, Curfs, & Hollins, 2007). Among the problems that staff identified were social, communication, emotional, and cognitive issues; issues related to symptom assessment and patient comprehension; ethical issues; and the impact on staff and other patients when a person with an intellectual disability was being cared for (Tuffrey-Wijne et al., 2007). The recommendation from this study was that "collaboration between palliative care services, disability service providers and carers is the most effective way to ensure optimal care for people with ID" (Tuffrey-Wijne et al., 2007). Reports of similar studies identifying problem areas and the educational and training needs of nursing and palliative care staff have appeared in the literature in the last five years (Millioud, Pont, & Berthouzoz, 2005; Read, Jackson, & Cartlidge, 2007; Sowney & Barr, 2006, 2007; Tuffrey-Wijne, 2002, 2003; Tuffrey-Wijne, Hollis, & Curfs, 2005; Tuffrey-Wijne, McEnhill, Curfs, & Hollins, 2007). These studies make important contributions to improving the practice of health care professionals in terms of end-of-life care for those with IDD.

One model for staff development, which was adapted by the Last Passages project and funded by the Administration on Developmental Disabilities and the Project on Death in America, was based on a model developed by New York State for end-of-life care for people with IDD (Botsford & Force, 2000). These materials have been disseminated in numerous venues to professionals and providers around the country. A Web site and additional resources supplement a curriculum that has been delivered in classroom-style training conducted at national, state, and local conferences for professionals, people with IDD, and their family members.

The Last Passages project convened a national task force consisting of health care professionals, medical ethicists, family members of and individuals with IDD, advocates, and providers who worked together for 3 years to collect and disseminate best practice materials, including a training manual, position paper, and case studies demonstrating best practices in end-of-life care for people with IDD. Representatives from the hospice community who participated in this effort created opportunities for national partnerships and future cross-training between hospice and disability service providers.

Family members and representatives from disability self-advocacy organizations collaborated with other members of the Last Passages project to insure that their input was included in all aspects of the discussion, planning, and development of materials. Their input included discussion of transplant and donor options, hospice and palliative care options, the impact of Medicaid funding streams, and end-of-life education for individuals with IDD. Representatives from state agencies were helpful in securing examples of best-practice policies from other states for adaptation or replication. The American Association on Intellectual and Developmental Disabilities (AAIDD, formerly AAMR) sponsored a national conference and many conference calls focusing on aging and end-of-life care for people with IDD. Finally, research and publications related to the Last Passages project continue to be disseminated in the form of journal articles and chapters in related publications (Botsford, 2004; Botsford & King, 2005; King, 2002; Kingsbury, 2004).

Dialogue and collaboration between providers of hospice, people with IDD and their families, nursing, hospitals, and community services are the most effective forces for impacting service delivery systems, particularly for persons with IDD who receive care in their own residences, family homes, or in isolated, rural communities across the country. As the general public and health care providers become more aware of hospice services and the use of palliative care, more opportunities arise for people with IDD to access hospice as an end-of-life care option.

EDUCATION OF PEOPLE WITH IDD AND THEIR FAMILIES

What is evident from recent studies of discussion groups with people with physical disabilities is the diversity of their opinions and preferences about their health care and end-of-life care (Asnor & Castanon, 2005; Fadem, Minkler, & Perry, 2003; Friedman & Gilmore, 2007; Gill & Voss, 2005; Thomas, 2008). In Fadem and colleagues' (2003) study of 45 people with physical disabilities,

> the central finding was that virtually all of the forty-five respondents expressed the desire for autonomy in life choices, and all but one respondent (based on religious beliefs) also expressed a desire to choose whether or not to end their lives if faced with a terminal disease or other significant life-changing situations. The commitment to and struggle for autonomy by study participants, if similarly found in larger representative studies, may provide an important key to depolarizing the debate. In this research study, the finding of a strong desire for choice was accompanied almost universally by an experience of disability-based discrimination. (Fadem et al., 2003)

The authors concluded that the findings "may be indicative of a community that deeply desires to air its views and to engage more openly in this debate" (Fadem et al., 2003). Despite the fact that they are often described as if they were a homogenous group, people with IDD and their families, like the general population, have differing views about health care and the end of life depending on factors such as culture, socioeconomic class, education, age, ethnicity, gender, their perception of their quality of life and degree of social support, and their values about individualism, autonomy, rights, and equality. For example, Gill and Voss (2005) developed a questionnaire to compare responses of people with various disabilities before and after a "balanced" informational presentation on legally assisted suicide and disabilities. Race, ethnicity, gender, and knowledge level were identified as important factors in participants' opinions (Matthew, 2008; Thomas, 2008).

What "disability" means to people with IDD and their diverse families, how demographic characteristics impact their access to health care and other services, how their culture defines who makes health care decisions within the family, their values about the end of life, and their perceptions of and relationships with professionals all have implications for their health care decisions and end-of-life decisions. This applies equally to the general population and minority groups. More research on these factors would contribute to growing knowledge and practice.

The role of education in preparing people with IDD for health care decision making is explored in Friedman and Gilmore's (2007) study, which found that some family members of adolescents with severe IDD changed their health care and end-of-life choices following a presentation of information about these choices. There are educational and informational materials available for use with individuals and groups, including individuals with IDD, to learn about and talk about health, illness, aging, and dying. Recent applications of person-centered planning concepts to end-of-life issues have also begun to demonstrate their usefulness as a method for engaging, educating, and involving people with IDD and their families in making health care and end-of-life decisions (Kingsbury, 2004, 2005).

POLICY REFORM

To promote equity in health care and end-of-life decision making for people with IDD, a uniform national HCBS Medicaid waiver policy is essential. The HCBS Medicaid waiver program, the primary option for the provision of support services, does not set consistent policy guidelines about end-of-life care options, and, as illustrated previously, states' policies are often unclear and inconsistent. Many states continue to treat the death of a person with IDD in an agency setting as cause for investigation rather than as a natural occurrence. Court-appointed guardians, particularly nonfamily members, are generally not provided with training or support for understanding the choices, process, and procedures for end-of-life care and decision making. Medicaid waiver programs' coverage of nursing care and other supports are inconsistent from state to state, which results in the forced relocation of individuals from their homes at the end of their lives. Fragmented care, potential conflicts of interest, and the dislocation of people from their homes and social supports create institutional and bureaucratic barriers to meaningful individual choices.

In addition, there are variations in state policies in regard to who can make and implement end-of-life care decisions and under what circumstances they can be made. Both individuals from the general population and people with IDD—who have not clearly identified a legal guardian and who may not be able to communicate their own health care and end-of-life care preferences due to age-related, accidental, or disease-related events—can be caught in legal limbo; this may result in over- or undertreatment and disregard of their preferences. The media attention devoted to cases like Terri Schiavo's has demonstrated the conflict, confusion, and controversy that can contort end-of-life care and decision making. A positive effect of the increased media attention is the heightened public awareness about the need for greater uniformity and clarity in the legal guidelines for people who, for a variety of reasons, are unable to speak for themselves (Bienen, Blanck, & Kirschner, 1997).

In a report on a roundtable discussion, sponsored by the U.S. Department of Health and Human Services and the Rand Corporation, the following observations and recommendations were delineated:

> Federal law generally defers to state law in defining and authorizing surrogate decision makers. However, the absence of default surrogate legislation in ten states leaves doubt about who may act as an appropriate surrogate for individuals lacking decision-making capacity. Within the context of the Medicare and Medicaid programs, the federal government could provide a default rule in the

absence of state legislation that defines who is an authorized decision-maker, following the priority model used by most states or some other approach. A default rule would eliminate uncertainty in those states without legislation, while allowing states to craft their own protocols. (U.S. Department of Health and Human Services, 2008)

This recommendation warrants serious consideration as a legislative proposal for eliminating a major area of confusion and inequity with far-reaching consequences for the individuals currently affected.

In her testimony on the "Consequences of Legalized Assisted Suicide and Euthanasia" before the U.S. Senate Committee on the Judiciary, Coleman made the following recommendations for improving end-of-life care for people with IDD:

- Public attention to and discussion of futility policies
- Review of Medicare and Medicaid laws regarding third-party decisions to withhold treatment
- Congressional examination of existing state futility policies
- A state-by-state review of laws and policies on guardianship and health care decision laws to prevent nonvoluntary and involuntary euthanasia
- Public education on the difference between end-of-life decisions and decisions to end the lives of disabled people who are not otherwise dying
- Passage of the Medicaid Community Attendant Services and Support Act to allow people with disabilities to live in the community rather than being forced into a nursing home, or congregate facility, thus compromising their quality of life (Coleman, 2006)

Her recommendations succinctly address the concerns that have been previously identified as major barriers to full health and end-of-life options and choices for people with IDD, as well as older people and minority groups. As such, they provide a clear agenda for policy reform by self-advocacy organizations, health care professionals, and legislators.

In the last decade, there has been broader inclusion of people with IDD and their families in community health care, health care decision making, and end-of-life decision making. However, professionals can do much better in supporting and empowering people with IDD and their families in health and end-of-life decision making by including them in policy reform, research, professional education, and professional practice. Professionals can also do much better by reducing barriers and providing access to services for individuals with IDD who are confronted with health care and the end-of-life decisions.

Active, ongoing discussions about end-of-life decision making are occurring in disability self-advocacy organizations and among individuals with IDD and their families; in disability service organizations, such as the Volunteers of America, The Arc, and AAIDD; in hospice organizations, such as the National Hospice and Palliative Care Organization; and among bioethicists, health care professionals, and legislators. There are numerous collaborative projects with representatives from a cross-section of organizations. New contributions to research, education, practice, and policy reform in the area of end-of-life care are emerging. Disability self-advocacy organizations provide the shared core values for uniting these efforts: the increased self-determination and independence of people with IDD. The overall goal is to insure that people with IDD have the full range of options and choices throughout their lives, including the end of life.

REFERENCES

Asch, A. (2005). Recognizing death while affirming life: Can end-of-life reform uphold a disabled person's interest in continued life? In B. Jennings, G. E. Kaebnick, & T. L. Murray (Eds.), *Improving end of live care: Why has it been so difficult?* (pp. 31–36). Garrison, NY: The Hastings Center.

Barbera, T., Pitch, R., & Howell, M. (1989). *Death and dying: A guide for staff serving adults with mental retardation.* Boston: Exceptional Parent Press.

Batshaw, M., & Silber, T. (2004). Ethical dilemmas in the treatment of children with disabilities. *Pediatric Annals, 33,* 752.

Behrman, R., & Field, M. (2003). *When children die: Improving palliative and end-of-life care for children and their families.* National Academies Press.

Beifus, J., & Yanok, J. (1993). Communicating about loss and mourning: Death education for individuals with mental retardation. *Mental Retardation, 31,* 144–147.

Bienen, L., Blanck, P., & Kirschner, K. (1997). Socially-assisted dying and people with disabilities: Some emerging legal, medical, and policy implications. *Mental and Physical Disability Law Reporter, 21,* 538–543.

Botsford, A. (2004). The status of end-of-life care in organizations and agencies providing services for older people with a developmental disability. *American Journal of Mental Retardation, 109,* 421–428.

Botsford, A., & Force, L. T. (2000). *End of life care: A guide for supporting older people with intellectual disabilities and their families.* Albany, NY: NYSARC.

Botsford, A., & King, A. (2005). End-of-life care policies for people with an intellectual disability: Issues and strategies. *Journal of Disability Policy Studies, 16,* 22–30.

Braddock, D., Hemp, R., & Rizzolo, M. (2008). *The state of the states in developmental disabilities 2008.* Washington, DC: American Association on Intellectual and Developmental Disabilities.

Castellani, P. (2005). *From snake pits to cash cows: Politics and public institutions in New York.* Albany, NY: State University of New York Press.

Charlton, J. I. (1997). *Nothing about us without us: Disability, oppression and empowerment.* Berkley: University of California Press.

Coleman, D. (2006, May 25). *The consequences of legalized assisted suicide and euthanasia.* Testimony before the U.S. Senate Judiciary Subcommittee on the Constitution, Civil Rights and Property Rights. Retrieved June 13, 2008, from http://judiciar.senate.gov/print_testimony.cfm?id=1916&wit_id=5379

Coppus, A., Evenhuis, H., Verbene, G.-J., Visser, F., van Gool, P., Eikelenboom, P., & van Duijin, C. (2006). Dementia and morality in persons with Down's syndrome. *Journal of Intellectual Disability Research, 50,* 768–777.

Fadem, P., Minkler, M., Perry, M., Blum, K., Moore L., & Rogers, J. (2003). Attitudes of people with disabilities toward physician-assisted suicide legislation: Broadening the dialogue. *Journal of Health Politics, Policy and Law, 28,* 977–1001.

Ferguson, P. (1994). *Abandoned to their fate: Social policy and practice toward severely retarded people in America, 1820–1920.* Philadelphia: Temple University Press.

Friedman, S., & Gilmore, D. (2007). Factors that impact resuscitation preferences for young people with severe developmental disabilities. *Intellectual & Developmental Disabilities, 45,* 90–97.

Gill, C., & Voss, L. (2005). Views of disabled people regarding legalized assisted suicide before and after a balanced informational presentation. *Journal of Disability Policy Studies, 16,* 6–15.

Hedger, C., & Smith, M. J. D. (1993). Death education for older adults with developmental disabilities. *Activities, Adaptation, and Aging, 18*, 29–36.

Janicki, M. P., Dalton, A. J., Henderson, C. M., & Davidson, P. W. (1999). Mortality and morbidity among adults with intellectual disability: Health service considerations. *Disability and Rehabilitation, 21*, 284–294.

Johnson, H. M. (2003a, February 16). Unspeakable conversations: The case for my life. *New York Times Magazine*, sec. 6. Retrieved June 8, 2008, from http://www.nytimes.com/2003/02/16/magazine/unspeakable-conversations.html?scp=12&s

Johnson, H. M. (2003b, November 23). The disability gulag. *New York Times Magazine*, sec. 6. Retrieved June 8, 2008, from http://www.nytimes.com/2003/11/23/magazine/the-disability-gulag.html?scp=19&sq=Harr

Kanner, L. (1964). *A history of the care and study of the mentally retarded.* Springfield, IL: Thomas.

Kauffman, J. (2005). *Guidebook on helping persons with mental retardation mourn.* Amityville, NY: Baywood.

Kennedy, E., Sed, C., & Sterns, H. (2000). *Person-centered planning for later life: Death and dying—A curriculum for adults with mental retardation.* Chicago: University of Illinois at Chicago, Rehabilitation Research and Training Center on Aging with Developmental Disabilities.

King, A. (2002, August). *End-of-life care.* Paper presented at the Qualified Mental Retardation Professionals Annual Program Meeting, Snowbird, UT.

Kingsbury, L. (2004). Person-centered planning in the communication of end-of-life wishes with people who have developmental disabilities. *Exceptional Parent, 34*(11), 44–46.

Kingsbury, L. (2005). Using person-centered planning to communicate healthcare and end-of-life wishes with people who have disabilities. *TASH Connections, 31*, 24–26.

Koyanagi, C. (2007). *Learning from history: Deinstitutionalization of people with mental illness as precursor to long-term care reform.* Washington, DC: Kaiser Commission on Medicaid and the Uninsured. Retrieved June 10, 2008, from http://www.kff.org/about/kcmu/cfo

Lillie-Blanton, M. (2008). *Addressing disparities in health and health care: Issues for reform.* Testimony before the Congress of the United States House of Representatives, Committee on Ways and Means Health Subcommittee, June 10, 2008. Kaiser Foundation, 1330 G Street NW, Washington, DC.

Matthew, D. B. (2008). Race, religion, and informed consent—lessons from social science. *Journal of Law, Medicine, & Ethics, 36*, 150–173.

Millioud, I., Pont, C., & Berthouzoz, B. (2005).Terminal care in an institution. *European Journal of Palliative Care, 11*, 167.

Read, S., Jackson, S., & Cartlidge, D. (2007). Palliative care and intellectual disabilities: Individual roles, collective responsibilities. *International Journal of Palliative Nursing, 13*, 130–435.

Rizzolo, M.C., Hemp, R., Braddock, D., & Pomeranz-Essley, A. (2004*). The state of the states in developmental disabilities: 2004.* Boulder: University of Colorado, Department of Psychiatry and Coleman Institute for Cognitive Disabilities.

Scheerenberger, R. C. (1987). *A history of mental retardation: A quarter century of promise.* Baltimore: Paul H. Brookes.

Sowney, M., & Barr, O. G. (2006). Caring for adults with intellectual disabilities: Perceived challenges for nurses in accident and emergency units. *Journal of Advanced Nursing, 55*, 36–45.

Sowney, M., & Barr, O. (2007). The challenges for nurses communicating with and gaining valid consent from adults with intellectual disabilities within the accident and emergency care service. *Journal of Clinical Nursing, 16*, 1678–1686.

Thomas, R. (2008). A literature review of preferences for end-of-life care in developed countries by individuals with different cultural affiliations and ethnicity. *Journal of Hospice and Palliative Nursing, 10*, 142.

Tuffrey-Wijne, I. (2002). The palliative care needs of people with intellectual disabilities: A case study. *International Journal of Palliative Nursing, 8*(5), 222–223.

Tuffrey-Wijne, I. (2003). The palliative care needs of people with intellectual disabilities: A literature review. *Palliative Medicine, 17*(1), 55–62.

Tuffrey-Wijne, I., Collins, S, & Curfs, L. (2005). Supporting patients who have intellectual disabilities: a survey investigating staff training needs. *Palliative Medicine, 11*(4), 182–188.

Tuffrey-Wijne, I., McEnhill, L., Curfs, L., & Hollins, S. (2007). Palliative care provision for people with intellectual disabilities: Interviews with specialist palliative care professionals in London. *Palliative Medicine, 21*, 493–499.

U.S. Department of Health and Human Services. (2008, August). *Advance directives and advance care planning: Report to Congress.* Retrieved July 29, 2009, from http://aspe.hhs.gov/daltcp/reports/2008/ADCongRpt

Watchman, K. (n.d.). *Let's talk about death: A booklet about death and funerals for adults who have a learning disability* (pp. 158–160). Edinburgh: Down's Syndrome Scotland.

Wolfensberger, W. (1972). *The principle of normalization in human services.* Toronto: National Institute on Mental Retardation.

Chapter 3

Ethical Foundations and Legal Issues

Judith Levy and Maureen van Stone

Introduction

The end of life can occur at any age. Furthermore, life can persist for days, weeks, months, or years after the diagnosis of a disease that has no cure. This is true for children as well as adults, those with intellectual and developmental disabilities (IDD), and those who have developed typically. As a rule, children and adults die from different causes. Adults die primarily from chronic diseases such as heart disease, cancer, or dementia; children die from congenital defects, prematurity, birth complications, and injuries (Institute of Medicine [IOM], 2003). In this chapter, we will use the term "end of life" to refer to life consistent with the following guidance from the National Institutes of Health State-of-the-Science Conference Statement:

> There is no exact definition of end of life; however, the evidence supports the following components:
>
> - The presence of a chronic disease(s) or symptoms or functional impairments that persist but may also fluctuate; and
> - The symptoms or impairments resulting from the underlying irreversible disease that require formal (paid, professional) or informal (unpaid) care and can lead to death. (National Institutes of Health, 2004)

In this chapter, we will include frequent references to two IOM reports—*Approaching Death: Improving Care at the End of Life* (1997) and *When Children Die: Improving End-of-Life Care for Children and Their Families* (2002). The latter grew out of the former, and so both apply to situations of end of life for both children and adults.

People with IDD are entitled to the same standards of medical care and treatment during their end-of-life period as all other human beings. In this chapter, we will examine end-of-life care for the population at large and apply it to our discussion of ethical and legal issues affecting people with IDD.

People with IDD, similar to the population in general, are living longer due to advances in health care at all phases of life. In 1996, according to a study in California, the difference in projected life expectancy for people with IDD was only 10 years less on average than that of the rest of the population (Strauss & Eyman, 1996). In the mid-1960s, increased attention was paid to issues for most people at the end of life, regardless of when that occurred (Dybwad, 1999). Unfortunately, due to attitudes toward people with IDD, these concerns and strategies were not applied in their health care until more recently. People with IDD are more vulnerable in all aspects of life compared to typically developing people because of their developmental issues as well as societal attitudes. However, they morally and legally require and are entitled to the same supports and services as anyone else throughout their life span, including the final stage of life, whenever that occurs.

VIGNETTES

Pediatric Vignette

Brianna is a 20-month-old girl with autism and moderate delays in all developmental domains. She lives with her parents and 8 siblings, the oldest being 19 years old. Her parents express strong religious faith, saying that they are "born-again" Christians. One day Brianna, her siblings, and her mother were outside playing as they took a break from their homeschooling. Her mother noticed that Brianna was not among them. They found her floating face down in the neighbor's swimming pool. Her mother pushed on her belly, forcing water out, 911 responded, and she was taken to a local hospital where she was resuscitated, intubated, and then taken by helicopter to a regional children's medical center. She was stabilized and monitored for the increased intracranial pressure. She was treated for hypertension, thermoregulatory instability, and seizures. She did not regain consciousness. Although she was not brain dead, according to the brain death exam, her pupils were fixed and dilated. She had no cough or gag reflex. She required tube feedings and ventilator support. After 2 weeks, she was transferred to a rehabilitation hospital, where she remained without change in status for several weeks. Her parents requested an herbalist friend to be allowed to intervene, and that was permitted on one occasion. The parents did not want to disconnect her from the ventilator saying that they did not "want to act like God," but they also said they would not do anything to keep her alive "if she's meant to die." Despite the fact that she remained in a coma and they were told there is little hope for recovery, they chose to have a Nissen fundoplication (tightening of the area between the upper part of her stomach and esophagus) to prevent aspiration of food into her lungs and potential pneumonia.

Adult Vignette

Anne is a 70-year-old woman with mild intellectual disability and osteoporosis. She was normally active for her age, lived in a home with the same two women for the past 25 years, and worked several days a week at a local church assisting the office staff. She has two nieces who maintain regular contact with her. She is her own guardian and up to this point has made most of her own medical decisions. She never had a serious illness until she experienced a stroke, fell down, and broke her hip. Since the incident, she has experienced significant pain, and her speech is difficult to understand due to the stroke. The doctors in the emergency department asked her to consent for hip repair and a cardiac procedure. However, she was anxious and disoriented from morphine given to her to treat the pain, so she refused. The staff at her home knew that this was very unusual behavior for her and was due to the acute situation. A house manager knew that she was close to her nieces, so she called to inform them of the situation. They arrived and talked with Anne about her complex condition. They asked the doctor to explain exactly what both surgeries would accomplish in simple but accurate language, and to explain the post surgical recovery, including physical therapy at a rehabilitation facility prior to going home. Of major interest to Anne was being able to return to her home and work. She was very relieved to hear that she would ultimately go home and resume her typical activities. She slowly calmed down and gave her consent for the surgeries.

ETHICAL CONCERNS AND PRINCIPLES

Ethics as a discipline attempts to organize our notions on what is morally permissible in a given situation. Ethical "concerns" in health care may be organized under four topics: medical indications, patient preferences, quality of life, and contextual issues (Jonsen, Siegler, & Winslade, 2006). Medical indications such as diagnosis and treatment are reviewed and considered in the context of the "fundamental ethical features . . . such as the goals of care and the possibilities for benefiting the patient" (p. 5). Patient preference refers to the right of an individual to make decisions about personal health care treatment. The issue of autonomy and self-determination of people with IDD is a much discussed topic in health care for people with disabilities. Quality of life varies from person to person, and it may be perceived differently by patients and their health care providers, especially when the patient has IDD. Contextual issues relate to family and provider influences on patient decision making, and financial, religious, cultural, confidentiality, resource allocation, legal, research, or conflict of interest issues.

These four topics can, in turn, be related to ethical "principles" developed by Beauchamp and Childress in their book *Principles of Biomedical Ethics* (2001), currently in its fifth edition. The authors discuss moral principles important to professional ethics. They state, "A set of principles in a moral account should function as an analytical framework that expresses the general values underlying rules in the common morality" (Jonsen et al., 2006, p. 139). They apply these principles to conflicts in moral perspectives and values occurring in health care situations. Unfortunately, these principles have not been applied fairly in all aspects of the lives of people with IDD due to the devaluing of these individuals' lives by others.

These ethical principles establish respect for the autonomy of persons with nonmaleficence, beneficence, and justice. Respect for the autonomy of others requires that we show respect for their views and decisions based on their personal values and beliefs. This principle relates to the concern for patient preferences and quality of life. Importantly, health care providers and others who help inform health care decisions must treat the patient in a manner that enables them to act autonomously. This is significant for people with IDD, who frequently experience environmental barriers to their optimal functioning in their everyday lives. Informed consent is the central method of respecting autonomy in health care settings. Historically, people with IDD of all types and levels of intellectual functioning were thought to be without the capacity for decision making. The term "person" is particularly important in that people with IDD were historically not considered persons with equal rights and entitlements. Even today a person in a persistent vegetative state may not be considered a person due to his or her lack of consciousness and inability to think rationally. Nonmaleficence refers to an obligation to do no harm. Harm is considered, in the broadest sense, anything that interferes with the legitimate interests of a person. A legitimate interest can range from preventing death, to avoiding a limb amputation so that an athlete can continue to play sports, to maintaining consciousness at the end of life despite pain so that a person can communicate with loved ones. Preventing people with decision-making capacity from exercising self-determination is harmful, as it interferes with their right to autonomy. On the other hand, failing to protect people from harm that they would inflict on themselves unwittingly (e.g., if they did not have the capacity to make an informed decision) would be harmful as well. The principle of beneficence requires that we work to benefit individuals and further their legitimate interests. In order to do this, we must engage in communication to learn about an individual's interests—something that may be difficult and time consuming for a person with IDD, both due to the fast-paced world of modern health care as well as the limitations some people with disabilities have in expressing their thoughts. A family practitioner who has known a patient for a lifetime may know this; however, a medical specialist who is consulting with and making recommendations about complex treatments to a new patient whose life is in the balance will have to spend time with the patient to learn about what is important to him or her. A difficulty with both nonmaleficence and beneficence is that our definitions of what is harmful and beneficial may differ from person to person based on our values. Frequently, based on their own personal values, interests, and ideas about what would be beneficial, physicians and family members want to make decisions for people with IDD. This is the concept of paternalism, which reflects an imposition of one person's values upon another. According to Beauchamp and Childress (2001), paternalism is at the heart of a fundamental ethical dilemma for physicians in choosing between the obligation to do what they feel is best and not harmful and the patient's autonomy. This dilemma is further accentuated when considering people who are vulnerable (e.g., because they are in an end-of-life situation and have limited decision-making capacity). It is critical to take into account both nonmaleficence and beneficence when considering medical interventions and quality of life. The notion of justice for all requires that we treat people equally according to their needs and do not discriminate against them due to a previous diagnosis or other characteristics unrelated to their current health care problem. However, in almost all situations, decisions are not made in a vacuum and "are influenced and constrained by contextual and external social, political, economic, and family considerations" (Jonsen et al., 2006, p. 159).

The Last Passages project, a project of the Center for Excellence in Aging Services at the State University of New York at Albany (SUNY–Albany), is funded as a project of national significance by the Administration on Developmental Disabilities. This project involves collaboration among SUNY–Albany, Volunteers of America, the New York State Association of Retarded Citizens, Inc., and Marist College. According to recommendations in the final project report, the authors agree with Ira Byock that end-of-life care must be based on a lifelong process of making choices in health care and experiencing the rituals and ceremonies, both subjective and individual, around death in a particular family, culture, and country of origin. Individuals with IDD must be included in the traditional rites surrounding the experience of dying and death itself. They must not be patronized or treated like children when they are adults.

Similarly, children with IDD should be made a part of these traditions when developmentally able to experience them. Life itself, and end of life, is rife with choices. All children must be exposed to situations where they are able to learn and make developmentally appropriate choices as they grow. Parents making end-of-life decisions for very small children, with or without IDD, must use their own life experiences and values to make decisions that a child may not be old enough to express. By law, parents may protect children from making unsafe or unwise decisions because parents have a duty to protect their children and look out for their best interests. However, it is morally wrong to exclude children from a decision-making process in which they are capable of participating—specifically regarding the initiation, withholding, or withdrawing of life-sustaining treatment. Children need to feel that they are part of the process and their opinions known and respected, but they also need to understand that the ultimate decision rests with their parents.

There are numerous barriers to the delivery of quality end-of-life care for individuals with IDD. First, health care providers and family members may overlook the decision-making capacity of the person with IDD and make choices without legal authorization or without taking the time to inquire carefully about an individual's preference in a particular situation. Furthermore, many end-of-life discussions include the inclination to see life-sustaining technology used by individuals with IDD as futile treatment during end-of-life situations. Many people with IDD live with tracheostomies, tube feeding, and even ventilator support. The following case illustrates the underestimation of this woman's capabilities and desires by her health care provider:

In January 1996, a 36-year-old California woman with Down syndrome (DS) received heart and lung transplants after initially having been denied, due to her diagnosis of DS and the physicians' assumption that she would not be able to manage her follow-up care and thereby "waste" a scarce resource. The physician changed his mind however after speaking with her and getting to know her better.

Health care professionals and family members need to obtain information about specific issues related to end-of-life care, including pain management and hospice for all individuals. Additionally, family members and service providers need to have knowledge of resources and training—on how to communicate with health care providers and to comprehend Medicaid regulations related to the end of life and the laws regarding health care decision making in their state—so that the playing field is level. Some of these legal issues will be discussed in greater detail later in the chapter.

Planning for the end of life is a major recommendation of the Last Passages project for those with IDD, just as it is for the population at large; however, very few people do it adequately to address all of their needs. People with IDD who are capable must be introduced to the idea of advance directives in order to make as many decisions and choices as possible for themselves and to rely on the person of their choice when they need assistance and possible protection. Advance directives may be defined narrowly or broadly depending on the preferences of the person, and the person may name one or more health care decision makers depending upon availability. Guardians of adults, just like guardians of children old enough to have expressed preferences, should always be held responsible for making decisions based on the person's values and beliefs as known to them. This is why it is imperative for a person to have in-depth, and sometimes very difficult, conversations with the people who may be making choices on his or her behalf. Some people with IDD will be able to create their own advance directives and make choices about future treatments; others will not be able to make such complex decisions but may be able to understand that some health care decisions will be beyond their comprehension. They may, however, be capable of identifying a health care agent (surrogate) whom they trust, such as a family member or friend, to make decisions for them using either the best interests (what produces the greatest benefit to the person) or substituted judgment (what the person would do if competent) standards. Some people will be unable to make decisions for themselves and will need the benefit of a surrogate decision maker identified by the court as their guardian.

"Decision-making capacity" is the term used to identify the ability of an adult person or a minor to understand and to make a decision about a particular question, including giving informed consent for health care. Two terms are used to apply in this situation: "mature minor" and "emancipated minor." The application of these terms differs from state to state, but they both generally imply that the individual has been granted the status of adult prior to the age of majority due to such life events as marriage, parenting a child, or serving in the armed forces. This status can also be granted if the minor has the ability to understand his or her condition, understand the risks and benefits, and participate in his or her medical decision making. States differ in their approaches to this issue, and neither status exists in all states.[1] These issues apply to all people with or without a disability as well as to children and adolescents who have had a lifelong illness or disability. Studies of children with diabetes have shown that as early as the age of four they have a remarkable ability to understand their disease and contribute to decisions about their own health care (Alderson, Sutcliffe, & Curtis, 2006). In adults, decision-making capacity is presumed unless proven otherwise and is not determined by age or diagnosis; it refers to actual functioning in a specific context and is affected by both cognitive abilities and affective states. It depends on functional demands and consequences and it can change for any number of reasons including injury, physical illnesses, psychological trauma, or other emotional and behavioral disorders.

These ideas regarding decision-making capacity are well described by Grisso and Applebaum (1998) in their book *Assessing Competence to Consent to Treatment*. The authors note that neither ethics as a discipline nor the law provides sufficient guidance to the practitioner in the trenches who is attempting to determine if a patient has the ability to give informed consent for health care treatment. According to the authors, the law's main concern is the effect of a person's mental or cognitive disorder on actual cognitive functioning. Ethics is concerned with protecting the patient's right to make decisions about his or her own health care and protecting the person from harm if he or she is inclined to make a decision that would cause harm. Appelbaum and Grisso demonstrate that if a person can understand information about a medical diagnosis and proposed treatment well enough to appreciate its personal significance, reason with the information, and express a voluntary choice, then that person should be able to make self-determined decisions in regards to his or her health care.

This understanding depends on the functional demands of the situation or, in other words, whether there is a match between the individual's abilities and specific decision-making demands (e.g., recommendation for antibiotics or surgery). If the consequences of

---

1. See the following reference for additional information on emancipation: http://www.peoples-law .org/children/emancipation/emancipation%20home.htm#What%20does

a decision are particularly serious, then the threshold for understanding is greater. Again, consider the young woman with Down syndrome who needs heart and lung transplants. Although she will surely die if she does not receive the transplant, she will also die if she cannot follow the postsurgical or medication regimens. Although the functional demands are high, they would equally be so for a typically developing person after such a serious surgery. Family members, nursing staff, and personal care providers could be brought into her home to assist her until she learns the regimens. Furthermore, consider the situation of the 70-year-old woman, described previously, who sustained a stroke and broken hip and whose decision-making capacity changed temporarily due to medication (morphine) and ensuing anxiety when she was alone after her accident. Helping her to understand the effects of medications, bringing in family members to help reduce her anxiety, and encouraging her physician to communicate a treatment plan in greater detail and in understandable terms would have increased her functional abilities and, to a certain extent, decreased the functional demands of her stressful situation. These ideas and procedures are commonly expected in health care situations involving people without IDD.

The Last Passages project recommends that decision makers have a prodisability attitude. Individuals with IDD have the same rights as others to make decisions to live a fulfilling life with a disability, to make choices that differ from the health care provider's recommendations, or to request what may be considered a futile treatment, such as nutrition and hydration when neither will cure the disease. Additionally, legally authorized proxies, family members, and friends must advocate—or help the individual with IDD advocate—for the full range of services and opportunities, including hospice care, pain management, and organ donation. Most, if not all, of these services and opportunities are included in advance directives, so the patient or proxy has an opportunity to consider and discuss these options when completing an advance directive. The following examples are illustrative of the need for justice, in the provision of health care to everyone, including people with disabilities:

In an article titled "The Case of Joanne Harris" (Edwards, 1997), the author asserts that people with disabilities are not entitled to organs per se, but are entitled to be screened for eligibility for a transplant due to organ failure, just as all other people at the end of life are screened. In the above-mentioned adult case study about Anne, the patient with mild intellectual disability and osteoporosis, the shared decision-making process is the context for good health care. Anne was treated with fairness, dignity, respect for her autonomy, and regard for her own well-being and quality of life as perceived by her. To have permitted Anne to refuse surgery without trying to help her come to a more informed decision would have been both physically harmful as well as an affront to her ability to make a choice in her best interest.

In his book by the same name, Ira Byock, a physician, coins the term "dying well" to describe a process that includes life as well as death, rather than using the popular term "good death," which seems to focus on the end result and gives us little information about the process itself and is therefore of limited value (1997). The concept of "dying well" can be applied to children and adults with IDD and their families. The author notes that this process is very individualized, and the actual specifics for a given person, child or adult, result from that person's unique characteristics. This is consistent with the principle of autonomy, which requires that we respect individuals' unique beliefs and preferences. Age, family relationships, culture, and country of origin, religious or spiritual beliefs, and achievements all play a part in how we approach and cope with our own death. Among other characteristics noted by individuals and their families involved in the dying process, Byock found that people who felt the best about the process were those receiving care and those involved in caregiving who talked and reminisced about relationships and "personal and spiritual matters" and who had the ability to use the time to "resolve and complete their relationships, and to get their affairs in order" (Byock, 1997, p. 31).

Aside from pragmatic issues such as education, transportation, housing, and employment, the overriding issues for individuals with IDD include self-determination and choice, fairness, and equality of opportunity in all aspects of life, including health care. Although some individuals with IDD may qualify for medical assistance or Medicare, these insurance programs do not cover many services needed by them when they are in the final stages of life (IOM, 1997).

Palliative and End-of-Life Care

Palliative care grew out of the need for new standards of care to deal the technological advances that keep people alive longer than was historically possible. It focuses on the

> prevention and relief of suffering through the meticulous management of symptoms from early through final stages of an illness; it attends closely to the emotional, spiritual, and practical needs of patients and those close to them. Other community, professional, and governmental responses include the development of hospice programs, bereavement support groups, and policies and programs that encourage communication about people's goals and preferences as they approach death. (IOM, 1997, p. 2)

Palliative care at the end of life can include both curative and life-prolonging treatment, but the focus is on preparing the individual for death. Palliative care individualizes each patient's needs and treatment, demonstrates respect for the patient and his or her family members within a care team, extends terminal care through bereavement, and provides information and support relative to making important decisions (IOM, 2003). Decision-making considerations for anyone would include the benefits and burdens of care, prognosis, avoidance of pain, and the patient's subjective experiences. In a crisis of life and death and in a world of increasingly diverse cultures with varying norms, values, beliefs, and principles, the opportunity for conflict among the players involved in the decision-making process increases exponentially. People with IDD are members of a culture that may view these situations differently than people without disabilities. For people with IDD and their family members, communication may be difficult because of intellectual and physical limitations; environmental barriers (e.g., the fast pace of health care, the setting of the conversation, and time allowed); and lack of emotional support. Given all of these issues, a tremendously complex situation exists.

Advances in medical care have increased concerns about continued use of life-sustaining technologies when death is predicted. However, life-sustaining treatments may be used to extend life after surgery or injury when recovery is expected. Furthermore, as noted previously, certain life-sustaining technologies such as ventilators, artificial nutrition and hydration, and tracheotomy are commonly accepted lifelong supportive treatments for people with cerebral palsy, spinal cord injuries, traumatic brain injuries, and other congenital and acquired disabilities. These interventions enable many to live and function optimally in their communities. These may be likened to the use of insulin for people with diabetes. Without insulin the person with Type 1 diabetes would die. But we do not generally think of insulin in the same category as tube feeding, for example, in the final stage of life. Curative treatments, as distinguished from life-sustaining treatments, include chemotherapy, radiation, antibiotics, and surgery, among others. Decisions to use these medical interventions must be made based on the balance of harm versus benefit to the individual and not solely on previously existing condition.

People without disabilities frequently make judgments and assumptions about the quality of life of a person with a disability, and this judgment is often different from the way the person and his family see it. If it is perceived that an individual with a disability is "suffering" by living with a disability or that there is little or no value to such a life, the approach to end-of-life care may be biased toward offering minimal treatment options. This attitude and resulting behavior interferes with the autonomy of the individual or his or her surrogate decision maker, is harmful and does not benefit the individual, and is unjust in that it treats the individual differently than others with the same illness. The surrogate decision maker for an individual who never made his wishes known must act in the patient's best interests. Jonsen and colleagues (2006) suggest that for individuals who have never had the capacity to understand and make their wishes known, one must assume the same interests in quality of life as would be assumed for any other individual. In this case, they would "have interests in the pursuit and securing of certain values" (p. 114) suited to their functional abilities. Health care agents or other surrogate decision makers must attempt to put themselves in the place of the individual patient and recommend "ethical evaluation" and "scrutinizing societally shared values" when challenges are made to best-interests decision making (p. 114).

Considering the previously mentioned woman with Down syndrome, the physician initially made a decision not to give her heart and lung transplants purely on the basis of her disabilities. In the case study regarding Brianna, the toddler with autism and moderate developmental delays who nearly drowned, the health care team respected her family's values, provided palliative care, including nutrition and hydration via tube, and provided information to assist the parents in their decision making—despite their own reservations about life-sustaining treatment.

It is important to note that it is universally agreed upon by ethicists and the general population alike that it is morally acceptable to withhold life support when death is deemed inevitable. However, the controversy persists regarding whether or not provision of artificial nutrition and hydration is medically or morally different from other life-sustaining interventions, as expanded in the discussions in chapter 10 (Smith & Hardt) and chapter 11 (Veatch). In fact, some research indicates that the latter interventions may be more burdensome than beneficial at end of life (Jonsen et al., 2006, p. 139). Most ethicists and judges agree that there is no significant difference between withholding and withdrawing treatment, assuming that palliative care is provided (President's Commission, 1983). However, for families having to make these decisions for their loved ones, the perception of withdrawal may be metaphorically similar to pulling the trigger, or at least more harmful than simply not providing treatment in the first place.

The question of futility also arises in discussions about treatment options. Futility, like the end of life, is difficult to define in clinical decision making. Edmond Pellegrino (2000) discussed coming to a decision about futility as a process of careful consideration and weighing of options, harms, and benefits specific to each individual's condition. Unfortunately, determination of futility may be influenced by the values of physicians and other health care providers as they provide care to people with disabilities whose lives they see as having limited value. Some treatments may have a double effect; that is, they have the intentional palliative effect of relieving suffering and improving the quality of life, such as the use of morphine for pain, but they also may have the unintended effect of hastening death (e.g., by suppressing respiratory function). This is referenced to as the Doctrine of Double Effect. Presently, this dichotomy is accepted in palliative care. Any of the previously mentioned treatments may promote conflicts of values, although palliative care supports the resolution of such conflicts without harming any of the parties.

The American Academy of Pediatrics opinion regarding palliative care for children may be summed up as focusing on the maintenance of quality in the child's remaining years, not just adding time to a child's life. This should be the focus of care for adults as well. Both children and adults, including those with IDD, should be informed about their conditions and treatment choices, and health care professionals should solicit their opinions and desires through developmentally appropriate conversations. In the case of children, it must be made clear that parents have the final decision-making authority, unless the child is emancipated from his or her parents.

Decision Making and Planning From an Ethical Perspective

The most important message for all people regarding the end of life, whether as a long-term strategy or an acute strategy based on the news of imminent death, is to have a plan based on their own desires. At one level, this includes advance directives and power of attorney for health care. At another level, it includes conversations with family members about their wishes and in some instances what they would like done in the next day, week, or month. When conflicts arise or planning is difficult in a hospital or hospice setting, the respective ethics committee or patient care advisory committee may be called upon to provide consultation and recommendations to mediate any differences and to guide discussions regarding medically sound, informed choices that reflect the individual's values.

Individuals with IDD are eligible for the same services as other people at the end of life. Palliative care, end-of-life care, and bereavement services are available in hospitals and nursing homes and may be provided in an individual's own home. Respite care for caregivers is available through state agencies and private nonprofit organizations.

Five Wishes is a template for an advance directive, accepted in at least 38 states. It differs from most advance directives in that it asks detailed questions about comfort, how people should treat the person, and specific information a person might want loved ones to know. It is available through Aging With Dignity (http://www.agingwithdignity.org) and was developed through a grant from the Robert Wood Johnson Foundation.

Similar to Five Wishes, Caring Conversations, developed by the Center for Practical Bioethics, assists individuals and family members in discussing important and personal topics prior to death and in developing a plan for care that is based on the desires and wishes of the individual at the end of his or life. Information is available through Center for Practical Bioethics at http://practicalbioethics.org/.

LEGAL ISSUES

Advances in medical technology over the last 40 years have created a new area of jurisprudence in the United States. The right to liberty protected by the 14th Amendment of the U.S. Constitution includes the right of a person to his bodily integrity in the absence of legally justified interference, including the right to refuse unwanted medical treatment. The right to refuse medical treatment includes the right to be informed by a physician of all information necessary to make a reasoned decision regarding one's medical care. The right to privacy in regards to the refusal of medical treatment is also protected by the U.S. Constitution. Some cases may raise competing interests under the Due Process Clause of the Constitution, including a person's right to refuse treatment and a person's right to life. Commonly, the cases that raise competing interests are the cases that are brought to the attention of the American public through the press and media.

Since the Supreme Court of the United States (Court) addressed the rights of surrogates to terminate life-sustaining medical care for incompetent patients in the seminal case *Cruzan v. Director, Missouri Department of Health*, significant change has occurred in state legislation on health care decision making (497 U.S. 261, 1990). In *Cruzan*, the Court upheld the Missouri Supreme Court's refusal to withdraw life support from Nancy Cruzan, a woman in a persistent vegetative state, because no clear and convincing evidence existed that would have supported the claim that Ms. Cruzan would have asked for the withdrawal of life support (*id.* at 284). The Court recognized that Ms. Cruzan held a general right to refuse life-sustaining treatment, and she did not lose that right by virtue of her incapacity. However, the Court focused on Ms. Cruzan's inability to exercise that right, namely by stating whether or not she would have chosen life-sustaining treatment (*id.* at 280). The Court held that it was constitutionally appropriate to demand clear and convincing evidence that the incapacitated person would have chosen to withhold life-sustaining treatment, which rejects the objective nature of the best interests standard commonly applied in these situations (*id.* at 281). The Court based its decision on the State's competing and compelling interest in preserving human life, as well as the interest to ensure that the decision to live or die is truly that of the incapacitated person and not his or her surrogate.

The Court in *Cruzan* left the broad outlines of legal doctrine on end-of-life medical decision making to the states, yet the presumption in favor of preserving life emerged (Miller, 2006). So, in response to the Court's holding in *Cruzan*, the National Conference of Commissioners of Uniform State Laws wrote the influential Uniform Health Care Decisions Act of 1993 (UHCDA), which was approved by the American Bar Association on February 7, 1994. The UHCDA carries a legislative power that enables an individual to accept or refuse medical treatment at will, specifically treatment that is considered to be life sustaining. The UHCDA permits competent individuals to appoint agents and to include preferences for end-of-life care decisions in a written advanced directive, which would result in no court interference (Miller, 2006). If an individual has no advance directive, the UHCDA grants surrogate decision-making power to a family member or close friend in a preferential order (e.g., spouse, child, and parent). The surrogate decision maker is required to make any decisions in the best interest of the individual and there are no limitations on end-of-life decisions (Miller, 2006). However, the UHCDA has limitations: it is not enforced in all states and it does not address individuals with IDD.

There are six components of the UHCDA, four of which focus on an individual's autonomy. First, the UHCDA acknowledges the right of a competent individual to decide all aspects of his or her own health care in all circumstances. An individual may broadly or narrowly define the scope of authority of an agency or institution. Second, the UHCHA enables an enacting jurisdiction to replace its existing legislation on the subject with a single statute. Since not all states have elected to do so, it is imperative to check the legislation in each state. Third, the UHCDA is designed to simplify and facilitate the making of advance health care directives and provides an optional form for doing so. Fourth, the UHCDA seeks to ensure that decisions about an individual's health care are governed by the individual's own desires and wishes to the extent known to the surrogate. Fifth, the UHCDA addresses compliance by health care providers and institutions, unless an instruction or decision requires the provision of medically ineffective care or care contrary to applicable health standards, or the instruction is declined by the physician for reasons of conscience. Lastly, the UHCDA provides a procedure for dispute resolution in which case the intervention of courts may be necessary (e.g., to enjoin an order, provide other equitable relief, or identify who is eligible to file a petition in court).

The definitions provided in the UHCDA are critical because individuals (lay people and health care professionals) commonly confuse or loosely interpret the meaning of terms. The UHCDA contains sections regarding advance health care directives and the revocation of an advance health care directive, the optional form, decisions by a surrogate, decisions by a guardian, obligations of health care providers, as well as information regarding health care information, immunities, statutory damages, capacity, and judicial relief. The UHCDA does not affect the right of individuals to make health care decisions when they do not have the capacity to do so, nor does it address the need of individuals with more severe IDD.

The law presumes competency in all persons (Callegary, 2005). There is no accepted legal definition of a never-competent individual; courts rely on the judgment of the physicians who examine the individual to determine whether the individual is competent to provide informed consent to treatment. Physicians may consider an individual's ability to absorb and comprehend information, to reason through alternatives, and to make and explain his or her decision. Most state legislatures mandate how a physician is required to demonstrate that an individual is not competent. For example, Maryland law provides that two physicians certify in writing (based on a personal examination) that the individual is incapable of making an informed decision regarding treatment (Callegary, 2005). Declaring an individual incompetent and assigning a court-appointed guardian should be the last resort, as it deprives a person of many rights and may or may not be in the person's best interest. The appointment of a health care agent is less restrictive and normalized; however, it is frequently overlooked when considering individuals with IDD. If an individual has the capacity to decide these issues, including whether to use life-sustaining procedures, whatever condition he or she is in, that person should have the opportunity to do so in absence of judicial interference.

States that adopted the UHCDA or a similar legislation typically address the following conditions: terminal condition, persistent vegetative state, and end-stage condition. The legislation assists individuals in making end-of-life medical decisions through statutes permitting living wills (a document outlining an individual's preferences regarding end-of-life treatment) and health care agents or proxies (surrogate decision makers) in the event the individual is not competent. The advantages to surrogate decision making are that it is determined by an episode of care, it is temporary, and it does not require court intervention. A living will or advance directive may help individuals to overcome evidentiary burdens and decline medical treatment without judicial interventions, which should be the goal for all individuals and families. A judge does not know the individual or his or her family and should not be making such decisions unless absolutely necessary. Many Americans realize that judicial proceedings may delay care and create significant stress and hardship for individuals and their loved ones, as evidenced by some recent Supreme Court cases covered by the press and media.

A Health Care Decisions Act contains patient safeguards, including the requirement that health care providers bring certain matters before their facility's ethics committee or file the petition in court (e.g., those providers who believe that an instruction to withhold or withdraw life-sustaining procedures is inconsistent with generally accepted standards of patient care). Family members and other qualified surrogates may file a lawsuit to enjoin allegedly unlawful actions, which must be expedited by the court (in an effort to delay care as previously mentioned). If a person does not comply with the act in good faith, that person may lose immunity (which is outlined in the Act) for decisions involving life-sustaining procedures. Finally, mercy killing, euthanasia, and assisted suicide are not authorized under any circumstances and may result in criminal penalties, as would be the case for the destruction, concealment, or forgery of an advance care directive.

It is apparent that end-of-life care for typically developing children and adults is very complex and may require judicial interference. End-of-life care for children and adults with IDD adds another layer of complexity, especially for the courts. The law requires a determination of whether or not the individual is competent to make a decision at that time, as well as a determination of whether or not the individual was previously competent. Only a court can make such a determination after reviewing the medical evidence provided by the individual's physicians. If the court determines that an individual is not competent, but was competent in the past, the individual's expressed wishes must be considered. Courts must consider expressed wishes even if those wishes do not appear to be rational. For never-competent individuals with more severe IDD, it may be very difficult for family members and caregivers to determine their wishes. In March of 2003, the State of New York passed a statute that specifically addresses never-competent individuals, whereas other states merely analogize to formerly competent individuals who left no instructions regarding their preferences and made no reliable statements while they were competent (Golden, 2003).

Never-Competent Individuals

There was a series of representative cases in which courts considered the expressed statements and actions of never-competent individuals in evaluating whether or not to discontinue medical treatment (Miller, 2006). In all of the cases, the individual had been adjudicated incompetent in a court of law, yet that did not mean that the individual did not have an opinion or preference. Unfortunately, their stated opinions or preferences did not rise to the level of informed consent as required by law, so the surrogate had to determine what weight to give the expression. In *Superintendent of Belchertown State Sch. v. Saikewicz*, the Supreme Court of Massachusetts considered a patient's physical resistance and noncooperation to the intravenous administration of chemotherapy drugs as one of six factors weighing against the treatment (Mass., 1977). The court in *Saikewicz* substituted its judgment for Saikewicz's by trying to anticipate his personal reaction to the chemotherapy, yet the court did not consider any physical expression of Saikewicz's will prior to or at the start of the treatment (*Id.* at 430). On the other hand, in *In re Storar*, the Court of Appeals for New York, ordered John Storar to undergo treatment despite his physical resistance and the expressed opposition of his guardian (N.Y., 1981). Mr. Storar had profound IDD and was diagnosed with inoperable bladder cancer at the age of 52. He required blood transfusions, which he physically resisted to the point that he required sedation. The court saw the transfusions as analogous to food and asserted they "did not involve excessive pain" (*id.* at 73). Mr. Storar's physical activities (e.g., feeding himself, showering, taking walks, and running) were seen as indirect evidence of his preference to live and the court found little relevance to his physical resistance (*id.*).

Other representative cases include a patient who repeatedly pulled out her feeding tube and another patient who pulled out her nasogastric tube. Both cases involved similar nonverbal expressions on the part of the incompetent persons; however, the courts' decisions were opposite based on their quality of life analyses. The Massachusetts court in *In re Heir* gave weight to Ms. Heir's expressions of opposition to the tube feedings and applied the substitute judgment doctrine, which provided them with justification for refusing treatment (Mass., 1984). Alternatively, the New York court in *In re O'Brien* set a higher bar for a nonverbal expression of refusing treatment and relied heavily on the state's interest in preserving the life of the incompetent (Sup. Ct. N.Y. County, 1986).

Finally, the Washington State Supreme Court ruled that even if a person was determined to be incompetent the court must consider a patient's expressed wishes. In *In re Guardianship of Ingram* (Wash., 1984), the court determined that Ms. Ingram, who suffered from dementia and throat cancer, verbally expressed her wish not to have throat surgery (because she would lose her ability to speak), which must be given substantial weight. The court also considered her ability to understand the problem and choices and the intensity of her preference (*id.* at 1371). In the end, the court applied the substituted judgment standard and considered all of the factors in the *Saikewicz* case, plus the expressed wishes of Ms. Ingram (*id.* at 1370). Ultimately, Ms. Ingram received radiation treatment rather than throat surgery and her personal autonomy was elevated above both her best interests and the state's interest in preserving her life (Miller, 2006).

Ultimately, the state's power over never-competent individuals is to protect them, as the person still retains his or her legal rights (Miller, 2006). Determining how to protect the rights of a never-competent individual in end-of-life care is extremely challenging for the courts. The principle of autonomy underlying the doctrines surrounding medical decisions requires an examination of the never-competent individual's preferences regarding treatment even when they do not meet the requirement of informed consent. A surrogate may reject those preferences if they are totally unreasonable; however, they must consider them in making a choice on behalf of that individual (Miller, 2006). Advocates, legal scholars, and the courts continue to debate the arguments for strong and weak surrogate decision makers.

The need for limits on the powers of decision makers is nowhere clearer than in a question as fundamental as life or death, because the consequences of abuse or misjudgment are both ultimate and irreversible. That is why there has been so much controversy and litigation over these issues in the U.S. courts. It is imperative that an individual chooses his or her health care proxy or agent wisely and chooses an alternative if the primary choice is unavailable. Whenever possible, the individual should discuss his or her preferences with any and all potential decision makers, as well as his or her spiritual advisor, if appropriate.

Legal Standards

Numerous states and the Supreme Court in *Cruzan* have endorsed a clear and convincing evidence standard for the withdrawal of life-sustaining treatment; therefore, any expression to the contrary would make it difficult to reach this standard (Miller, 2006). Some courts have also held that when evidence of intent is equivocal it is best to err in favor of preserving life. However, the lack of public awareness of the clear and convincing evidence standard is pervasive and the legal standard is inconsistently enforced and overlooked (Golden, 2003). Some health care professionals and attorneys may subjectively construe the facts of the cases to avoid strict application of the standard; that is, life-and-death decisions may be made without the benefit of clear legal guidance (Golden, 2003). It is important to note that physicians do not need to provide medically ineffective treatment—which will neither prevent or reduce the deterioration of the health of the individual nor will prevent the impending death of an individual—or any treatment that is not within the range of morally acceptable alternatives. Individuals and families may or may not understand the physician's obligation, so the discussion as to whether a treatment can be administered by the health care professional is an important discussion when planning for the end of life. The courts emphasize the general principle that caution should be exercised when substituting a third party's judgment for another individual's on the issue of life-sustaining treatment. Because the law is evolving, both individuals and their families may be subject to its uncertainties (Golden, 2003).

Future Planning

Individuals with IDD and their families should plan for the future and avoid some of the legal obstacles previously identified. They should meet with an attorney who can help frame the legal issues and understands the array of options available to them. Some considerations include current and future needs, current financial assets and resources of the individual and family, distribution of assets upon death, personal and medical decision making, specifics regarding end-of-life care decisions, access to records, and financial decision making (Greenbaum, 2007). Individuals with IDD who are listed in wills and receive direct inheritances need to understand how the amount of the inheritance may affect their ability to access public benefits, and, in some cases, may cause them to become ineligible. The solution is not to disinherit the individual because public benefits will not cover all necessary living expenses; nor is the solution to disclaim the amount due to the individual. It is imperative that individuals with IDD and their families discuss the distribution of assets upon death and not assume that another family member will take care of the individual with IDD.

For some families, a third-party supplemental-needs trust (or a special needs trust) is an alternative to ensure that assets never belong to the individual with a disability and the person was never directly entitled to the money or other assets. The trust is drafted by an attorney (not a financial advisor) and names a trustee who is responsible for managing and using the funds for the benefit of the individual with a disability (known as the beneficiary). The trustee has broad discretion to manage the property on behalf of the beneficiary, which may become critical in some end-of-life care situations. The trust may include money, life insurance policies, retirement benefits, and joint bank accounts, all of which must be properly titled. A third-party supplemental-needs trust may be established for an individual of any age; however, it is important to note that the trust is irrevocable. The trust may be created during someone's lifetime or upon death and does not require any prior state approval or authorization. In some cases, the Social Security Administration or Medicaid may request to review the document to ensure that it complies with their agency requirements. All of these issues are extremely complex and may have serious implications, which is why it is absolutely critical that an individual with a disability and his or her family choose an experienced attorney with whom they are confident and comfortable.

Some individuals with disabilities handle their finances by themselves, whereas others may need limited assistance or have total dependence upon another individual or an entity (Greenbaum, 2007). Individuals with more severe disabilities should authorize a representative payee to receive their cash benefit (e.g., Social Security Disability Insurance or Supplemental Security Income), which requires the completion of forms by the representative payee and the health care professionals working with the individual with a disability. These procedures do not require an attorney; however, an attorney may be necessary if they receive unanticipated funds that would make them ineligible for these benefits. In these cases, an attorney may advise the individual of ways to spend down the money or create a trust. Financial planning for individuals with IDD is critical to ensure that their needs are met throughout their life, especially the end of life when parents or other caregivers may not be available.

Commonly, individuals with IDD have extensive educational, medical, and, in some cases, legal records. It is imperative that the individual or his or her caregiver has access to all the records, especially in the case of an emergency. If the individual does not have the capacity to make informed decisions, then the surrogate decision maker should have access to any and all pertinent records. Attorneys who advocate on behalf of children with disabilities and their families advise families to keep organized records outlining all important information, including a list of all the child's schools and dates attended; the location of important documents (e.g., birth certificate, social security card, and immunization records); contact information for all health care professionals; and a list of medications (Greenbaum, 2007).

There is a federally mandated Protection and Advocacy (P&A) System and Client Assistant Program (CAP) in every state and territory, as well as a Native American P&A. These programs work to protect the human, civil, and legal rights of individuals of all ages and with all types of disabilities. Individuals and their families may wish to access the advocacy and legal services of their local P&A, specifically for resources and materials regarding future planning. It is critical that individuals and families choose an attorney who understands the complexity of these cases. Proactive individuals and families who appropriately plan for the future decrease the likelihood of any type of court involvement and increase the probability that medical, financial, and legal decisions will be made in the individual's best interest.

LEGAL OBSTACLES

Both medical technology and the increased mobility of all Americans (including individuals with IDD) have contributed to this area of jurisprudence. For example, a Health Care Decisions Act in one state may conflict with a statute in another state, which may result in a court proceeding. Years ago, individuals with IDD were often housed in state institutions (presumably near their families); today, this is rarely the case. Many individuals with IDD live in states other than those of their families or they move and travel. It is imperative for mobile individuals, especially individuals with IDD, to determine whether or not the advance directive or living will be upheld in their new state of residence. Individuals must also ensure that copies of the advance directive are furnished to their health care providers in their new state of residence.

There are some individuals with IDD in community living arrangements with no legal guardian, and they may be unable to provide informed consent to medical treatments (Botsford, 2004). Health care professionals and hospital staff providing community-based services are reluctant to serve adults with IDD who do not have legal guardians. In some cases, they have accepted their choice of legal guardian in the past but refuse to do so as they become older (Botsford, 2004). It is imperative that individuals with IDD and their families plan early so that an individual with IDD does not find him or herself as an elderly person with no guardian and an inability to receive proper care. Chapter 18 (Kingsbury) discusses person-centered planning as a way to allow an individual with IDD to make choices about end-of-life care.

LEGISLATIVE ISSUES

Developing and disseminating positive policy models and lobbying for change in existing policies that negatively impact end-of-life care should be the goals for professional, organizational, parental, and consumer advocacy groups across the county. Both Medicaid and Medicare benefits for individuals with IDD receiving end-of-life care need to reach every state, and those services need to be provided consistently across the country (Botsford, 2004). Finally, state legislatures need to carefully scrutinize their Health Care Decisions

Act and required forms to ensure that they provide meaning and benefits to as many individuals as possible—including individuals with IDD—who may have the capacity to make health care decisions on their own behalf, especially if the language of the advance directive is simple and understandable to them.

RESOURCES

As the result of the IOM reports referred to in this chapter, two free publications have been developed summarizing the reports. Their intent is to assist people to work through end-of-life situations for themselves and loved ones, and they suggest ways that individuals may contribute to the growth of palliative care services at the end of life in our society. These publications include *Working Together: We Can Help People Get Good Care When They Are Dying* (IOM, 2000) and *When Children Die: Improving Palliative and End-of-Life Care for Children and Their Families* (IOM, 2003).

REFERENCES

Alderson, P., Sutcliffe, K., & Curtis, K. (2006, November/December). Children's competence to consent to medical treatment. *Hastings Center Report*, p. 25.

Beauchamp, T. L., & Childress, J. F. (2001). *Principles of biomedical ethics* (5th ed.). New York: Oxford University Press.

Botsford, A. L. (2004). Status of end of life care in organizations providing services for older people with a developmental disability. *American Journal on Mental Retardation, 5*, 421–428.

Byock, I. (1997). *Dying well*. New York: Riverhead Books.

Callegary, E. (2005). Consent & competency. In *Best Practices in Developmental Disabilities: A Maryland Resource* (pp. 7–18). College Park, MD: Office of External Affairs, University of Maryland.

Cruzan v. Dir., Missouri Department Health, 497 U.S.261 (1990).

Dybwad, G. (1999). Introduction. In S. Herr & G. Weber (Eds.), *Aging, rights, and quality of life*. Baltimore: Brookes.

Edwards, S. (1997, Spring). The case of Joanne Harris. *Newsletter of the Network on Ethics and Intellectual Disabilities, 2*(2).

Five Wishes, Aging With Dignity. P.O. Box 1661, Tallahassee, FL 32302-1661. Retrieved November 12, 2008, from http://www.agingwithdignity.org

Golden, B. (2003). New law gives guardians authority to end futile treatment for adults with retardation. *New York State Bar Journal, 75*, 16.

Greenbaum, J. (2007). Life planning for adults with developmental disabilities: A guide for parents & family members. Oakland, CA: New Harbinger.

Grisso, T., & Applebaum, P. S. (1998). *Assessing competence to consent to treatment*. New York: Oxford University Press.

In re Guardianship of Ingram, 689 P.2d 1363 (Wash. 1984).

In re Heir, 464 N.E.2d. 959 (Mass. App. 1984).

In re O'Brien, 517 N.Y.S.2d. 348 (Sup. Ct. N.Y. County, 1986).

In re Storar, 420 N.E.2d 64 (N.Y. 1981).

Institute of Medicine (IOM). (1997). *Approaching death: Improving care at the end of life*. Washington, DC: National Academies Press.

Institute of Medicine (IOM). (2000). *Working together: We can help people get good care when they are dying*. Washington, DC: National Academies Press.

Institute of Medicine (IOM). (2003). *When children die: Improving end of life care for children and their families*. Washington, DC: National Academies Press.

Jonsen, A., Siegler, M., & Winslade, W. (2006). *Clinical ethics* (6th ed.). New York: McGraw-Hill.

Miller, E. (2006). Listening to the disabled: End-of-life medical decision making and the never competent. *Fordham Law Review, 74*(5), 2889–2925.

National Institutes of Health. (2004). *National Institutes of Health State-of-the-Science Conference statement on improving end-of-life care.* Washington, DC: U.S. Government Printing Office. Retrieved November 12, 2008, from http://consensus.nih.gov/2004/2004EndOfLifeCareSO S024html.htm

Pellegrino, E. D. (2000). Decision to withdraw life-sustaining treatment: A moral algorithm. *Journal of the American Medical Association, 283*(8), 1065.

President's Commission. (1983). *Deciding to forego life-sustaining treatment.* Washington, DC: U.S. Government Printing Office.

Strauss, D., & Eyman, R. K. (1996). Mortality of people with mental retardation in California with and without Down syndrome. *American Journal of Mental Retardation, 100*(6), 643–53.

Superintendent of Belchertown State Sch. v. Saikewicz, 370 N.E.2d 417, 432 (Mass. 1977).

Uniformed Health-Care Decisions Act (1993), National Conference of Commissioners on Uniform State Laws. Approved by the American Bar Association, Kansas City, Missouri, February 7, 1994.

PART II

Medical Conditions and Management

Chapter 4

Complex Medical Problems Affecting Life and Life Span in Children

SANDRA L. FRIEDMAN

INTRODUCTION

This chapter will focus on a specific group of children with intellectual and developmental disabilities (IDD) who have multiple associated medical problems. These children present with severe to profound IDD, an often unpredictable course of medical problems, and shortened life span (Chaney & Eyman, 2000; Strauss, Shavelle, Reynolds, Rosenbloom, & Day, 2007). While life expectancy for many children and adults with IDD has markedly improved, and usually closely follows that of the general population, some continue to experience life-threatening illnesses at a higher rate (Hayde, Kim, & DePaepe, 2005; Hutton & Pharoah, 2006; Katz, 2003; Patja, Iivanainen, Vesala, Oksnen, & Ruoppila, 2000; Patja, Molsa, & Iivanainen, 2003; Strauss, Cable, & Shavelle, 1999). At times, these children will recover from an acute episode, return to their baseline level of functioning, and continue to live for many years. At other times, they may recover yet return to a baseline that is somewhat lower than previously experienced—a process that may recur with future illnesses. There are situations in which these children undergo a gradual decline in functioning with age, without concomitant acute medical episodes. There are also times when an unanticipated acute episode occurs with a rapid decline in functioning that may lead to death (Friedman, Choueiri, & Gilmore, 2008; Klick & Ballantine, 2007).

It has been well documented that the presence of developmental disabilities in children, particularly children with intellectual disabilities, has a significant impact on health and general functioning (Boulet, Boyle, & Schieve, 2009). Medically fragile children with severe IDD present with a number of common medical problems, although certainly each child has his or her own constellation of health-related issues. These problems need to be addressed on an ongoing basis in order to maintain baseline level of functioning. As medical conditions worsen, so do the problems associated with severe IDD, and therefore adjustments are made to best meet the goals of care put forth by families and their medical team. These children are unique in that many of the treatments provided may be viewed as "extraordinary" for some in the general population and yet are "ordinary" in these situations because they are provided during periods of relative stability in order to maintain a baseline level of functioning. Conditions that the medical team may encounter while caring for these children will be reviewed using a systems approach; certainly not all children with severe IDD experience all of these problems. This overview is not intended to be an exhaustive review of the issues, but rather to provide an overview of the complexity of issues that need to be considered when providing medical care. Medical treatment and management at the end of life, when death is soon anticipated, are addressed in chapter 6.

Palliative care is often associated with care at the end of life when treatment is changed from goals of cure to goals of comfort. However, palliative care encompasses more than just pain management and medical treatments. It also provides assistance to the patient, family, and caregivers in the form of education, spiritual support, respite, and other ancillary therapies and services (American Academy of Pediatrics [AAP], 2000), which are addressed in other chapters of this book. Unfortunately, this type of care may not always be provided in a timely manner because prognosis may remain uncertain (Davies et al., 2008). This is particularly true for children who require multiple medical treatments and have experienced frequent hospitalizations throughout their lifetime. However, palliative care may also be provided to people with chronic medical problems who continue to be treated aggressively for acute illnesses when death is not imminent. Palliative care should be integrated within the overall care plan for a child and should be provided on an ongoing basis, whether the anticipated outcome is cure or death (AAP, 2000; Back, Arnold, & Quill, 2003; Graham & Robinson, 2005). Comfort should always be a goal of care no matter what the anticipated outcome of an illness or condition.

ETIOLOGIC FRAMEWORK

Extensive review of the etiology of neurological and associated medical problems is beyond the scope of this chapter. However, to provide a framework for understanding the issues faced by children with significant, special health care needs and IDD, it is helpful to understand the diversity of this group with regards to etiology of their medical and cognitive presentations. The presence of IDD reflects structural and/or functional changes to the central nervous system (CNS). Brain development begins early in the embryonic period and continues after birth. There are different stages of brain development, each with different vulnerabilities to injury. The timing, duration, and type of insult potentially affect developmental outcomes differently. The same insult that occurs at 20 weeks of gestation will have different effects than if it occurs at 36 weeks, 40 weeks, or even after birth. These insults may result in various changes in brain structure and function, including neuronal cell death, impairment of migration of the cells in the developing brain, specific lesions, and/or disruption of maturation.

More is being learned about insults to the developing brain with regards to timing of these episodes, resultant lesions or abnormalities in brain growth, associated changes in brain chemistry, and gender differences in response to insults. Premature infants are particularly vulnerable to adverse effects such as infection, metabolic abnormalities, and hemodynamic instability (Eklind et al., 2001; Volpe, 2003). We are not yet at the point in which treatments are available to reverse these insults; however, more is being learned about the physiologic mechanisms that occur, with exploration of potential interventions (Felling et al., 2006; Kumral et al., 2003). The brain continues to develop in the postnatal period, with interaction of the environment affecting brain development as well. Chemical or psychosocial environmental factors may positively or negatively affect both the structure and function of the CNS, with etiology sometimes complex or uncertain (Kaufman, Plotsky, Nemeroff, & Charney, 2000; McEwen, 2000).

Etiologic periods have been divided into those that occur in the pre-, peri-, or postnatal periods. Those insults that occur before birth are termed congenital, and generally those that occur after birth are acquired. However, there may be some conditions that are prenatally determined yet do not manifest themselves until later in life. The types of etiologic factors may be further characterized as due to factors such as hypoxia-ischemia, trauma, infection, genetics, metabolism, toxicity, deprivation, multiple factors, or unknown insults. The type of insult for each of the categories may be different based on the timing of the event: for example, deprivation in the prenatal period may take the form of placental insufficiency that deprives the fetus of essential components in the maternal blood, whereas deprivation in a young child may take the form of inadequate intake of essential dietary nutrients. These etiologic insults occur across the spectrum of cognitive abilities, although there are generally more neurological and associated medical problems with more severe IDD. There are common medical problems that are seen in this group of children, notwithstanding the clearly identifiable or presumed etiologic factors.

COMMON MEDICAL CONDITIONS

Children with severe IDD and complex medical problems may present with a multitude of medical conditions that require ongoing care in order to maintain health. The presence of significant neurological abnormalities, regardless of the etiology, is associated with a greater likelihood of other associated medical conditions, affecting most organ systems. Common areas that may require chronic and acute treatments include the pulmonary, gastrointestinal (GI), and neurological systems. In addition, these children are more vulnerable to infections and their potential negative sequelae. Children with intellectual disabilities also have an increased incidence of congenital anomalies affecting multiple organ systems, which increase with the severity of the disability (Petersen, Bourke, Leonard, Jacoby, & Bower, 2007). Therefore, other problems that occur with increased frequency may involve the endocrine, cardiac, and urologic systems. Metabolic problems may occur as inborn errors of metabolism, such as phenylketonuria (PKU), or acquired abnormalities, such as those associated with liver failure or certain toxins. Sensory problems are common, such as vision and hearing loss. While these sensory deficits do not affect life span by themselves, they may be associated with other medical conditions that do influence mortality. The presence of significant disabilities also has an impact on behavioral functioning, which may manifest as affective symptoms such as anxiety and depression, self-injurious behaviors, or aggression. A child who is nonverbal is not as able to report his or her symptoms; therefore, subtle indicators of illness need to be identified and treated expeditiously.

It is important to note that these medical issues need to be considered in the context of an individual child's medical stability, quality of life, and goals of care. These issues often change with time, and therefore ongoing medical review and communication between the health care team and family with regards to treatment and management decisions are crucial. There are times in which it is appropriate to choose aggressive medical management, times when it is ethically appropriate to choose different options of care, and times when aggressive procedures and treatments may not be recommended.

Neurological

Changes in structure of the brain, either congenital or acquired, are associated with an increased risk of epileptic seizure disorders. There also are conditions that may lower the seizure threshold, such as fever, acute illness, low blood sugar, electrolyte imbalance, psychosocial stress, and pain. The risk of epilepsy in the general population is approximately 1%, while those with IDD have an increased risk that has been reported to range from approximately 14 to 40%, depending on the population studied and the type of disability evaluated (Bowley & Kerr, 2000; McDermott et al., 2005; Morgan, Baxter, & Kerr, 2003). Seizures represent abnormal electrical activity in the brain with distinctive manifestations that may include abnormalities in muscle movements, tone, consciousness, and higher cortical functioning. Epileptic seizures represent a pattern of seizures that are recurrent and have distinct types of presentations, prognostic factors, and responses to certain treatments. It is important to identify the type of epilepsy in order to provide appropriate treatment and prognostic information.

Treatment with anticonvulsant medications is common, with many medications used to treat different types of seizure disorders. While these medications may be useful to reduce seizure frequency, patients need to be followed closely for side effects and complications related to medication use. Management of children on medications includes assessment of a child's mental status and behavior, as well as periodic evaluation of drug levels, liver function, or hematologic tests. Ideally, one wants to use the fewest number of medications to achieve acceptable seizure control (Alvarez, 2006). At times when seizure control is difficult to attain despite use of various medications, other treatment modalities may include use of the ketogenic diet or a vagal nerve stimulator. In certain situations, surgical interventions may also be considered (Vasconcellos et al., 2001).

Some children may have complicated and difficult to control seizure disorders, and so the goals of care become reduction of seizure frequency rather than total cessation of seizure activity (Alvarez, 2006). While it may be desirable for an individual to experience no seizure activity at all, it may not be possible unless that person is significantly sedated with reduced interaction with the environment. There should be a plan to rapidly intervene during periods of status epilepticus—situations in which seizures are prolonged or repetitive—that may prevent the need to seek treatment at an emergency room or hospital (Treiman & Walker, 2006; Wusthoff, Shellhass, & Licht, 2007). Medications such as rectal Valium have been used to abort continuous seizures, and there are times when intravenous medications are administered when other interventions fail. In these situations, care must be taken to monitor the respiratory status of the patient to avoid respiratory depression that may also be associated with use of these medications. Additional medical conditions, such as illness, fever, or metabolic changes that may contribute to increase in seizure frequency, may also need to be ruled out (Baumer, 2004).

Neurophysiologic testing should be performed to identify and characterize seizures. If testing is negative and there continues to be a high index of suspicion for a seizure disorder, repeat electroencephalograms or long-term monitoring should be performed.

Individuals with IDD have a high incidence of other behaviors that may appear to be seizures, such as movement disorders, idiosyncratic behaviors, and psychiatric disorders. Therefore, care must also be given to evaluate other medical conditions such as pain, anxiety, or additional mood issues (Wusthoff, Shellhaas, & Licht, 2007). Gastroesophageal reflux (GER) associated with movements of the extremities and trunk, known as Sandifer syndrome, may appear to give the false impression of a seizure. These behaviors need to be differentiated from seizures in order to be treated appropriately and to reassure caregivers.

Children with significant neurological dysfunction are also at risk for thermoregulatory instability. Autonomic instability may also be associated with abnormalities in blood pressure and heart rate. Periods of low or high temperature may occur without an obvious cause for this change. Exposure to an increase in ambient temperature or being clothed or wrapped heavily may result in elevation of body temperature. Treatment may simply require a change in the environment or removing excess clothing or covers. More commonly, children may experience hypothermia when temperature falls lower than 96 degrees Fahrenheit. Hypothermia may be associated with reduced responsiveness. Bundling with more clothing or blankets may be adequate to increase a child's temperature. When this type of intervention is not adequate, warming devices such as the T-pump may be necessary. Additional evaluation and laboratory tests would be required if the temperature instability appears to be associated with other signs or symptoms of infection or metabolic disturbance.

Abnormalities in muscle tone are common, particularly for those with cerebral palsy. Spasticity may contribute to a number of other medical conditions, including problems in the structure and function of the tendons, muscles, bones, and skin integrity. These issues are discussed in the next section.

Orthopedic and Bone Health

While the neurological condition associated with cerebral palsy or static encephalopathy may not be progressive, the changes in the neuromuscular and orthopedic systems may progress over time. Significant increase in muscle tone may contribute to discomfort and pain, as well as difficulties with seating, positioning, and providing daily care (Houlihan, O'Donnell, Conaway, & Stevenson, 2004). To address these issues, muscle relaxants, such as Valium and Baclofen, have been used orally or per gastrostomy tube (G-tube). Medication may also be administered intrathecally, such as with a Baclofen pump. At times, injections of Botox or Phenol are administered, followed by serial casting. In situations in which there is severe impairment, surgical interventions to improve motor function are used, such as selective dorsal root rhizotomy (Krigger, 2006; Winter & Kiely, 2007).

Significant abnormalities in muscle tone may contribute to the development of scoliosis or other spine abnormalities. Severe scoliosis not only interferes with positioning and seating, but it also reduces lung capacity and hinders respiratory function. Children may be treated with orthotic devices, such as soft spinal orthoses, or undergo surgical intervention, such as spinal fusion, to stop progression of the scoliosis. Recovery from these procedures may be difficult, and the determination as to which of these procedures are used must take into account the patient's overall medical condition and stability.

Similarly, increase in muscle tone may be associated with stress on joints, leading to contractures, subluxations, and dislocations. In addition to medical management of the spasticity, conservative treatment may include orthotic devices such as splints or alterations in seating systems. Surgery to release muscles or tendons may also be performed on children with significant spasticity, reducing discomfort while improving function or positioning (Deluca, 1996).

Children with cerebral palsy are at increased risk for osteopenia and osteoporosis, even with adequate nutritional intake, including calcium and Vitamin D. There are some genetic disorders, such as homocystinuria, that are associated with reduced bone mass. Endocrine disorders—such as growth hormone deficiency, hyperparathyroidism, hyperthyroidism, and sex hormone deficiency—may also be associated with low bone mass. Other factors that contribute to fragile bones include reduced mobility and weight bearing, nutritional deficits, chronic disease and cytokine release associated with inflammation, medications such as antiepileptic drugs and glucocorticoids, and delays in pubertal development (Munns & Cowell, 2005; Sheth, 2004). These changes in bones result in an increase risk for bone fractures compared to the general population (Stevenson et al., 2006). Fractures may occur due to everyday movements rather than significant trauma, such as with transferring a person from bed to wheelchair. In situations in which patients present with crying of uncertain cause, close examination needs to be done to rule out the presence of fracture.

It is important to obtain laboratory tests including blood chemistries—such as liver function tests, calcium, phosphorus, alkaline phosphatase; hormone levels such as thyroid-stimulating hormone (TSH) and parathyroid hormone (PTH); Vitamin D levels, as well as additional studies as indicated (Henderson, Kairalla, Barrington, Abbas, & Stevenson, 2005). Bone density testing, such as with the dual energy X-ray absorptiometry (DXA) scan, should also be considered when practical. Weight bearing is generally recommended, with standers being used even for individuals who are not able to stand or walk independently. Intravenous treatment with bisphosphonates has been used to treat osteoporosis, particularly for those who have had fractures previously (Steelman & Zeitler, 2003).

Pulmonary

Chronic and acute respiratory problems are relatively common in children with severe IDD. Chronic issues may develop from a child's inability to adequately expand lung tissue or clear secretions due to immobility and respiratory muscle weakness with associated reduced respiratory effort (Seddon & Khan, 2003). Children may have an inadequate cough mechanism with poor protection of the airway from secretions that may also pool in upper and lower airways (Morton, Wheatley, & Minford, 1999). Mucous plugging may also occur due to a collection of thick secretions in the lower airway, as well as with medications that may be used on occasion to reduce copious oral secretions in a child with excessive drooling. Poor nutrition and frequent recumbent positioning may also contribute to reduced respiratory effort.

Recurrent aspiration of saliva or food is a relatively common problem in children with severe IDD. Aspiration may occur because of reduced oropharyngeal tone and coordination and/or GER. Aggressive management of these problems may be needed to prevent serious lower respiratory tract infections, chronic lung changes, and/or changes to the upper esophagus that includes bleeding, stricture, and precancerous mucosal changes. Feeding tubes (gastrostomy and jejunostomy) also may need to be considered to allow for adequate nutrition in a safe manner.

The presence of kyphoscoliosis in children with cerebral palsy may result in restriction of chest wall structure and function. Chronic restrictive lung disease and reduced lung volume increase the potential need for supplemental oxygen, particularly in times of respiratory illness. Reactive airways disease, or wheezing, that may be associated with chronic lung changes is also common. Reduced ambulation and independent movement may also contribute to atelectasis, a medical condition in which portions of lung tissue collapse.

Some children also present with respiratory problems more specific to the medical condition associated with their intellectual disability. For example, children who are born very premature and with very low birth weight may be at risk for chronic lung changes, referred to as bronchopulmonary dysplasia. Some children with neurodegenerative disorders exhibit a progressive loss of respiratory effort. In most situations, however, the children require frequent chest percussion, suctioning, and/or postural drainage to maintain patent airways. Chronic airway and pulmonary problems may necessitate use of oxygen, bronchodilators, multiple medications, and even tracheostomy to promote stable respiratory status (Carron, Derkay, Strope, Nosonchuk, & Darrow, 2000). At times, noninvasive, positive pressure ventilation, such as CPAP (continuous positive airway pressure) and BiPAP (bilevel positive airway pressure), or mechanical ventilation are used in order to maintain adequate oxygenation and stable respiratory functioning (Ullrich & Mayer, 2007). As with many other types of interventions, consideration must be given to the child's medical condition, stability, and goals of care before initiating these treatments. Low-dose morphine has also been effectively used to improve refractory respiratory distress (Abernethy et al., 2003).

There are also individuals who have problems with apnea—or periods in which breathing stops—that place them at greater risk for respiratory distress. There are two types of apnea: central and obstructive. Central apnea refers to a failure in the brain activity that triggers the breathing mechanism and it frequently occurs during sleep. These children may require use of the ventilator for naps or overnight sleep to assure continued respiratory effort. Obstructive apnea occurs when there is some type of mechanical reason that the airway may be blocked, particularly during sleep. This may occur because of enlarged tonsils or adenoids, variation in the structure or function of the upper airway, or obstruction secondary stenosis of the airway. There often are medical and surgical interventions that can be used to overcome these mechanical obstructions. Obstructive apnea may respond to using a nasopharyngeal airway, weight loss, removal of tonsils and adenoids, repositioning of the tongue or mandible, or tracheostomy (McKenna, 2006).

A tracheostomy may also be recommended in medical situations associated with upper airway obstruction, craniofacial anomalies, prolonged intubation, neurologic impairment, trauma, and vocal fold paralysis (Carron et al., 2000). It is important that the family and medical team carefully consider the child's condition and the overall care plan when considering whether to go forward with this recommendation. For those who undergo the procedure, care must be taken to maintain a patent airway with suctioning and regular tracheostomy changes. Close monitoring is also required, as the tube may be inadvertently extruded, plugged, or compressed (McKenna, 2006).

Acute respiratory illnesses—such as bronchitis, asthma, pneumonia, and even significant upper respiratory tract infections—may provide an added stress on the existing chronic respiratory problems. It is important to identify these problems early, to assess the cause for the distress, and to treat them aggressively to avoid significant deterioration in respiratory status (Waltz & Katz, 2006). Antibiotics, bronchodilators, chest physiotherapy, frequent suctioning, supplemental oxygen, and an increase in other means of respiratory support may all be necessary to return a child to his or her baseline level of pulmonary functioning (Brook, 1996).

Gastrointestinal

Gastrointestinal disorders—not the least of which are disorders related to nutritional problems—frequently occur in children with severe IDD. Some children with significant neurological disorders may present with growth failure or be malnourished, while others may be overweight (Mascarenhas, Meyers, & Konek, 2008). Eating by mouth provides pleasure and improves the quality of life. However, problems that may affect the intake of nutrition may include acute illnesses, food-medication interactions, caregiver involvement, nutrient adequacy, and absorption of nutrients (Cohen, Piazza, & Navathe, 2006). For individuals with severe IDD and concomitant medical problems, feeding also may be associated with discomfort and an excessive amount of time to finish meals. Nutritional losses may occur from frequent emesis, as well as caloric expenditure higher than expected for those with cerebral palsy who ambulate compared to the expenditure of typically developing children. On the other hand, children who are nonambulatory tend to expend less energy. For those who receive enteral tube feedings, it is important to meet nutritional needs without excessive caloric intake that may cause a child to become overweight.

Feeding disorders may be caused by sensory and/or motor problems affecting chewing and swallowing. Dysphagia, or difficulty swallowing, may involve abnormal function in several phases of the swallowing process, including taking in and preparing the food in the oral phase, beginning of the reflexive swallow, and the pharyngeal phase (Fishman & Bousvaros, 2006). A child may need to be observed feeding, and additional tests such as a chest X-ray and videofluoroscopy may need to be performed to identify the problem and to provide feeding recommendations. Changes in food or fluid consistency may be required, and sometimes it is recommended that oral feeding actually be discontinued to avoid recurrent aspiration that may lead to significant lower respiratory tract problems.

GER is also common due to loosening of the juncture between the stomach and lower esophagus, allowing for a back flow of gastric secretions and food into esophagus (Del Giudice et al., 1999). Chronic GER may lead to changes in the mucosal lining of the lower esophagus, such as esophagitis with associated bleeding, esophageal strictures, or to precancerous changes as seen in Barrett's esophagitis. GER may be uncomfortable and associated with anemia due to occult or frank bleeding. Assessment for GER may include a pH probe study in which the acidity of the lower esophagus is evaluated for the presence of acid from the stomach to determine whether a person is experiencing gastroesophageal reflux. Medical management with medications may be required to neutralize or reduce the secretion of gastric acids and/or increase gastric motility. Various medications have been used to treat these symptoms (Fishman & Bousvaros, 2006), such as prokinetics (metoclopramide), H2 antagonists (ranitidine), and proton pump inhibitors (omeprazole).

A child may initially be able to take all of his nutrition orally, but over time the ability to take in adequate nutrition decreases due to increased problems with oromotor function, GER, or changes in medical status. Vomiting and weight loss may also occur. Surgical interventions may be recommended when medical management proves to be inadequate. A fundoplication is a procedure in which the area between the lower esophagus and stomach is tightened, preventing reflux of stomach contents into the esophagus. The use of an enteral tube may also be considered when a child is unable to take oral nutrition either because of poor oromotor function or significant GER and associated aspiration. Consideration may be given to a tube inserted into the stomach (gastrostomy or G-tube) or into the jejunum (jejunostomy or J-tube). Open surgical and laparoscopic procedures have been used for fundoplications and for enteral tube placement. In a study that assessed the outcome for children who underwent laparoscopic antireflux surgery, there were no postoperative complications or mortality. However, about half of the patients studied continued to have respiratory problems, with some children reexperiencing GER and requiring another fundoplication (Kawahara et al., 2004). Therefore, while these procedures have some benefit, many children remain symptomatic. As with other medical interventions that may be recommended, it is important to evaluate the whole child, considering his or her medical status, stability, and goals of care when considering these procedures.

Previous studies have also shown that children with cerebral palsy who were fed via gastrostomy tube continued to have a high death rate (Sleigh & Brocklehurst, 2004; Strauss & Shavelle, 1998). However, mortality has decreased even in children with enteral tubes in recent years (Strauss, Shavelle, Reynolds, Rosenbloom, & Day, 2007). It has been surmised that more experience with management of medical and nutritional problems related to G-tube use has contributed to the improvement in outcomes over time. With a feeding tube, a child still may be able to eat some food orally, or experience "taste treats," while the rest of his or her nutrition is provided via enteral tube to assure adequate nutritional intake.

Abnormalities in smooth muscle function contribute to problems in gastric motility and delayed gastric emptying (Santucci & Mack, 2007). Reduced mobility of the gastrointestinal tract may require changes in feeding to allow for slower administration of nutrition. Vomiting and retching may occur, requiring changes in administration of feedings (Richards, Milla, Andrews, & Spitz, 2001). Gastrostomy tube feeding may not be tolerated in their usual amounts or rates during times of illness. Bolus feeds may need to be changed to continuous feeds, and continuous feeds may need to be changed to a rate that is slower than usual. While slower, continuous feeds may be better tolerated, they also limit the time that a child is not connected to the gastrostomy tube.

Constipation is another very common problem among children with severe to profound IDD. The reason for the high rate of this condition is not entirely clear, although a number of contributing factors have been implicated. Reduced mobility, decreased intake of dietary fiber, inadequate fluids, use of some medications, and abnormalities in smooth muscle function and motility may contribute to this condition. In addition, there are specific medical conditions that occur in children with IDD that cause an added risk for constipation. Some of these conditions may be classified as anatomical, such as those that may occur in children with congenital anomalies that include the GI tract, specifically the anal area. Neuromuscular conditions may also contribute to constipation, such as myelomeningocele and other abnormalities of the spinal cord. Metabolic conditions, such as thyroid abnormalities and celiac disease, have been implicated, as well as certain medications, such as some pain and anticonvulsant medications (Fishman & Bousvaros, 2006). Inadequately treated or recognized constipation may present with reduced feeding tolerance, nausea, vomiting, obstruction, and discomfort. Dietary means should be used to prevent constipation, but adequate dietary intake of fluids and foods containing fiber may not be enough to prevent it. Treatment should be done in a stepwise fashion to avoid dependence of high doses of stimulant laxatives. For some children, however, daily medication is necessary to assure regular bowel movements.

Infections

Pneumonia has long been a common cause of mortality in people with IDD. More aggressive treatment of pulmonary infections, improvement in antimicrobial agents, and treatment of conditions that contribute to infections—such as aspiration of feeds—have reduced the morbidity and mortality associated with pulmonary infections. However, respiratory problems continue to be a relatively common occurrence and require aggressive management. While these types of infections continue to be the most common, other infections include those related to the head, neck, and urinary tract. Poor communication skills may also interfere with identification of early symptoms related to illness; therefore, it is important to be able to identify subtle indicators of illness, such as facial grimacing, reduced appetite, increased agitation, increase seizures, and thermoregulatory instability, to name a few.

Anatomical impairments, such as those of the head and neck have been implicated as increasing the risk for some infections. Children with Down syndrome and with cleft palate are at increased risk of ear infections. The presence of a neurogenic bladder, with stasis of urine in the urinary tract and/or need for recurrent bladder catheterization has been associated in urinary tract infections. In addition, impaired immune responses, abnormalities in ciliary kinetics, and disorders in smooth muscle function may all increase the risk of infection in children with IDD (Keyserling, 2006). Children who are medically fragile may have difficulty fighting common infections and therefore are at greater risk for complications from influenza and even common cold viruses, such as rhinovirus. Children with special health care needs should be vaccinated from childhood illnesses, as set forth by the American Academy of Pediatrics guidelines, as well as receive the influenza vaccine on an annual basis. In addition, prophylaxis should be provided to children exposed to influenza.

Genitourinary

Children with IDD may present with a number of either congenital or acquired disorders of the genitourinary (GU) system. Anomalies of the GU tract may be associated with some genetic syndromes. Congenital abnormalities of kidneys may be associated with abnormalities in lung development (Martín et al., 2004). Abnormalities in the kidneys or urinary collecting system, such as narrowing at the juncture between the kidneys and collecting system, may result in obstruction leading to changes in structure and function of the kidney. These changes may increase susceptibility to infection or, more concerning, permanent renal impairment. Some syndromes may also be associated with absent, partially functioning, or abnormally formed kidneys. There are some syndromes in which renal problems may not initially be present but require monitoring because of the increased risk of developing renal problems or tumors, such as Wilms tumors for those diagnosed with Beckwith-Wiedemann syndrome.

Spinal cord abnormalities that may affect the urologic system may be congenital, such as with myelodysplasia or spina bifida. Trauma to the spinal cord may also affect urological functioning. Just as smooth muscle dysfunction may affect the gastrointestinal tract, it also may affect the genitourinary tract. Neurogenic bladders may reduce the frequency of urination, increasing the need for catheterization and the risk of infections. In addition to the neurogenic causes of bladder dysfunction, some incontinence may reflect cognitive level of functioning. Incontinence of stool and use of a diaper may also make these children more prone to ascending infections caused by common gastrointestinal flora.

Metabolism

Inborn errors of metabolism (IEM) refer to a group of disorders in which abnormalities exist in biochemical pathways in the body. They occur relatively infrequently in the general population and are comprised of a diverse group of disorders with varying inheritance, timing of presentation, clinical symptoms, morbidity, and mortality (Kayser, 2008). Some IEM are associated with significant intellectual and developmental disabilities if undetected or untreated in a timely manner. Phenylketonuria (PKU) is an aminoacidopathy that requires early identification and ongoing treatment to avoid profound cognitive and other developmental problems. There are some IEM for which no treatment exists or efficacy of treatment is limited, such as with the gangliosidoses like Tay-Sachs disease.

Some of these disorders may be identified prenatally via amniocentesis. Newborn screening programs have resulted in identification of a number of these disorders, such as with PKU and hypothyroidism (Schulze et al., 2003; Simpoulos, 2009). Some IEM are not identified initially but later present with progressive neurological deterioration and in association with symptoms such as abnormalities in muscle tone, lethargy, seizures, loss of developmental milestones, apnea, vomiting, and feeding intolerance. Some disorders, such as Leigh syndrome, worsen with physiologic stress and may not even be identified until after a stressful event, such as use of anesthesia for a relatively minor procedure. It is important to be able to identify the problem, as some inborn errors of metabolism may respond to diet restrictions, vitamin cofactors, supplements of the deficient factor or enzyme replacement, and at times organ or bone marrow transplant (Kamboh, 2008).

Other types of metabolic problems may be acquired. Anticonvulsant medications are commonly used in children with severe IDD. However, some of these medications affect the metabolism of liver enzymes, in addition to affecting electrolyte balance, blood cells, and platelets. Drugs may be metabolized in the body via the cytochrome P450 enzymes, whereby enzymes may be inhibited or induced and therefore affect the level of certain medications in the body (Cupp & Tracy, 1998). Care must be taken to determine if one drug affects the metabolism of another, which may either lead to undesirable toxic or subtherapeutic levels of a needed medication. There are also times in which fulminant sepsis (infection in blood stream) may result in metabolic dysfunction of the liver or kidneys, potentially leading to failure of these organs.

Endocrine

Endocrine disorders occur with relative frequency in children with IDD. Some endocrinologic disorders actually may cause or contribute to the neurological conditions, although with better screening and medical management the outcomes of these problems can be improved significantly. The incidence of congenital hypothyroidism has dramatically diminished as a result of screening. Some children with IDD may present with endocrinologic disorders requiring supplementation therapy as part of their specific syndrome, such as thyroid hormone for children with Down syndrome; thyroid, growth, and/or estrogen hormone therapy for girls with Turner syndrome; and testosterone therapy for boys with Klinefelter syndrome (Botero & Fleishman, 2006). Medical management of these children requires close monitoring for these disorders with appropriate hormone therapy as indicated.

The pituitary gland is responsible for secretion of hormones associated with growth and the regulation of fluids and electrolytes. Panhypopituitarism may be congenital or acquired and may be seen in children with severe IDD. Congenital panhypopituitarism may be seen in certain genetic syndromes, such as septo-optic dysplasia. Panhypopituitarism also may be the result of infections (e.g., meningitis) or brain trauma. It has significant impact on metabolism, growth, and development and has the potential of being life-threatening in certain situations. This condition may be associated with hypothyroidism, which may affect growth, development, temperature stability, mood, mental status, menstruation, and bowel patterns. Growth hormone and sex hormones may also be affected. Disruption also may cause the syndrome of inappropriate antidiuretic hormone (SIADH), in which sodium imbalance may occur. Laboratory testing may include monitoring for electrolytes, glucose, hormone levels, with adjustments in fluid intake, medications, or supplemental hormones, as imbalance in some situations may be life threatening. Certain medications, such as the antiepileptic medication carbamazepine, may also present with low serum sodium levels consistent with SIADH. Some children require fluid restriction or medication such as desmopressin (trade name DDAVP) for SIADH.

Congenital and acquired abnormalities in the structure of the central nervous system itself may also be associated with abnormalities in pubertal development (Botero & Fleishman, 2006). Central precocious puberty is a relatively common occurrence in children with severe IDD. Analysis of growth parameters, bone age, secondary sexual characteristics, gonadotropins, and sex hormones needs to be done. Imaging studies of the central nervous system and/or of the genital tract may be important to perform in order to clarify the diagnosis and determine the course of treatment. Hormone therapy with oral, enteral, or intramuscular use of Provera has been used to suppress menstruation and associated cramping and discomfort.

Other children, such as those with Prader-Willi or Down syndrome, may have problems with glucose intolerance or they may develop diabetes mellitus. Problems with very high or very low glucose may also be life threatening and require immediate intervention.

Cardiac

Congenital heart disease (CHD) may be present in certain genetic disorders, such as Down, Williams, DiGeorge, and CHARGE syndromes. Even for children without specific syndromes associated with developmental disorders, the presence of CHD is also associated with abnormalities in the CNS (Padula & Ades, 2006). In addition, other factors—such as hypoxia, hemodynamic instability, prolonged heart-lung bypass, and use of multiple medications—occurring before, during, or after surgical interventions may predispose a child to developmental delays, although usually not in the severe to profound range.

Previously, children with CHD associated with a genetic syndrome or multiple congenital anomalies did not regularly undergo cardiac surgery. Currently, however, heart surgery is generally offered to these children except in situations when survival of the child is not anticipated. Prior to surgery, heart failure is managed with medications and adequate nutritional support (Dooley, 2006). Residual problems after surgery may require the use of medications to address the underlying cardiac abnormality (e.g., insufficiency of the mitral or tricuspid valves) and diuretics. Fluid management and electrolyte balance needs to be monitored closely in these cases.

Sensory

Children with severe IDD have an increased risk of being visually or hearing impaired. They may also have sensory processing difficulties that make tolerance of different types of sensory input difficult. While deficits in hearing and vision are not associated with increased risk of dying—just as sensory aversion is not associated with life-threatening conditions—it is important to acknowledge these issues to better care for the individual.

Ophthalmologic problems are also common in children with certain congenital or genetic disorders. Congenital cataracts, glaucoma, degenerative changes to the retina, optic atrophy, and strabismus are just some of the problems that may affect a child's vision (Fulton, Mayer, Miller, & Hansen, 2006). Some of these problems respond to treatment, such as cataracts, while others do not, such as optic atrophy. Prematurity has been associated with retinopathy of prematurity. Congenital infections, such cytomegalovirus, or perinatal infections, such as herpes, can also affect visual acuity and functional use of vision. Identification of some of these abnormalities may actually provide important diagnostic information about the cause of a child's developmental disability. Identification is also needed to determine appropriate medical treatment and educational interventions.

Similarly, hearing loss may be associated with specific genetic or congenital disorders, such as Down syndrome, CHARGE syndrome, some congenital infections, and certain mitochondrial disorders. Children who undergo extracorporeal membrane oxygenation (ECMO) management for problems such as congenital heart disease or congenital diaphragmatic hernia are at increased risk of developing progressive sensorineural hearing loss in the first few years of life (Fligor, Neault, Mullen, Feldman, & Jones, 2005). Because hearing is important for the development of language and for interaction with the environment, it is essential to identify the presence and type of hearing loss, as well as determine if medical intervention is indicated.

Sensory processing abnormalities have also been associated with some developmental disorders. Sensory aversions or sensory-seeking behaviors may be present. Some children may require desensitization against certain stimuli, as well as require particular sensory input in order to calm. While soft music may be soothing to some, if a child is not able to hear it then other means to comfort may need to be employed, such as massage or soft touch. There are techniques and systems that employ different sensory interventions for calming purposes or for increasing responsiveness to the environment. These methods may be used every day, during illness, and at the end of life.

Behavior

Behavioral presentation of a person with or without IDD may be affected by a number of physiologic or external influences. If someone is not feeling well because of physical symptoms, he or she may be more apt to become agitated, upset, depressed, sad, or anxious. The consequences of those symptoms, such as inability to participate in preferred activities, may also affect mood or behavior. In addition, some people may also have an underlying psychiatric condition that affects behavior and interaction with others.

People with IDD have a greater incidence of psychiatric disorders compared to the general population (Emerson, 2003). The term "dual diagnosis" refers to the presence of intellectual and psychiatric disabilities. While some people do need medication and respond well to treatment of a concomitant psychiatric disorder, it is important to be able to identify changes or problems in behavior, rule out potential causes for changes in behavior, and address those potential causes before automatically assuming the need for medication to treat the behavior.

People with IDD may present with aggression or self-injurious behaviors (SIB), which may reflect illness, pain, boredom, or self-stimulatory behavior. Change in mood similarly may be influenced by environmental changes or losses, as well as medical problems, such as new onset abnormalities in thyroid metabolism.

MAKING DECISIONS

The following is a vignette that illustrates some of the issues involved in making difficult decisions regarding the medical care of a child with severe IDD and complex medical problems.

Emma is a 9-year-old girl born with a chromosome abnormality. She lives at home and receives educational instruction and therapies through the public school system. Her parents provide much of her care, although she does receive home nursing support overnight.

Emma had a prolonged course in the neonatal intensive care unit (NICU) as a newborn. She was born premature and required a ventilator for several months. She later developed stridor secondary to granulation tissue in her upper airway because of the prolonged need for intubation. Emma also has a history of failure to thrive and poor oral intake. Feeding evaluation revealed both motor and sensory issues that interfered with oral intake. She had poorly coordinated suck and swallow abilities and an aversion to objects in her mouth. Videofluoroscopic evaluation also indicated significant aspiration of fluids. She underwent Nissen fundoplication and G-tube placement and gained weight once enteral feedings were initiated.

She has been followed by multiple medical providers, including neurology to treat her seizure disorder, physiatry to treat spasticity, orthopedics to monitor her back and joints, pulmonary for her chronic lung disease, and gastroenterology because of issues related to feeding and nutrition.

Over the past several years, she was hospitalized at least 3 or 4 times per year, primarily for respiratory problems. A sleep study revealed both obstructive and central sleep apnea, with associated hypoxic episodes. It was recommended that she undergo tracheostomy placement and use the ventilator at night. She usually is on room air, although she may require supplemental oxygen during episodes of lower respiratory tract infection and/or wheezing. After the tracheostomy and the nighttime ventilator were initiated, she appeared to be more alert and responsive to others.

Emma's muscle tone has increased over time. She receives physical and occupational therapies, wears hand splints, and orthotics on her lower extremities. She takes muscle relaxants, and consideration is being given to surgery because of her worsening scoliosis.

Between her illnesses, she appears to be happy and responds to others, particularly family members. Although she was given the flu vaccine in late autumn, she developed a febrile illness associated with upper and lower respiratory tract symptoms. Testing indicated a strain of influenza not well covered by the vaccine. Her respiratory status deteriorated rapidly, requiring admission to the intensive care unit (ICU). She was placed on a ventilator on a continuous basis to support respiration. Emma had not exhibited this degree of illness since her neonatal period. She also was treated with antiviral agents and rigorous pulmonary toilet. Chest X-ray revealed pneumonia for which she also received antibiotics. In addition, Emma exhibited an increase in seizure frequency, requiring adjustment of her anticonvulsant medications.

Her medical team had concerns that Emma would not recover from this illness. The palliative care team was consulted. Goals of care were discussed with her family, who desired aggressive treatment of her medical condition and full resuscitation in the event of cardiopulmonary arrest. Medications were also given to promote comfort. Emma recovered from the illness to her usual baseline and was discharged home after 6 weeks.

The situation with Emma illustrates the complexity of her medical problems and the issues that must be addressed on a daily basis in order to maintain her health and well-being. Illnesses that may be considered relatively common in the general population and are tolerated without significant morbidity may be life threatening in children with complex medical problems and severe disabilities. Families are periodically faced with events in which they need to consider their child's status, the potential outcome of their child's illness, available treatment options, and the possibility that their child may not survive. In the example cited earlier, although there was a possibility that Emma may have succumbed to influenza, with appropriate supportive treatment she did recover.

One may consider how events would have transpired if her condition took another course. She may have recovered, but her baseline of functioning may have been lower than it was before her illness. For example, she may have required more oxygen at home, longer periods on the ventilator, and more frequent pulmonary treatments. Each subsequent, acute illness may have resulted in a smaller decrease in baseline functioning, more periods of instability, and less frequent episodes of positive interaction with her environment. These are all factors that her family would need to consider when decisions are revisited about aggressive medical management and resuscitation status in order to balance the degree to which treatments become more of a burden than a benefit.

What if Emma did not respond to the supportive treatment? Despite aggressive ventilatory support and pulmonary treatments, she could have not been able to maintain adequate oxygenation. She may have begun to demonstrate metabolic abnormalities of her liver and kidney function, leading to failure of these organs. In order to tolerate all of her treatments, she may have needed heavy sedation so that her interaction with others would have been quite limited. At some point, her family in conjunction with her medical team may have decided that the burdens outweighed the benefits of aggressive treatment. They may no longer have wished for resuscitation effort to be provided in the event of cardiopulmonary arrest. Management would then shift to making her as comfortable as possible, using pain medications, while also trying to allow some periods in which she would be able to sense the presence of her family. She would be provided with some oxygen and gentle suctioning for comfort, but not for treatment of her pulmonary condition. Monitors may then be removed, with blood work and invasive procedures discontinued. At some point, when her gastric motility was significantly reduced and her abdomen became more distended, fluid may be discontinued but her lips could be moistened with glycerin swabs. Her family would have been able to comfort and remain with her until she died.

The monitoring and treatment of medical problems affecting the various organ systems may change as one approaches the end of life. While aggressive treatments may continue, at some point it may be determined that treatment offers no benefit and recovery is not possible. Table 4.1 illustrates the different approaches that may be taken for a child with multiple and complex medical problems during routine care compared to management when death is soon anticipated. It is understood that there are different approaches to managing some of these medical issues based on the medical situation of individual patients and the wishes of decision makers.

At end of life, respiratory function is often more depressed, either because of reduced respiratory effort, infection, reduced ability to clear secretions, and diminished respiratory drive secondary to changes in oxygen and carbon dioxide levels. Monitoring of oxygen, carbon dioxide, and other blood gases would be discontinued, although oxygen and suctioning may be provided to provide comfort. Neurologically, there may be reduced responsiveness or alteration in mental status due to change in metabolic functioning, infection, or respiratory status. Sedative medication may be reduced to potentially improve interaction with others while maintaining adequate pain management. Seizure frequency and/or duration may be different because of change in seizure threshold due to these same metabolic, pulmonary, or infectious factors and would require continued treatment. Cardiac function may be affected by pulmonary or metabolic status, although cardiac monitors may not be used and cardiopressor medications would not be administered. The child may develop an ileus, in which the normal peristaltic action of the GI tract significantly slows down resulting in intolerance of enteral or oral feeds with abdominal distension. Nutrition and hydration may be progressively reduced and then stopped in order to provide comfort. Narcotics would be provided for pain, which may slow gut motility and cause constipation that also requires treatment. The liver may no longer be able to metabolize routine medications and may actually begin to fail, as may the kidney, further affecting a person's mental status and ability to interact with the environment. Active correction of metabolic abnormalities would not occur. Intubation and use of the ventilator would not be initiated for those who have Do-Not-Resuscitate (DNR) orders and have changed from goals of care to comfort only. At some point the family may choose to discontinue use of the ventilator for those receiving mechanical ventilation.

There are no easy ways to address these issues, and families often approach decisions about the type, intensity, and duration of treatments quite differently. It is always

Table 4.1
Medical Management Considerations

Medical problem	Type of treatment	Decision to treat	
		Chronic	*End of life*
Cardiopulmonary	Check O2 saturation	Y	N
	Chest physiotherapy	Y	Y/N
	Start ventilator	Y/N	N
	Provide O2	Y	Y
	Monitor vitals	Y	N
	Withdraw ventilator	N	Y
Seizures	Treat seizures	Y	Y
	Consider alterative (diet, surgery)	Y	N
	Monitor AED levels	Y	N
GI	Nutrition/hydration	Y	Y/N
	Treat constipation	Y	Y/N
	Treat GER	Y	Y/N
	Withhold N&H	N	Y/N
Pain	Pain relief	Y	Y
	Frequent use of narcotics	N	Y
	Concern about prolonged narcotics	Y/N	N
Infection	Treat all	Y	N
	Treat only for comfort	N	Y/N
	No treat	N	Y/N
	Monitor lab work	Y	N
Metabolism	Monitor chemistries	Y	N
	Check drug levels	Y	N
	Correct imbalances	Y	N

Key: O2 = oxygen; AED = antiepileptic drug; N&H = nutrition and hydration;
GER = gastroesophageal reflux.

important for accurate information to be presented to families on a proactive and ongoing basis, with opportunities for families to express their values, wishes, and concerns. Respect for the life of a child and for a family's hopes are always important. There are times, however, when our knowledge, expertise, and skills cannot stop the inevitability of death. At those times, we must continue to support the comfort and dignity of the patient and remember that he or she is part of a larger social and family network that also requires our support.

References

Abernethy, A. P., Currow, D. C., Frith, P., Fazekas, B. S., McHugh, A., & Bui, C. (2003). Randomised, double blind placebo controlled crossover trial of sustained release morphine for the management of refractory dyspnoea. *British Medical Journal, 327*, 523–528.

Alvarez, N. (2006). Epilepsy. In I. L. Rubin & A. C. Crocker (Eds.), *Medical care for children and adults with developmental disabilities* (pp. 255–270). Baltimore, MD: Paul H. Brookes.

American Academy of Pediatrics Committee on Bioethics and Committee on Hospital Care. (2000). Palliative care for children. *Pediatrics, 106*(2), 351–357.

Back, A. L., Arnold, R. M., & Quill, T. E. (2003). Hope for the best, and prepare for the worst. *Annals of Internal Medicine, 138*(5), 439–443.

Baumer, J. H. (2004). Evidence based guideline for post-seizure management in children presenting acutely to secondary care. *Archives of Disease in Childhood, 89*(3), 278–280

Botero, D., & Fleishman, A. (2006). Endocrinology. In I. L. Rubin & A. C. Crocker (Eds.), *Medical care for children and adults with developmental disabilities* (pp. 387–398). Baltimore, MD: Paul H. Brookes.

Boulet, S. L., Boyle, C. A., & Schieve, L. A. (2009). Health care use and health and functional impact on developmental disabilities among U.S. children, 1997–2005. *Archives of Pediatric and Adolescent Medicine, 163*(1), 19–26.

Bowley, C., & Kerr, M. (2000). Epilepsy and intellectual disability. *Journal of Intellectual Disability Research, 44*, 529–543.

Brook, I. (1996). Treatment of aspiration or tracheostomy-associated aspiration pneumonia in neurologically impaired children: Effect of antimicrobials effective against bacteria. *International Journal of Pediatric Otorhinolaryngology, 35*(2), 171–177.

Carron, J. D., Derkay, C. S., Strope, G. L, Nosonchuk, J. E., & Darrow, D. H. (2000). Pediatric tracheostomy: Changing indications and outcomes. *Laryngoscope, 110*, 1099–1104.

Chaney, R. H., & Eyman, R. K. (2000). Patterns of mortality over 60 years among persons with mental retardation in a residential facility. *Mental Retardation, 38*(3), 289–293.

Cohen, S. A., Piazza, C. C., & Navathe, A. (2006). Feeding and nutrition. In I. L. Rubin & A. C. Crocker (Eds.), *Medical care for children and adults with developmental disabilities* (pp. 295–306). Baltimore, MD: Paul H. Brookes.

Cupp, M. J., & Tracy, T. S. (1998). Cytochrome P450: New nomenclature and clinical implications. *American Family Physician, 57*(1), 107–116.

Davies, B., Sehring, S. A., Partridge, J. C., Cooper, B. A., Hughes, A., Philp, J. C., et al. (2008). Barriers to palliative care for children: perceptions of pediatric health care providers. *Pediatrics, 121*(2), 282–288.

Del Giudice, E., Staiano, A., Capano, G., Romano, A., Florimonte, L., Miele, E., et al. (1999). Gastrointestinal manifestations in children with cerebral palsy. *Brain and Development, 21*(5), 307–311.

Deluca, P. A. (1996). The musculoskeletal management of children with cerebral palsy. *Pediatric Clinics of North America, 43*(5), 1135–1150.

Dooley, K. J. (2006). History and management of congenital heart disease. In I. L. Rubin & A. C. Crocker (Eds.), *Medical care for children and adults with developmental disabilities* (pp. 373–378). Baltimore, MD: Paul H. Brookes.

Elkind, S., Mallard, C., Leverin, A. L., Gilland, E., Blomgren, K., Mattsby-Baltzer, I., et al. (2001). Bacterial endotoxin sensitizes the immature brain to hypoxic-ischaemic injury. *European Journal of Neuroscience, 13*(6), 1101–1106.

Emerson, E. (2003). Prevalence of psychiatric disorders in children and adolescents with and without intellectual disability. *Journal of Intellectual Disability Research, 47*, 51–58.

Felling, R. J., Snyder, M. J., Romanko, M. J., Rothstein, R. P., Ziegler, A. N., Yang, Z., et al. (2006). Neural stem/progenitor cells participate in the regenerative response to perinatal hypoxia/ischemia. *Journal of Neuroscience, 26*(16), 4359–4369.

Fishman, L. N., & Bousvaros, A. (2006). Gastrointestinal issues. In I. L. Rubin & A. C. Crocker (Eds.), *Medical care for children and adults with developmental disabilities* (pp. 307–324). Baltimore, MD: Paul H. Brookes.

Fligor, B. J., Neault, M. W., Mullen, C. H., Feldman, H. A., & Jones, D. T. (2005). Factors associated with sensorineural hearing loss among survivors of extracorporeal membrane oxygenation therapy. *Pediatrics, 115*, 1519–1528.

Friedman, S. L., Choueiri, R., & Gilmore, D. (2008). Staff carers' understanding of end of life care. *Journal of Policy Practice in Intellectual Disabilities, 5*(1), 56–64.

Fulton, A. B., Mayer, D. L, Miller, K. B., & Hansen, R. M. (2006). Eye and vision care. In I. L. Rubin & A. C. Crocker (Eds.), *Medical care for children and adults with developmental disabilities* (pp. 343–352). Baltimore, MD: Paul H. Brookes.

Graham, R. J., & Robinson, W. M. (2005). Integrating palliative care into chronic care for children with severe neurodevelopmental disabilities. *Journal of Developmental and Behavioral Pediatrics, 26*(5), 361–365.

Hayde, M. F., Kim, S. H., & DePaepe, P. (2005). Health status, utilization patterns, and outcomes of persons with intellectual disabilities: Review of the literature. *Mental Retardation, 43*(3), 175–195.

Henderson, R. C., Kairalla, J. A., Barrington, J. W., Abbas, A., & Stevenson, R. D. (2005). Longitudinal changes in bone density in children and adolescents with moderate to severe cerebral palsy. *Journal of Pediatrics, 146*(6), 769–775.

Houlihan, C. M., O'Donnell, M., Conaway, M., & Stevenson, R. D. (2004). Bodily pain and health-related quality of life in children with cerebral palsy. *Developmental Medicine and Child Neurology, 46*(5), 305–310.

Hutton, J. L., & Pharoah, P. O. D. (2006). Life expectancy in severe cerebral palsy. *Archives of Disease in Childhood, 91*, 254–258.

Kamboh, M. (2008). Clinical approach to the diagnosis of inborn errors of metabolism. *Pediatric Clinics of North America, 55*, 1113–1127.

Katz, R. (2003). Life expectancy for children with cerebral palsy and mental retardation: Implications for life care planning. *NeuroRehabilitation, 18*(3), 261–270.

Kaufman, J., Plotsky, P. M., Nemeroff, C. B., & Charney, D. S. (2000). Effects of early adverse experiences on brain structure and function: Clinical implications. *Biological Psychiatry, 48*(8), 778–790.

Kawahara, H., Okuyama, H., Kubota, A., Oue, T., Tazuke, Y., Yagi, M., & Okada, A. (2004). Can laparoscopic antireflux surgery improve the quality of life in children with neurologic and neuromuscular handicaps? *Journal of Pediatric Surgery, 39*(12), 1761–1764.

Kayser, M. A. (2008). Inherited metabolic diseases in neurodevelopmental and neurobehavioral disorders. *Seminars in Pediatric Neurology, 15*(3), 127–131.

Keyserling, H. L. (2006). Infectious disease. In I. L. Rubin & A. C. Crocker (Eds.), *Medical care for children and adults with developmental disabilities* (pp. 607–612). Baltimore, MD: Paul H. Brookes.

Klick, J. C., & Ballantine, A. (2007). Providing care in chronic disease: The ever-changing balance of integrating palliative and restorative medicine. *Pediatric Clinics of North America, 54*(5), 799–812.

Krigger, K. W. (2006). Cerebral palsy: An overview. *American Family Physician, 73*, 91–100.

Kumral, A., Ozer, E., Yilmaz, O., Akhisarglu, M., Gokmen, N., Duman, N., et al. (2003). Neuroprotective effects of erythropoietin on hypoxic-schemic brain injury in neonatal rats. *Biology of the Neonate, 83*(3), 224–228.

Martín, C., Darnell, A., Duràn, C., Bermúdez, P., Mellado, F., & Rigol, S. (2004). Magnetic resonancy imaging of the intrauterine fetal genitourinary tract normal anatomy and pathology. *Abdominal Imaging, 29*, 286–302.

Mascarenhas, M. R., Myers, R., & Konek, S. (2008). Outpatient nutrition management in neurologically impaired children. *Nutrition in Clinical Practice, 23*, 597–607.

McDermott, S., Moran, R., Platt, T., Wood, H., Isaac, T., & Darai, S. (2005). Prevalence of epilepsy in adults with mental retardation and related disabilities in primary care. *American Journal on Mental Retardation, 110*(1), 48–56.

McEwen, B. S. (2000). Effects of adverse experiences for brain structure and function. *Biological Psychiatry, 48*(8), 721–731.

McKenna, M. A. (2006). Ear, nose, and throat care. In I. L. Rubin & A. C. Crocker (Eds.), *Medical care for children and adults with developmental disabilities* (pp. 365–372). Baltimore, MD: Paul H. Brookes.

Morgan, C., Baxter, H., & Kerr, M. (2003). Prevalence of epilepsy and associated health service utilization and mortality among patients with intellectual disabilities. *American Journal on Mental Retardation, 108*, 293–300.

Morton, R. E., Wheatley, R., & Minford, M. J. (1999). Respiratory tract infections due to direct and reflux aspiration in children with severe neurodisability. *Developmental Medicine and Child Neurology, 41*, 329–334.

Munns, C. F., & Cowell, C.T. (2005). Prevention and treatment of osteoporosis in chronically ill children. *Journal of Musculoskeletal and Neuronal Interactions, 5*(3), 262–272.

Padula, M. A., & Ades, A. M. (2006). Neurodevelopmental implications of congenital heart disease. *NeoReviews, 7*, e363–e369.

Patja, K., Iivanainen, M., Vesala, H., Oksnen, H., & Ruoppila, I. (2000). Life expectancy of people with intellectual disability: A 35-year follow-up study. *Journal of Intellectual Disability Research, 44*, 591–599.

Patja, K., Molsa, P., & Iivanainen, M. (2000). Cause-specific mortality of people with intellectual disability in a population-based, 35-year follow-up study. *Journal of Intellectual Disability Research, 45*, 30–40.

Petersen, B., Bourke, J., Leonard, H., Jacoby, P., & Bower, C. (2007). Co-occurrence of birth defects and intellectual disability. *Paediatric and Perinatal Epidemiology, 21*, 65–75.

Richards, C. A., Milla, P. J., Andrews, P. L., & Spitz, L. (2001). Retching and vomiting in neurologically impaired children after fundoplication: Predictive preoperative factors. *Journal of Pediatric Surgery, 36*(9), 1401–1404.

Santucci, G., & Mack, J. W. (2007). Common gastrointestinal symptoms in pediatric palliative care: Nausea, vomiting, constipation, anorexia, cachexia. *Pediatric Clinics of North America, 54*, 673–689.

Schulze, A., Linder, M., Kohlmüller, D., Olgemöller, K., Mayatepek, E., & Hoffmann, G. F. (2003). Expanded newborn screening for inborn errors of metabolism by electrospray ionization-tandem mass spectroscopy: Results, outcomes, implications. *Pediatrics, 111*, 1399–1406.

Seddon, P. C., & Khan, Y. (2003). Respiratory problems in children with neurological impairment. *Archives of Disease in Childhood, 88*(1), 75–78.

Sheth, R. D. (2004). Bone health in pediatric epilepsy. *Epilepsy and Behavior, 5*, 30–35.

Simpoulos, A. P. (2009). Genetic screening: Programs, principles, and research—thirty years later. *Public Health Genomics, 12*, 105–111.

Sleigh, G., & Brocklehurst, P. (2004). Gastrostomy feeding in cerebral palsy: A systematic review. *Archives of Disease in Childhood, 89*, 534–539.

Steelman, J., & Zeitler, P. (2003). Treatment of symptomatic pediatric osteoporosis with cyclic single-day intravenous pamidronate infusions. *Journal of Pediatrics, 142*(4), 417–423.

Stevenson, R. D., Conaway, M., Barrington, J. W., Cuthill, S. L., Worley, G., & Henderson, R. C. (2006). Fracture rate in children with cerebral palsy. *Pediatric Rehabilitation, 9*(4), 396–403.

Strauss, D., Cable, W., & Shavelle, R. (1999). Causes of excess mortality in cerebral palsy. *Developmental Medicine and Child Neurology, 41*(9), 580–585.

Strauss, D., & Shavelle, R. (1998). Life expectancy of adults with cerebral palsy. *Developmental Medicine and Child Neurology, 40*, 369–375.

Strauss, D., Shavelle, R., Reynolds, R., Rosenbloom, L., & Day, S. (2007). Survival in cerebral palsy in the last 20 years: Signs of improvement? *Developmental Medicine and Child Neurology, 49*, 86–92.

Treiman, D. M., & Walker, M. C. (2006). Treatment of seizure emergencies: Convulsive and nonconvulsive status epilepticus. *Epilepsy Research, 68*, 77–82.

Ullrich, C. K., & Mayer, O. H. (2007). Assessment and management of fatigue and dyspnea in pediatric palliative care. *Pediatric Clinics of North America, 54*, 735–756.

Vasconcellos, E., Wyllie, E., Sullivan, S., Stanford, L., Bulacio, J., Kotagal, P., & Bingaman, W. (2001). Mental retardation in pediatric candidates for epilepsy surgery: The role of early seizure onset. *Epilepsia, 42*(2), 268–274.

Volpe, J. J. (2003). Cerebral white matter injury of the premature infant—more common than you think. *Pediatrics, 112*, 176–180.

Waltz, P. A., & Katz, E. S. (2006). Pulmonology. In I. L. Rubin & A. C. Crocker (Eds.), *Medical care for children and adults with developmental disabilities* (pp. 325–342). Baltimore, MD: Paul H. Brookes.

Winter, S., & Kiely, M. (2007). Cerebral palsy. In I. L. Rubin & A. C. Crocker (Eds.), *Medical care for children and adults with developmental disabilities* (pp. 233–248). Baltimore, MD: Paul H. Brookes.

Wusthoff, C. J., Shellhaas, R. A., & Licht, D. J. (2007). Management of common neurologic symptoms in pediatric palliative care: Seizures, agitation, and spasticity. *Pediatric Clinics of North America, 54*, 709–733.

CHAPTER 5

Medical Conditions in Adults Near the End of Life

MARC T. EMMERICH

INTRODUCTION

In the past half century, individuals with intellectual and developmental disabilities (IDD) have enjoyed a marked improvement in their medical care. As a result, the vast majority now lives into adulthood and therefore is at risk of facing the same medical problems that all adults face, including irreversible medical conditions that ultimately result in death. Clinicians for adults in the general population often view cognitive impairment itself as an indication for limiting aggressive medical interventions and changing the focus of care to comfort only. This chapter discusses an approach to shift this paradigm for adults with IDD when considering medical care decisions in specific circumstances near the end of life.

The chapter includes the following discussions: life expectancy of adults with IDD; criteria for determining when an individual is approaching the end of life and how these criteria can be understood in the presence of an intellectual disability; when it is appropriate to forego routine medical procedures; and medical problems common among adults with IDD near the end of life.

LIFE EXPECTANCY

Pertinent to the discussion of whether or not it is appropriate for an individual's medical care to be shifted to end-of-life treatment is an understanding of that individual's life expectancy. In the 1950s, prior to many medical advances that prolonged life, most individuals with IDD were "warehoused" in institutions that provided minimal developmental support or medical care. The life expectancy of individuals with IDD was markedly shorter than that of the general population at that time, as well as that of people with IDD who are living today (Marino & Pueschel, 1996; Sutton, Factor, Hawkins, Heller, & Seltzer, 1993). Previously, physicians routinely informed mothers of infants with significant IDD that their babies would die within the first 6 months of life. As a result, many people have come to believe that adults with IDD have already long outlived their life expectancies. Consequently, they might believe that it is reasonable to ignore any medical issue that adults with IDD encounter.

However, many of those dire predictions of physicians in the mid-20th century have proven to be erroneous. Indeed, many of the individuals predicted to die within the first 6 months of life are still alive today, some now in their late 90s. In addition, more physicians now advocate for aggressive interventions for reversible, life-threatening conditions in infants with severe developmental and medical problems (Wolraich, Siperstein, & Reed, 1991), resulting in an even further increase in life expectancy for individuals with IDD.

What is the current life expectancy of individuals with IDD? Strauss and Shavelle (1998) published an important study that evaluated factors that impacted life expectancy in adults with cerebral palsy. In more than 24,000 individuals with cerebral palsy, it was found that the etiology of cerebral palsy was not a significant factor in determining life expectancy, nor was the degree of intellectual disability. The only issues that significantly affected life expectancy were mobility and feeding method. It was noted that mobility needed to be quite severely impaired in order to have an effect on life expectancy (see Table 5.1).

From the data in Table 5.1, it can be seen that individuals who were independent in feeding orally and able to roll over or sit up on their own had life expectancies within approximately 10 years of those of the general population. Over the past 20 years, life expectancies for children with severe IDD and gastrostomy-fed adults have increased by about 5 years (Strauss, Shavelle, Reynolds, Rosenbloom, & Day, 2007). It is no longer acceptable to assume that treatment of an acute illness in an individual with IDD would be futile based on the argument that he or she has already outlived his or her life expectancy. Likewise, when an individual with IDD develops a severe, acute illness or a potentially ominous disease, such as cancer, it is not automatically appropriate to implement end-of-life care.

Table 5.1
Life Expectancy (Additional Years) by Age and Cohort

Sex/age	Cannot lift head			Lifts head			Rolls/sits			General population
	TF	FBO	SF	TF	FBO	SF	TF	FBO	SF	
Female										
15y	15.4	21.3	—	21.1	27.7	43.4	25.0	39.2	52.7	65.0
30y	13.4	23.8	—	16.2	28.1	33.0	21.5	34.1	40.1	50.4
45y	—	20.4	—	16.1	20.6	23.6	23.3	24.1	29.4	36.2
Male										
15y	11.7	16.9	—	16.7	22.8	38.8	20.3	34.3	48.7	58.3
30y	12.0	22.0	—	14.7	26.2	31.0	19.8	32.1	38.0	44.5
45y	—	17.5	—	13.6	17.7	20.6	20.3	21.0	26.3	31.1

Tube fed (TF); fed by others, without feeding tube (FBO); self-feeds (SF) = group too small for reliable computation of life expectancy or confidence interval.

Note. From "Life Expectancy of Adults with Cerebral Palsy," by D. Strauss & R. Shavelle, 1998, Developmental Medicine and Child Neurology, 40, p. 369–375. Table III. Copyright 1999 Wiley Publishers, United Kingdom. Reprinted with permission.

Given this argument, when is it appropriate to implement end-of-life care for an individual with IDD? In the 1980s, after consent decrees forced improved care, every effort was made to provide medical care and maintain health and life regardless of an individual's condition. In some facilities around that time, a Do-Not-Resuscitate (DNR) order was considered inappropriate for any resident. As a result, there were residents, such as those with Down syndrome, who developed end-stage Alzheimer dementia with severe swallowing problems and recurrent aspiration pneumonia. Eventually they deteriorated to the point of no longer being ambulatory, conversant, or even aware of their surroundings. Yet all measures continued to be taken to aggressively treat any illness. When they "finally" succumbed to one of their numerous episodes of aspiration pneumonia, lifesaving protocols, including cardiopulmonary resuscitation (CPR), were implemented in an attempt to keep the individual alive for another day. Implementation of CPR imposed the risk of painful rib fractures in these elderly, frail individuals and resulted in intubation (a tube put down the throat to force air into the lungs) and at times electric shocks in an attempt to cardiovert them back to life. All this was done even though the clinicians knew that there was minimal chance of survival despite the efforts made (Awoke, Mouton, & Parrott, 1992). The lack of the option to implement a DNR order at this end stage of life resulted in aggressive medical interventions. Some would now consider these interventions to be cruel compared to a calm, peaceful death with family and friends at their side.

As a result of these same consent decrees to provide improved care, there were younger individuals with profound IDD who indeed benefited from the improvements in medical services. Similar to the individuals with end-stage dementia, they may have had comparable and significant limitations in their motor, feeding, communication, and social interaction abilities. But they were younger and more vibrant. If they became acutely ill, it seemed appropriate, not cruel, to impose aggressive medical intervention to combat the acute illness.

Where does one draw the line? For whom are aggressive medical interventions considered to be cruel? How does one decide when end-of-life care should be implemented? When does the end of life begin?

When Does the End of Life Begin?

In the general population, several criteria are used to help patients and their families decide when it might be appropriate to withhold aggressive medical interventions and to shift the focus of care toward the comfort and quality, rather than the duration, of life. Criteria that are often considered include poor prognosis regarding the outcome of an illness, a treatment regimen with risks that outweigh the anticipated benefits, new physical disability that results in increased dependence, refractory pain, and cognitive dysfunction.

Consider an individual who was the head of her household, who was able to work, who provided for her family, and who had meaningful conversations with family members and acquaintances. As she aged and developed disabilities—perhaps from strokes, end-stage dementia, or terminal cancer—she was rendered incapable of providing support or companionship to others. She was no longer capable of enjoying life and relationships, and there was no reasonable hope that this situation would significantly improve in the future. At that point, this individual, if capable, and her family members would likely want to avoid aggressive, potentially uncomfortable, and invasive medical interventions aimed at prolonging life. Instead, they may favor striving for comfort and improved quality of life, whether this may result in a slightly shorter life span. When health care personnel experience these situations repeatedly, they generally become comfortable with accepting, and helping families to accept, a limitation of expectations for what medical care can provide. There is recognition that decreased medical intervention may be a preferable plan of care (Besdine, Rubenstein, & Snyder, 1996).

As a result, it is fairly common for health care personnel to see an acutely ill individual who happens also to have severe IDD and immediately place him in a similar category as the individual described earlier. After all, the individual with IDD may have cognitive dysfunction with an inability to have meaningful conversations with family and acquaintances; may have a physical disability and dependence on others; may have behaviors such as self-injury that suggest that the individual is not able to enjoy life and relationships with others and/or may have refractory pain; and may have a prognosis that fails to indicate any potential for improvement in these chronic conditions. Since medical care will not likely improve the underlying problems, then some health care providers might argue that it is inappropriate—even cruel—to impose medical interventions on such an individual, even if the intervention may effectively treat an acute, reversible illness that is superimposed on the chronic disability. Some might even argue that routine screening for common maladies is inappropriate because no matter what reversible, treatable problem may be found, the underlying, untreatable disability will remain. Furthermore, some might argue, medical illness and death would "put him out of his misery," referring to the misery of a life with IDD.

This type of attitude may lead to a severe deterioration in trust between the health care provider and the family members who have cared for, loved, and received love from the individual with the disability for decades. Health care providers need to understand that it is usually not appropriate to place individuals with long-term, stable disabilities into the same category as those with new-onset, irreversible, progressive, degenerative conditions. An individual with a new onset, irreversible, progressive, degenerative condition is functioning below his former baseline, to which there is no reasonable hope for return. It is anticipated that this disability is *not* at a stable baseline but rather will exacerbate as the underlying degenerative illness relentlessly progresses. In contrast, the stable level of functioning of a person with IDD represents his or her baseline.

If an individual with IDD is acutely ill but there is a reasonable chance that medical interventions may result in return to his or her stable baseline, then it is probably appropriate to recommend treatment of the acute illness in order to return to the stable baseline regardless of the level of baseline functioning (Emmerich, 2006). However, this recommendation is made with the caveat that some medical interventions might not be tolerated well, therefore requiring the use of sedation, with its risk of adverse effects. When there is a higher risk of adverse effects in people with IDD compared to the general population, the risk-benefit ratio of providing the intervention must be adjusted. However, the benefit side of that equation should not be diminished simply because the individual has IDD (Service & Hahn, 2003). The degree of benefit remains the degree to which it is likely that the individual will return to his or her baseline level of functioning, no matter where that baseline level is and regardless of whether or not he or she has IDD.

This framework for evaluating the appropriateness of medical interventions allows for withholding invasive medical procedures in individuals with IDD who also have a super-imposed irreversible, progressive, degenerative illness, such as those with Down syndrome who have developed end-stage Alzheimer dementia. Even though the individual may have an underlying IDD, it may still be appropriate to withhold medical intervention based on the level of cognitive functioning. In this case, if it is determined that the advanced dementia precludes a return to that individual's baseline, and that further deterioration in cognitive function is expected, it may be appropriate to consider withholding aggressive, invasive medical interventions. Regardless of whether or not an individual has IDD, the discussion about withholding medical treatments and implementing end-of-life care must include an evaluation of the degree to which these interventions may potentially return the individual to his or her baseline level of functioning, regardless of what that level may be.

In general, the more acute and aggressive the irreversible deterioration of function is, the more appropriate it is to recommend avoidance of aggressive intervention. The gradual deterioration of motor function that sometimes accompanies severe cerebral palsy is generally not reason enough to warrant recommendations to avoid aggressive treatment for acute illness or to withhold routine screening procedures. Even though there is no reasonable likelihood that the individual with cerebral palsy will ever return to the level of motor function he or she had when younger, the individual's deterioration is so gradual that it is usually appropriate to recommend aggressive treatment of acute illness if there is a reasonable chance that he or she will return to a recent baseline.

Individuals with IDD and their relatives or caregivers sometimes complain that clinicians are uncaring (Molloy, Knight, & Woodfield, 2003), such as when recommending the limitation of therapy for an individual. The clinician's perspective may be that the recommendations are rooted in deep caring, warmth, and concern for the individual. For example, consider an oncologist who spends a large amount of time and energy working with patients and families to accept and prepare for the end of life. From the oncologist's perspective, it is appropriate—even desired—to encourage individuals and their families to accept the limitations that cancer has imposed upon them and to make decisions based on an acceptance of those limitations. The oncologist is likely to consider it a profound disservice to give patients and families false hope and to encourage aggressive medical interventions that will not reverse the course of the cancer to a significant degree. In the situations that oncologists face every day, one of their most important and beneficial tasks is to help individuals and their relatives avoid a poor-quality end-of-life experience ruined by overaggressive medical intervention. However, when an oncologist is then faced with an individual with severe IDD, he may have the same intense disdain for the thought of aggressive medical intervention for an acute illness knowing that it will not improve the underlying severe disability. The clinician may believe that treatment of the acute illness will be imposing uncomfortable medical interventions that are futile (in terms of their inability to cure the IDD) and would simply cause discomfort to an individual who would not be able to understand the reason for the discomfort.

The issue arises about whether it is necessary or beneficial to understand the reason for discomfort from a medical intervention. A few years ago, I had a severe earache. I noted swelling in my ear canal and lost hearing in that ear. Recognizing that I might have a potentially life-threatening abscess in the ear, I did not waste time calling my primary care physician. Instead, I went directly to the emergency department of the Massachu-setts Eye and Ear Infirmary, a tertiary hospital for the most complicated diseases of the eyes and ears. The emergency physician examined my ear, handed me a prescription for eardrops, and informed me that I had otitis externa, a minor infection of the ear canal. Otitis externa is one of the most common diagnoses I make among my patients who are adults with IDD. What a revelation it was for me to think how often my patients suffer with the same symptoms that sent me running frantically to a tertiary hospital emergency room. Luckily for my patients, most do not know that their symptoms might be that of a rare, life-threatening abscess, so they don't have to worry about it. They simply accept their symptoms and deal with them the best they can, perhaps trying to communicate about them, until someone hopefully notices and gives them treatment that will help dis-sipate the discomfort.

Many clinicians express concern about the ability of people with IDD to live with the discomfort of a particular disease or to tolerate certain invasive treatments or adverse effects of medications, such as chemotherapy. Their limited ability to understand the rea-son for the chemotherapy is presumed to make it harder for them to tolerate the adverse effects. In fact, it may be that a limited ability to understand cancer and chemotherapy makes it much *less* anxiety provoking. In my experience, individuals with IDD often toler-ate intense illness *better* than most individuals in the general population would! Therefore, it is not necessarily appropriate to withhold treatment from individuals solely because their lack of understanding is presumed to make the administration of that treatment a hardship for them. An individual's limited understanding may actually make it easier for him or her to tolerate a procedure or treatment.

Avoidance of Routine Medical Procedures

When is it appropriate to recommend the avoidance of routine medical procedures?

For the purposes of this discussion, "routine" medical procedures are those in which the benefit clearly outweighs the risk and ones that most clinicians would perform on any patient in a particular medical circumstance. This includes screening procedures, such as measuring blood pressure or colonoscopy for those over age 50, as well as tests done only in special situations, such as esophagogastroduodenoscopy (EGD, or upper endoscopy) after a patient presents with hematemesis (vomiting blood). For this discussion, these are all considered "routine" because they would be done for anyone who meets the criteria for needing them.

However, there are circumstances in which it would not be appropriate to perform such procedures. Consider an individual with end-stage gastric cancer who is at risk for hematemesis and who receives hospice care. This person has indicated that invasive pro-cedures are no longer desired because, although there may be a short-term benefit, the long-term prognosis does not justify any significant interventions. In this case, an EGD would not be considered a routine procedure for this individual.

An EGD is a routine procedure for those with evidence of upper gastrointestinal bleeding, but it would be appropriate to avoid in the end-of-life case described earlier. Similarly, a Pap smear is considered to be a routine procedure for all women. However, is it ever appropriate to avoid this procedure, other than in end-of-life situations? A Pap smear is an invasive procedure that is often not well tolerated by some women with IDD. It may require the administration of significant amounts of sedation or even general anesthesia in order to complete. It is used to screen for cervical cancer, for which some women are at higher risk. If a woman with IDD is at low risk for cervical cancer, and if she would require general anesthesia for a Pap smear to be performed, then the risk of performing the Pap smear may outweigh the benefit and it may be reasonable in her case to recommend avoiding it. Avoidance of Pap smears in this case is not being done as part of a comfort-only end-of-life plan. It is simply the avoidance of one particularly discomforting procedure while all other medical procedures might still be implemented for that individual in order to maintain the goal of extending the duration of life.

Some clinicians would consider *any* procedure that is performed on someone who is not completely cooperative and who does not fully understand what he or she is going through to be a nonroutine procedure. Such medical providers might, therefore, recommend that no procedure be performed on such individuals, no matter what the benefit might be. However, it is more appropriate to weigh the risks versus the benefits for each procedure for each individual. It is usually appropriate to perform a procedure for an illness that can potentially be treated and carries a reasonable chance of recovery to baseline functioning, unless the performance of the procedure itself imposes risks that outweigh the benefits.

MEDICAL CONDITIONS NEAR THE END OF LIFE

Dementia

Dementia is a term referring to a group of illnesses that all manifest in memory loss. By far the most common type is Alzheimer disease, which is probably a group of several diseases with differing etiologies that all manifest in similar pathological and clinical characteristics. Dementia is one of the most common conditions affecting individuals with IDD at the end of life. One reason for the high prevalence of dementia in this population is its almost universal prevalence in Down syndrome. Autopsy studies have revealed that 100% of individuals with Down syndrome exhibit the pathological brain changes of Alzheimer disease by the time they are 20 years old. However, the clinical manifestations of Alzheimer dementia, though presenting at earlier ages than in the general population, do not generally begin until the 40s to 50s. Some individuals with Down syndrome even live into their 60s without any clinical evidence of dementia. However, the vast majority of individuals with Down syndrome who do not die from some other illness earlier in life will eventually develop Alzheimer dementia.

Early signs of dementia are primarily related to short-term memory loss. This early stage may not be recognized, especially in nonverbal individuals. If an individual has never been able to express his recent memories, then the lack of such expression will not be recognized as a change in function. In that case, a change might not be recognized until the individual has more severe memory loss resulting in interruption of familiar routines. For example, an individual who previously was able to move independently from any room in the house to the bathroom but who now gets lost on the way, as if forgetting where he or she was going, might be suffering from dementia. It is important to recognize, however, that other clinical conditions may result in similar presentations and some of those conditions are reversible with appropriate treatment. Before assuming that an individual has irreversible, progressive Alzheimer dementia, it is important to rule out potentially reversible causes of dementia, such as hypothyroidism, Vitamin B12 deficiency (both of which are common in Down syndrome), depression, adverse effects of medication, hypercalcemia (high blood calcium), a brain tumor, and others.

The course of Alzheimer dementia is quite variable, and deterioration from clinical onset to death may last for over a decade or may only span a couple of years. Given that the diagnosis of dementia in individuals with IDD is often delayed until its later stages, the time from diagnosis to death is likely to be shorter compared to that of the general population. It is not easy to predict how long an individual will live when the diagnosis is first made. But a year or two after the diagnosis, a retrospective assessment of the rapidity of decline may provide an indication of the rate of future decline. Medications for the memory loss in Alzheimer disease are generally of limited benefit and for a limited number of individuals; they are usually more useful in the earlier stages of Alzheimer disease. Since many individuals with IDD cannot be diagnosed in the earlier stages, the usefulness of medication for memory loss in this population is even more limited than it is in the general population. However, medications for problems associated with Alzheimer disease, such as sleep disorder, mood disturbance, and seizures, may be quite helpful (Janicki & Wisniewski, 1985).

Many individuals with Alzheimer dementia develop epileptic activity usually manifesting initially in myoclonic jerks, some of which can become so frequent and intense that they interfere with daily activities. Epileptic activity can also manifest as full body, tonic-clonic seizures. This is especially notable in individuals with Down syndrome because, compared to other individuals with IDD, those with Down syndrome have a lower prevalence of seizure disorder. However, once individuals with Down syndrome develop Alzheimer disease, they are then much more likely to exhibit seizures. The myoclonic activity may sometimes be abated by long-acting benzodiazepines, such as clonazepam (Klonopin), at the risk of increasing lethargy and decreasing cognitive function. The tonic-clonic seizures can sometimes be managed with traditional antiepileptics. Low-dose phenobarbital has also been quite effective with—at least in some clinicians' experience— no more apparent impairment of cognitive function (at this stage of Alzheimer disease) than might be seen with newer antiepileptics (N. Alvarez, personal communication, 1994). Despite this treatment, however, once seizures associated with Alzheimer disease occur, it usually is a marker for a more rapid decline in function with accelerated decrease in ambulation, activities of daily living skills, and even ability to eat. Reduction in eating results both from decreased ability to get the food to the mouth independently and from progressively increasing dysphagia (impaired swallowing). The dysphagia predisposes to recurrent aspiration, and ultimately the actual cause of death is often either recurrent aspiration pneumonia and/or failure to thrive secondary to limited nutritional intake. At this stage, an individual is generally considered to be in end-stage Alzheimer disease.

It is usually recommended that a feeding tube *not* be placed to bypass the dysphagia associated with end-stage Alzheimer disease because there is no hope, even with placement of a feeding tube, that there will be recovery to a stable, baseline level of functioning. A feeding tube will not prevent the relentless, progressive, irreversible deterioration of the underlying Alzheimer disease. Rather, it is usually recommended that eating by mouth be optimized with changes in food texture, bolus volumes, and positioning to allow the individual to continue to enjoy that aspect of life as much as possible, thereby focusing care more on the quality rather than the duration of life.

Other forms of irreversible dementia present much less frequently in individuals with IDD. In the general population, multi-infarct dementia is the second most frequent form of dementia. It is a result of recurrent cerebrovascular accidents (strokes), each of which cause the death of a group of brain cells. With each episode, there may be a decline in function associated with the brain cells lost. Therefore, when dementia develops in relation to multiple infarcts, it is usually stepwise. It is characterized by a stable level of functioning for a while, then a sudden decrease with stabilization at that level for a while, then another sudden decrease with stabilization at that level. This type of trajectory with multi-infarct dementia renders it much more difficult to provide a prognosis. After diagnosis, an individual may remain stable for years before the next infarct. Or the next infarct may occur less than a year later and be in a critical area of the brain, causing severe disability or sudden death.

Much less frequent in the general population is Lewy-body dementia in which new-onset hallucinations and Parkinsonian-type motor dysfunction are noted along with or after the diagnosis of dementia. This timeline helps to distinguish this disease from the dementia associated with Parkinson disease in which the Parkinsonian features (and/or hallucinations related to anti-Parkinson medications) precede the dementia. It is possible that in individuals with IDD, the later recognition of dementia may alter the timeline in which manifestations are recognized in Lewy-body dementia, resulting in the finding of motor dysfunction and, perhaps, hallucinations prior to the diagnosis of dementia. Therefore, in individuals with IDD, it may be more difficult to distinguish Lewy-body dementia from the dementia associated with Parkinson disease. In any case, because of the high prevalence of Alzheimer disease associated with Down syndrome, the Lewy-body and Parkinsonian dementias make up only a small fraction of the dementias that are seen in adults with IDD.

Gastrointestinal Issues

Gastrointestinal conditions are remarkably common in people with IDD. These include gastroesophageal reflux disease (GERD) and dysphagia with associated risk of aspiration, often resulting in pneumonia. Therefore, it is appropriate to include aspiration pneumonia in the category of gastrointestinal issues because the underlying problem that leads to the aspiration may be dysphagia, with or without GERD. Other prominent gastrointestinal issues in this population include constipation and enteral feeding via gastrostomy or jejunostomy tubes.

Dysphagia with recurrent aspiration pneumonia is often a cause of death. Aspiration pneumonia is probably the most common reason for hospitalizations of adults with IDD. It is usually recommended that a speech pathologist and/or occupational therapist evaluate a person with dysphagia, sometimes with the aid of a videofluoroscopy-swallowing evaluation (modified barium swallow), to determine the best textures and bolus sizes for swallowing. The most appropriate seating and head positions may also be determined to optimize the ability to swallow and avoid aspiration. The imaging study may also help identify silent aspiration in which the individual does not cough, choke, or make any attempt to clear the aspirated material from his or her throat (larynx), trachea, or lungs. This silent aspiration is the most dangerous, as there may be a delay in identifying the aspiration that causes hypoxia and/or pneumonia, and therefore may be much more difficult to manage. Sometimes a chest X-ray or computed tomography scan of the chest will reveal evidence of recurrent aspiration in individuals not previously known to experience aspiration.

To the extent that the swallowing evaluation may provide recommendations to minimize aspiration, the individual may be able to continue eating by mouth. For example, they might be advised to eat only finely chopped solids and/or to thicken all liquids to nectar- or honey-thick consistency. However, sometimes the aspiration is found to be so severe that a feeding tube is recommended to bypass the swallowing apparatus altogether. In some cases, feeding tubes are used for liquids while solids can still be swallowed via the mouth. Feeding tubes allow liquid nutritional formula to be inserted directly into the gastrointestinal tract without having to be swallowed. Usually, if a permanent feeding tube is needed, a gastrostomy tube (to the stomach) is placed. However, depending on the amount of gastroesophageal reflux an individual may have, a jejunostomy tube (to the jejunum) may be indicated to avoid reflux of liquids or solid food from the stomach up into the esophagus.

When an individual becomes acutely ill and cannot tolerate eating or drinking, then he or she would generally be hospitalized and hydrated with intravenous (IV) fluid. When the individual recovers from the acute illness, it is typical to restart feeding with clear liquids in small amounts with a gradual increase in volume as tolerated. They subsequently are advanced to full liquids, then gradually to solids as tolerated. However, when an individual has a feeding tube and then is restarted on feeding after a period of only IV hydration, hospital clinicians often mistakenly restart immediately with full-strength formula feeding at full volume through the tube. This often results in ileus (lack of bowel motility) and vomiting with the risk of aspiration. This reaction should not be construed as an end-stage event with inability to tolerate feeding even through a tube. Rather, it should be recognized as a normal reaction to a bolus feeding after a period of time without any feeding. The resumption of feeding through the tube should be done in a similar way to the resumption of feeding by mouth: start with clear liquids in small volumes, increase volume as tolerated, and then gradually add feeding formula.

Casarett, Kapo, and Caplan (2005) suggest that placement of a feeding tube is almost never appropriate. The authors, however, seem to be referring to individuals near the end of life, which was not stated. The criteria for the placement of a feeding tube should be similar to those for any other medical procedure after weighing the risks and benefits of the procedure for that individual. For individuals with impaired swallowing who are otherwise stable, recommendation of a feeding tube in order to maintain adequate nutrition would be appropriate. However, if the swallowing problem is part of a progressive, degenerative illness with no hope for return to a former stable baseline, then, depending on the anticipated aggressiveness and rapidity of the degenerative illness, it may be appropriate to recommend avoidance of feeding tube placement and to just optimize intake by mouth as much as possible. Withdrawal of a feeding tube, just like withdrawal of any other therapy, is considered ethically equivalent to avoidance of feeding tube placement in the first place. In other words, if a feeding tube is already in place, the discontinuation and withdrawal of that tube may be recommended if the same criteria are met as described earlier for the recommendation to avoid placement of a feeding tube altogether.

Constipation is another remarkably prevalent condition in individuals with IDD. Even among those individuals with IDD who are ambulatory and have no apparent motor or physical disabilities, constipation is still significantly more common than in the general population (Emmerich, 1993). The reasons for this are unclear; perhaps it is related to bowel training issues and/or emotional issues (Schonwald & Rappaport, 2004). In any case, many individuals with IDD receive multiple laxatives of various forms and still require rectal suppositories and/or enemas on a regular basis to help manage their bowel movements. Because some of these individuals are unable to communicate (or perhaps even recognize) when they are having difficulty with bowel movements, it is often important for caregivers to be aware of this potential problem and, if possible, to monitor frequency of bowel movements.

Bowel dysfunction may become profound in rare instances, usually in individuals with the most severe physical limitations. Bowels may become nearly unresponsive to significant doses of even the most powerful laxatives and suppositories. Management with a variety of enemas and rectal tube placements may also have limited effect. Since this most severe form of constipation is most likely to occur in individuals with severely limited motor function, including limited function of their swallowing apparatus, such individuals often have dysphagia with risk of aspiration. Tube feeding often has to be curtailed as the bowel immobility causes gastroesophageal reflux and aspiration. Over time, the individual may either succumb to recurrent aspiration pneumonia, or feeding may have to be limited to such an extent that the individual cannot maintain adequate nutrition and hydration. At that point, the individual can be recognized to have an irreversible, progressive, degenerative, end-stage illness, and it may be appropriate to recommend limiting interventions to comfort measures only.

Seizure Disorders

By definition, individuals with IDD have some kind of central nervous system dysfunction. Compared to the general population, individuals with IDD have a much higher prevalence of epileptic seizure disorders. While some adults may not have seizures, others may present with a rare episode of epileptic activity, others with periodic seizures that are well controlled with antiepileptic medication, and others with frequent seizures that are not well controlled despite a combination of antiepileptic therapies. Among individuals with IDD, those with Down syndrome have a relatively lower incidence of seizure activity.

The clinical presentation of seizures does not always reflect the degree of epileptic activity seen on an electroencephalogram (EEG). Many asymptomatic individuals, even in the general population, may have occasional epileptic spikes on an EEG that are of no clinical significance and require no treatment. However, there may also be subtle clinical presentations of epileptic activity (absence seizures) that might not be obviously observed by others but that do affect the individual symptomatically, for example with a temporary lapse in awareness. There also may be focal seizures that are clinically obvious but that only affect a localized part of an individual's motor function, such as an arm tremor or turning the head and eyes to one side without affecting other parts of the body. Sometimes epilepsy manifests as complex partial seizures with a series of behaviors that might be seemingly purposeful, but of which the individual has no apparent awareness or voluntary control. There are also pseudoseizures, in which an individual (usually one who also has true epileptic seizures) has episodes of behavior that resemble typical seizure activity and that may be behaviorally reinforced by the reaction they provoke in others witnessing the event. Although there still may be no outright voluntary, conscious control of these pseudoseizures, the individual usually remains aware of the activity and the surroundings during the seizure and there is no epileptic activity on an EEG that is correlated with the timing of the seizure. All of these types of seizures are ones that are *not* likely to be associated with a life-threatening event.

The classic full-body, tonic-clonic seizure, formerly called "grand-mal," is one that may result in a life-threatening episode. Even among those who manifest this type of seizure, the disorder is usually controllable with antiepileptic medications and when a seizure does occur, the incidence of sudden death is rare. The more intense the seizure is and the longer it lasts, the greater the likelihood that an individual will have sudden death. Those individuals with severe epilepsy manifesting in profoundly intense, full-body, tonic-clonic seizures that are intractable to a variety of antiepileptic therapies—including medications, vagal nerve stimulation, and even brain surgical procedures—may be at risk for sudden death during a seizure. Even in this circumstance, however, the prediction of death is only a vague one and it is extremely difficult to establish a timeline of deterioration or life expectancy. A DNR might be appropriate in such situations, but it is otherwise unlikely that one would plan for a period of palliative care prior to death in this case.

On the other hand, there are situations in which seizure activity might be indirectly associated with a plan for palliative care. An intense seizure may result in a temporary loss of oxygen to the brain resulting in brain damage with subsequent decrease in cognitive or motor function. This deterioration in function may lead to a discussion about the limitation of life-sustaining treatment. That discussion might be similar to the one about multi-infarct dementia described earlier, since the progression (periodic, unpredictable, stepwise, sudden losses of brain function) is similar.

Another situation in which epileptic activity might be indirectly associated with palliative care is when it is a consequence of another irreversible, degenerative process. As noted in the discussion of people with Down syndrome and Alzheimer dementia, the onset of seizure activity often is associated with a predictable decline in future function.

Cardiopulmonary Disease

Some individuals with IDD also have congenital anomalies such as cardiac malformations that result in specific cardiopulmonary symptoms with age. These anomalies are now frequently treated surgically in infancy, with significantly less frequent, persistent, long-term consequences. However, there continues to be a population of individuals who did not undergo early treatment and/or had lesions that are not surgically correctable. Their cardiac abnormalities may predispose them to end-stage cardiopulmonary failure. Generally, chronic hypoxia can be managed with long-term oxygen supplementation. Often the deterioration in cardiopulmonary function in these situations is extremely gradual and an individual may live for years on oxygen therapy. However, over time the cardiopulmonary status deteriorates to a point in which treatment with oxygen is not effective and the patient's condition is incompatible with life. The approach to end-of-life care in these situations is similar to that of end-stage cardiac disease, which is discussed later.

Congenital anomalies can also result in chest wall deformities, which are relatively common in cerebral palsy. This may lead to restrictive lung disease in which the lungs have limited space in which to expand. There is potential for increasing restriction as a kyphosis or scoliosis (anterior or lateral curvatures of the spine) worsens. Those individuals who undergo surgical placement of spinal rods to stabilize their curvatures and prevent worsening kyphoscoliosis are less likely to experience the consequences of progressively increasing restrictive lung disease. Ultimately, in those whose kyphoscoliosis does continue to progress, respiratory failure may gradually develop and the approach to end-of-life care is similar to that of end-stage cardiac disease.

As individuals with IDD receive markedly improved medical care compared to half a century ago, they are enjoying longer lives and therefore also have the same medical problems that the general population develops as they age. Aside from dementia, the life-threatening problems of the elderly are primarily cardiopulmonary disease and cancer. The difference for individuals with IDD is not in the physiological manifestations of the diseases but rather in the clinical presentation. Many individuals with IDD, even if verbal, have limited ability to reliably describe their symptoms, especially pain. The diagnosis of disease therefore may be delayed.

After the diagnosis is made, a person may have a limited ability to describe symptoms, thus limiting the optimal management of the disease. For example, an individual with coronary artery disease manifesting in angina (usually intense chest pressure) who cannot report about that angina might not be treated until more obvious clinical signs present— such as more intense chest pain, respiratory compromise, or syncope (fainting)—at which point more heart damage may have occurred than would have been the case had the angina been treated earlier. These considerations must be taken into account when making decisions about how aggressive to be in managing cardiac disease. People with cardiac disease are at risk of experiencing a catastrophic event over time. These occurrences may result in death, severe impairment, and/or gradual decline in cardiac function, with progressively decreased exercise capacity, increased need for supplemental oxygen, and potentially progressive impairment in cognitive ability. As these problems progress, they result in end-stage cardiac disease, and decisions need to be made about whether or not it is appropriate to pursue aggressive measures to prolong life.

With end-stage cardiac disease, a DNR is usually considered appropriate. After resuscitative efforts for a sudden death that occurs outside the hospital, the overall chance of survival to hospital discharge is only 6.4% (Nichol et al., 1999). Survival in those with underlying end-stage cardiac disease is probably even lower, and survival is not necessarily accompanied by a return to baseline. Therefore, many consider it cruel to implement CPR—pressing on a chest, risking rib fractures, applying painful electric shocks, forcing air down the throat (with some air inadvertently blowing into the stomach)—at the last moment of life when the chances of recovery are so minute. With end-stage cardiac disease, the risk of resuscitative efforts so clearly outweighs the benefit that it eases the burden of deciding to withhold those efforts. However, it may be much more burdensome to decide about the interventions for cardiac failure *before* sudden death, such as when considering whether or not one should be intubated (have a tube placed through the mouth into the throat, in which case the individual cannot speak) and placed on a ventilator for assisted breathing when necessary to maintain life. If the acute exacerbation is potentially reversible, with recovery to baseline likely, then such interventions might be thought to be appropriate. Unfortunately, sometimes the positive pressure of a ventilator pushing air into the lungs (as opposed to the negative pressure that normally sucks air into the lungs) causes adverse consequences, such as lowering of blood pressure. This reaction then results in the need for more invasive procedures, such as intravenous catheters that enter the heart to measure pressures there, which then increases the risk of arrhythmias, bleeding, or other subsequent issues. An individual's inability to reliably communicate his or her symptoms makes these situations even more perilous.

It is sometimes not easy to predict whether any of these adverse consequences are likely to occur when someone is placed on a ventilator. It is important for clear communication to occur between the individual (as much as possible), his or her advocates, and the medical clinicians caring for the individual about the risks versus the benefits of any procedures. Again, it is recommended that the likelihood of returning to that individual's stable baseline be the primary parameter on which to base decisions about interventions.

Cancer

Cancer is a word that used to be practically synonymous with death. In fact, it was not that long ago that a patient with cancer would never be told his or her diagnosis in order to prevent discouragement over an inevitable demise within the year. Furthermore, despite the progress made in the treatment of several forms of cancer, there are still many cancers that remain lethal within a year or two of diagnosis. One of the primary roles of oncologists is to assist patients and their families to deal with the end of life. However, it is important to recognize that not all diagnoses of cancer result in inevitable death in a short period of time. Better screening and treatments have resulted in prevention, cure, or at least remission of some cancers for such a long period that death might occur from other causes before the cancer takes its toll. Thanks to advances in adjunct therapies (Kris et al., 2006), many cancer treatments are now much better tolerated than they were in the past. Therefore the risk-benefit ratio of treatment has often shifted significantly in favor of treatment. Furthermore, progress continues to be made, and some cancers that today are considered incurable may be able to be much better controlled in the near future.

Individuals with IDD who are given a diagnosis of cancer are often presumed to be doomed as they are expected to be unable to cooperate with or to tolerate treatment with adverse effects that they cannot understand. This presumption may be appropriate in many situations. However, there are cancers that are potentially treatable without a significant burden on the patient. The wide variety of cancers and their treatments makes it incumbent upon clinicians and caregivers of individuals with IDD to refrain from categorizing all "cancers" into a single paradigm. Screening for breast cancer with mammograms, prostate cancer with PSA tests and digital rectal exams, or cervical cancer with Pap smears may lead to a rapid and relatively simple curative procedure, perhaps with easily tolerated medication.

Screening or treatment procedures sometimes need to be modified somewhat to accommodate an individual with IDD, such as avoidance of radiation therapy due to inability to stay still for a long enough period of time. Mammography generally cannot be done on an individual under general anesthesia, so if sedative premedication is not adequate, then sometimes screening for breast cancer must be done by physical exam alone, without the added benefit of mammography. Although individuals with Down syndrome have an increased risk of hematologic malignancies, they have a decreased risk of solid tumors, such as breast cancer, compared to the general population. If a woman with Down syndrome has a severe intellectual disability and cannot cooperate for a mammogram, she may require fairly heavy sedative premedication, with a likely limited value mammographic image. The risk-benefit ratio for this screening procedure may therefore be quite different from that of the general population.

On the other hand, given the potential curability of cervical and breast cancer, it is reasonable to at least consider screening for these in individuals with IDD, despite the recognized difficulties that may be involved with the screening tests. It is not appropriate to automatically reject all cancer screening and treatment outright just because an individual has IDD. As with any other medical procedure, the risks and benefits must be weighed for each procedure and for each individual.

Treatment of cancer needs to be addressed with just as much consideration as given to the screening procedures. Oncologists spend a significant amount of time and energy discussing with patients and their caregivers the management of cancer and its associated problems near the end of life. At some point in the treatment of a cancer, an oncologist may sit with the patient and caregivers and encourage a change of course from aggressive efforts to fight the cancer—regardless of the adverse effects—to backing off of the aggressive fight, avoidance of adverse effects, and focusing on comfort and quality, rather than on duration, of life. In many cases, the point at which this switch is made is when the patient's cognitive function has declined to a point at which he or she is no longer able to comprehend his or her situation or environment. The patient might be considered to be unable to understand the value of therapy that is causing adverse effects, and therefore it may be considered cruel to impose such therapy.

When an individual with IDD presents to an oncologist, the level of cognitive function may be interpreted as an indication to avoid aggressive therapy with adverse effects. Again, it is important to distinguish the stable, nondeteriorating level of cognitive function of an individual with IDD from the progressive, degenerative cognitive decline that might be associated with an end-stage cancer. If an individual with IDD develops cancer, then the decision about treatment should be based on the same paradigm described earlier: if there is reasonable hope that treatment can return that individual to his or her stable baseline, then it is usually appropriate to recommend treatment. It must be recognized that, for some individuals, the limited ability to cooperate (e.g., with radiation therapy, as noted earlier) and the adverse effects of treatment may be so significant that such therapy might not be in their best interest. However, many clinicians would be surprised at what individuals with IDD are able to tolerate that even individuals in the general population would have difficulty tolerating. Intellectual disability alone is not a reason to avoid interventions for the treatment of cancer or any other malady. Risks and benefits of usual treatments must be considered along with other options for the management of the individual and his or her acute disease. If, given all the options available, there is little reasonable hope for the individual's return to his or her stable baseline, then it is appropriate to consider the withholding of interventions and to recommend care that promotes comfort and quality, rather than duration, of life.

Severe, Acute Illness

When an individual with IDD, who has limited ability to communicate about his symptoms, arrives in an emergency ward with a marked change in behavior, it may be difficult to ascertain the reason for the behavior. The diagnostic work-up may require conversations with a number of caregivers, preferably those who have known the individual for a long period of time as well as those who witnessed the recent course of events. It may require several "shot in the dark" tests, including perhaps multiple imaging studies that may be difficult to obtain if the individual is not cooperative, especially when in acute discomfort. These extra requirements, coupled with unfamiliarity with individuals with IDD in general, may discourage an emergency department clinician from engaging in a diagnostic work-up. It may be easier for the clinician to fall back on the (mistaken) assumptions that the individual has already lived beyond his or her life expectancy and has little to offer the world anyway. Therefore, in the clinician's mind, an extensive work-up would be a waste of time. It is usually beneficial if an advocate for the individual helps to educate the emergency department clinician about the individual, the value of his relationships with those who know him, and about how to assess medical problems in individuals like him or her. It is especially helpful if the primary care clinician converses with the emergency clinician to clarify how the current presentation compares to previous ones.

When an acute problem requires an invasive procedure, such as surgery or endoscopy, the decision whether or not to proceed is complicated by the added difficulties of performing the procedure urgently. An individual with IDD might require general anesthesia in order to cooperate with a procedure and, depending on the presence of underlying issues such as congenital anomalies, the risks of anesthesia in an urgent setting may be even greater than it otherwise would be. Often a surgeon will be reluctant to proceed with a surgical procedure because of the anticipated inability of the individual to cooperate with postoperative care, such as pain management, avoiding the removal of dressings, or participating in required rehabilitative maneuvers. These are all concerns that must be accounted for when deciding on a course of action.

However, a person with IDD may be able to tolerate discomfort, procedures, and their aftermath as easily, if not more easily, than any other individual due to his or her limited ability to fully understand the extent of the problem. As with any medical condition, the decision whether or not to proceed with interventions needs to be individualized around the patient and the procedure. The primary issue is whether or not the individual is likely to recover from the acute illness and return to his or her stable baseline level of functioning.

CONCLUSION

Adults with IDD now have much longer life expectancies compared to just a few decades ago; except for those individuals with the most significant limitations of movement and eating, their life expectancies now approach those of the general population. While diagnostic and therapeutic plans often need to be modified to accommodate an individual's special needs, individuals with IDD can often tolerate much more than might be expected. No matter what an individual's baseline level of functioning may be, if a treatment is likely to return that individual to his or her stable, baseline level, then it is usually appropriate to recommend that treatment. However, even in the presence of a stable disability, if an irreversible, progressive, degenerative process is superimposed over that disability, then it may be appropriate to avoid aggressive intervention and change the focus of therapy to promote comfort and quality, rather than duration, of life.

REFERENCES

Awoke, S., Mouton, C. P., & Parrott, M. (1992). Outcomes of skilled cardiopulmonary resuscitation in a long-term-care facility: Futile therapy? *Journal of the American Geriatrics Society*, *40*(6), 593–595.

Besdine, R., Rubenstein, L., & Snyder, L. (1996). *Medical care of the nursing home resident, What physicians need to know*. Philadelphia: American College of Physicians.

Casarett, D., Kapo, J., & Caplan, A. (2005). Appropriate use of artificial nutrition and hydration—Fundamental principles and recommendations. *New England Journal of Medicine*, *353*(24), 2607–2612.

Emmerich, M. T. (1993). *Constipation in adults with developmental disabilities*. A Bold New Approach, Abstracts of Presentations for 117th Annual Meeting of the American Association on Mental Retardation, Washington, DC.

Emmerich, M. T. (2006). Community practice for adults. In I. L. Rubin & A. C. Crocker (Eds.), *Medical care for children and adults with developmental disabilities* (2nd ed., pp. 79–88). Baltimore, MD: Brookes Publishing.

Janicki, M., & Wisniewski, H. (1985). *Aging and developmental disabilities, issues and approaches*. Baltimore, MD: Brookes Publishing.

Kris, M. G., Hesketh, P. J., Somerfield, M. R., Feyer, P., Clark-Snow, R., Koeller, M., et al. (2006). American Society of Clinical Oncology guideline for antiemetics in oncology: Update 2006. *Journal of Clinical Oncology, 24*(18), 2932–2947.

Marino, B., & Pueschel, S. (1996). *Heart disease in persons with Down syndrome*. Baltimore, MD: Brookes Publishing.

Molloy, D., Knight, T., & Woodfield, K. (2003). *Diversity in disability: Exploring the interactions between disability, ethnicity, age, gender and sexuality* (pp. 118–119). Leeds, UK: Published for the Department of Work and Pensions by Corporate Document Services. Retrieved August 2, 2008, from http://www.dwp.gov.uk/asd/asd5/rrep188.pdf

Nichol, G., Stiell, I. G., Laupacis, A., Pham, B., De Maio, V., & Wells, G. A. (1999). A cumulative meta-analysis of the effectiveness of defibrillator-capable emergency medical services for victims of out-of-hospital cardiac arrest. *Annals of Emergency Medicine, 34*, 517–525.

Schonwald, A., & Rappaport, L. (2004). Consultation with the specialist: Encopresis assessment and management. *Pediatrics in Review, 25*(8), 278–283.

Service, K. P., & Hahn, J. E. (2003). Issues in aging: The role of the nurse in the care of older people with intellectual and developmental disabilities. *Nursing Clinics of North America, 38*(2), 291–312.

Strauss, D., & Shavelle, R. (1998). Life expectancy of adults with cerebral palsy. *Developmental Medicine and Child Neurology, 40*, 369–375.

Strauss, D., Shavelle, R., Reynolds, R., Rosenbloom, L., & Day, S. (2007). Survival in cerebral palsy in the last 20 years: Signs of improvement? *Developmental Medicine and Child Neurology, 49*, 86–92.

Sutton, E., Factor, A., Hawkins, B., Heller, T., & Seltzer, G. (1993). *Older adults with developmental disabilities, Optimizing choice and change*. Baltimore, MD: Brookes Publishing.

Wolraich, M. L., Siperstein, G. N., & Reed, D. (1991). Doctors' decisions and prognostications for infants with Down syndrome. *Developmental Medicine and Child Neurology, 33*(4), 336–342.

CHAPTER 6

Medical Treatment and Management at the End of Life

JULIE HAUER

INTRODUCTION

Planning for end-of-life care is best approached as an ongoing process in a person's life that begins well in advance of a terminal illness. This includes assuring access to and utilization of high quality end-of-life care for all individuals with intellectual and developmental disabilities (IDD). Barriers to meeting this goal are many and include attitudes toward people with disabilities, uncertainty of prognosis, and lack of clinical training and experience with this population. Areas and skills that have been identified as being in need of improvement include communication with the patient and family and training in the assessment of pain and other distressing symptoms in individuals with IDD (Graham & Robinson, 2005; Tuffrey-Wijne, McEnhill, Curfs, & Hollins, 2007).

Surrounding end-of-life care are the debates actively taking place within society that are guided and influenced by ethics, morality, religion, personal values, justice, and quality of life. Case reports in the literature highlight the consequences of this debate with examples of systems that provide more interventions, possibly in order to avoid the impression of discrimination based on disability (Lohiya, Tan-Figueroa, & Crinella, 2003), as well as those that do not offer treatment based on an assumption of poor quality of life (Tuffrey-Wijne, 2003). As our society wrestles with these challenges, we should actively avoid bringing this debate to the bedside. We need to take into account individual and family preferences and be guided by knowledge of the legal and ethical constructs that influence our care decisions.

To assist with the goal of attaining quality end-of-life care, this chapter will outline a framework for guiding medical decisions when there is uncertainty, and it will offer an outline for end-of-life symptom management. A list of suggested resources is provided at the end of the chapter.

DR is a 25-year-old woman with cerebral palsy and intellectual disability. She is nonverbal and nonambulatory. She receives fluid and nutrition by a gastrostomy feeding tube. Other

---

With gratitude to Dr. Lawrence Charnas for his support and guidance with this chapter.

associated problems include neuromuscular scoliosis, history of a fracture, and recurrent pul-
monary illnesses. She has experienced an increased frequency of respiratory exacerbations over
the years, with treatment including antibiotics and prednisone during acute illnesses, which
now occur every 1 to 2 months. Her daily chronic treatment includes nebulizer treatments
of inhaled steroid as well as bronchodilators as needed, chest physiotherapy and a vest for
bronchial drainage, and Trendelenburg positioning to allow maximal clearance of oral and
pulmonary secretions. She receives supplemental home oxygen as needed.

Following repeat hospitalizations, her caregivers shared their concern that hospitalizations
were providing less benefit and were distressing for DR: "We know her better and know how to
care for her better than can be provided in the hospital." They also describe her days as enjoy-
able between respiratory illnesses with distress during acute exacerbations. One of her home
care nurses described an episode when DR turned blue "so quickly" that it made it difficult to
provide all interventions available. They are not ready to "give up on her," and they worry that
there will be criticism if something happens to her at home.

THE FRAMEWORK

An Approach to the Challenge of Prognosis, Uncertainty, and Decision Making

The literature summarizing life expectancy provides a context but does not guide the decisions that families face. Uncertainty of prognosis has been identified as the most common
barrier to palliative care and optimal end-of-life care for seriously ill children (Davies et
al., 2008). Palliative care is a model of interdisciplinary care that emphasizes "the active
total care of patients whose disease is not responsive to curative treatment" (World Health
Organization, 1998). It seeks to improve the quality of life for patients and their families
and to prevent and relieve suffering by promptly identifying and treating pain and other
problems, whether they are physical, psychosocial, or spiritual (Working Party of Association for Children's Palliative Care [ACT] and Royal College of Paediatrics and Child
Health [RCPCH], 2003). Interdisciplinary palliative care teams often include a palliative
care physician, an advanced practice nurse, a chaplain, and a social worker. Hospice and
Palliative Medicine is also a recognized medical subspecialty with trained experts who
may lead such interdisciplinary teams. Early introduction of palliative care assures the use
of interventions to address physical and emotional suffering (Wolfe, Klar, et al., 2000).
Parents have reported this type of intervention as being helpful, even though the information may be upsetting (Mack, Wolfe, Grier, Cleary, & Weeks, 2006), and does not
lessen their hope (Mack et al., 2007). Physician communication about what to expect in
the end-of-life care period, as well as the parental perception of preparedness, have been
identified as components of high-quality care (Mack et al., 2005).

There is limited literature regarding how to best address this type of uncertainty for
those who care for individuals with IDD. Steele (2005a, 2005b) studied the experience
of families with children dying from neurodegenerative conditions, describing how they
navigate "uncharted territory" and use strategies such as seeking and sharing information,
focusing on the child, reframing the experience, and promoting the child's health. At
times of more serious illness, factors influencing parental decisions to limit or discontinue
specific medical therapies include assessments of the child's quality of life, the child's likelihood of improvement, the perception of their child's suffering, the perception of their
child's will to survive, previous experience with death and end-of-life decision making for

or with others, financial resources, and concerns regarding lifelong care. Parents express the desire to do what is in the best interest of their child while struggling with guilt and managing a unique type of chronic sorrow (Meyer, Burns, Griffith, & Truog, 2002; Scornaienchi, 2003; Sharman, Meert, & Sarnaik, 2005).

Hypothetical Disease Trajectory

Figures 6.1 and 6.2 are intended to provide a hypothetical framework for reflecting on and anticipating the health and functional trajectory of an individual with severe IDD. The figures are also intended to guide families through uncertainty and decision making by using a reflection on the past as an introduction to a possible future. Knowledge of associated health problems, such as recurrent respiratory exacerbations from chronic pulmonary aspiration, allows identification of interventions intended to improve or maintain the individual's current health and functional status. By reflecting on the prior benefit of interventions, the probable and possible future benefit can be anticipated (Back, Arnold, & Quill, 2003).

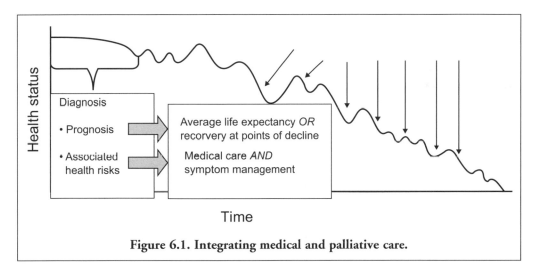

Figure 6.1. Integrating medical and palliative care.

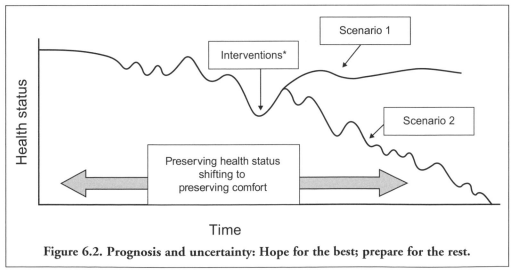

Figure 6.2. Prognosis and uncertainty: Hope for the best; prepare for the rest.

Some examples of interventions are the following: gastrostomy feeding tube, treatment of gastroesophageal reflux, antireflux surgery, treatment of acute respiratory exacerbations, and medication changes for intractable epilepsy

The hypothetical disease trajectory highlights that many health problems of individuals with severe IDD progress gradually with initial treatment benefit and then return to health and functional baseline. Over time, less return to baseline occurs from the interventions available. Parents may request intensive interventions and predict a positive outcome from an acute event, when, subsequently, an actual decline in health status occurs rather than a return to baseline. This attitude may reflect a "pressure of past success" (Graham & Robinson, 2005). Asking parents of a child with IDD to make a decision to limit interventions before the child has had any decline in health can be disorienting without context. They may feel like the emphasis is on limiting interventions because of the disability instead of on focusing on the anticipated health risks that are associated with the disability. By identifying associated health problems, monitoring for changes in health status, and noting any decreased benefit from treatments, we can identify individuals with IDD who have life-limiting conditions and are at risk of experiencing life-threatening events.

The best guide to the future is a combination of this knowledge along with a reflection on the past. It allows us to consider what is likely to happen and what may happen. Questions to consider and review to assist with this reflection include the following:

- Have goals of care been identified as a guide to decisions?
- Have options that meet these goals been offered, or have medical interventions been presented as "required" for the problem identified?
- How will the course look with or without the treatment available?
- Will an intervention bridge to a goal and provide sufficient recovery or prolong a process?
- Do we continue to see a benefit from chronic and acute treatment options with maintenance or return of health and functional status?
- Are we seeing less benefit over time with less return to prior baseline, longer periods of illness, or a shorter time between each illness?
- What percentage of each day or week is "good" or "quality" time, and how does today compare with 1 year ago, 6 months ago, and so on?
- What percentage of each day or week is spent in suffering?
- When will these interventions maintain or improve health instead of prolong a process of decline or suffering?

Palliative Care as a Model of Care: Tools and Techniques

Table 6.1 outlines examples of the communication tools used in palliative care. Defining goals of care is a critical part of guiding decision making by identifying interventions and care that meet identified goals rather than treat a medical problem in isolation. Palliative care recognizes that it is distressing for parents and physicians to encounter the limits of medicine. At such times, people often do more out of a sense that they need to do something. Palliative care identifies other options, such as symptom management, and recognizes that there is always care to provide as goals shift from treatment and cure to quality of life and comfort. Medical treatment and palliative care are ideally integrated together

Table 6.1
Communication Tools Used in Palliative Care

Objectives	Suggested language
Determine goals of care as a guide to decision making	• We will always review how the interventions available meet the goals you've identified. • Goals commonly include comfort and quality of life, might shift to providing care at home when less benefit or greater burden is seen from care in the hospital, might shift to comfort only when limited benefit is identified from the treatment available, and can be a specific activity such as maintaining current health status for a family trip.
Focus on parental expertise	• Though I will honestly reflect on changes in your daughter's health and functional status, you are the expert in how these changes look and affect her quality of life. • Though we bring expertise in evaluating and managing health problems in children, you are the expert in how such problems look in your daughter.
Anticipate worries	• We know that worries of parents at such times often include the following: Is my child suffering? Will my child get better? Is there more we can do? We will talk through these worries. • We can talk through some of the "what ifs" so as to address any worries you may have, so you know what to expect, to assure that we have a care plan in place, and to allow you to focus on loving your daughter
Reflect on the past as a guide to the future	• I wonder if we are seeing less recovery and less time between each illness. • Do you think we are seeing fewer good days now compared to 6 and 12 months ago? • Your daughter's story will guide us along the way. Our job as parents and care providers is to watch, listen, and reflect honestly on what the story is telling us.
Acknowledge the limits of interventions	• I can only imagine how hard it is to be seeing fewer good days. I wish we had interventions that could reverse this. • Your daughter continues to receive exceptional care at home. My observation is that we are seeing fewer benefits from the treatment we have available. What have you observed?

(continued on next page)

Table 6.1
Communication Tools Used in Palliative Care (*continued*)

Objectives	Suggested language
Limiting treatment does not mean limiting care	• I worry that your daughter's body is getting tired out despite the best treatment available.
	• It might make sense to identify what we won't do if her body becomes too tired to sustain adequate breathing. We won't limit treatments that have reasonable benefit but will protect her from interventions that may harm or prolong suffering.
	• We will always provide care that maximizes comfort throughout her life.
Hope for the best; prepare for the rest	• We know families often hold simultaneously their hope for the best possible outcome with their realistic understanding of the severity of the problem.
Offer continuity with a safety net	• We may not know when your daughter will have more problems, but you will always have a team available to help guide and support you on this journey.
Identify decision making as a dynamic process	• What might seem like the "right" decision today could change. Your decisions are never final and can change as the clinical course changes.
	• Withholding and withdrawing treatment are ethically and legally equivalent but can feel different emotionally.

for children with life-limiting conditions (American Academy of Pediatrics [AAP] Committee on Bioethics and Committee on Hospital Care, 2000; Himelstein, Hilden, Boldt, & Weissman, 2004; Klick & Ballantine, 2007).

Areas of need as a result of slow decline include planning for future problems, avoiding interventions of limited benefit, and assisting long-term caregivers (Dy & Lynn, 2007). Planning ahead may be incorporated into discussions to allow families time to prepare— even when the timeline is difficult to determine. Figures 6.1 and 6.2 provide frameworks for allowing physicians to discuss "what if" while giving permission to parents to maintain hope. Discussions that assist parents in preparing help lessen suffering and can provide positive benefits to later bereavement (Mack et al., 2006, 2007; Valdimarsdottir et al., 2007; Wolfe, Klar, et al., 2000). Discussion can also identify the location of end-of-life care as another goal to guide decision making and thus introduce hospice as a resource to meet this goal. We can reassure parents and loved ones along the way that these discussions whether to use hospice as a resource are not about "giving up" on today's care but about future needs and are not about stopping care but of supporting care. Supportive care also includes attending to siblings as parents often worry about how to prepare their other children. Child life specialists or therapists can provide this through palliative care and hospice programs.

Discussing resuscitation requires an honest assessment of the likelihood of benefit and possible burden. It is important that we assume responsibility for this assessment so as not to imply parental or guardian responsibility for the decision. This includes sharing observations if we are seeing less benefit from interventions available and assurance that comfort will always be maintained. This is also a time to review that future decline in health is not a result of the decisions made or the care provided at home; rather, certain health problems cannot be "cured" or "fixed." Families need reassurance that interventions will be used as long as they maintain sufficient benefit to quality of life and comfort.

In the case of DR, goals of care were reviewed and identified. A goal was identified to continue home treatment without further hospitalizations. A home care treatment protocol for future respiratory illnesses was offered to meet this goal. They continue to hope for as many good days as possible and believe this plan will help meet that goal. Discussion did not involve asking, "Do you want DR intubated?" To prevent further hospitalizations, however, it was recommended that Do Not Resuscitate (DNR) be documented, to which the family agreed. As DR appears in distress during respiratory illnesses, interventions for comfort were explained and offered.

END-OF-LIFE CARE: MANAGING PAIN AND OTHER DISTRESSING SYMPTOMS

Providing comfort to patients is always a part of medical treatment. There are times, however, when comfort becomes the foremost goal of care. This section will focus on the primary role of medical treatment and management at the end of life, namely, the assessment, evaluation, and management of pain or other distressing symptoms.

Assessment

The usual components of the pain history can be difficult to assess in an individual with IDD and may not be possible in a nonverbal individual. These components include the following:

- Description of pain (Is the pain sharp, stabbing, dull, burning, or tingling?)
- Location of pain (Where does the pain spread or travel?)
- Intensity of pain (How would you rate your pain on a scale of 1 to 10?)
- Duration of pain (Is the pain constant or does it come and go?)
- Frequency of pain (How often does the pain happen?)
- Factors that worsen or relieve pain (Is there anything that makes the pain better or worse?)

Pain Assessment in Individuals with IDD

The assessment of pain in individuals with IDD falls into two main categories: assessment through self-report and assessment through observation. The underlying IDD may alter affective processing, memory, or the ability to communicate information about pain. Assessment that utilizes reporting and rating of pain must be appropriate to the individuals' cognitive level. Understanding of the child or adults' functional level should be sought from parents and care providers, often indicated as a developmental age. Clinicians should use a validated pain-rating system appropriate for the level of intellectual function.

Pain assessment tools involve the concept of placing and understanding things in order of magnitude. Children from 5 to 6 years of age develop the ability to create a series in order of size but only through trial and error. Pain rating tools appropriate for this functional age include poker chips and the Oucher, a scale with facial pictures showing increasing levels of pain (Beyer & Aradine, 1986). Children from 7 to 10 can more reliably use tools to quantify pain, including use of the Wong-Baker FACES pain-rating scale (Wong, Wilson, Hockenberry-Eaton, Winklestein, & Schwartz, 2000). Adolescents develop the ability to use a numerical rating scale, such as a 0 to 10 scale, to rate their pain without any tool being present.

Individuals with IDD may have an ability to indicate the following:

- Presence of pain (Does anything in your body hurt? Do you have pain anywhere?)
- Location of pain (Please point to the place in your body that hurts.)
- Rating of pain (How much does it hurt?)

Observational tools are available for individuals unable to report pain. Specific distress behaviors have been associated with pain and are very helpful in quantifying pain in children unable to provide self-report. Behavioral measurement must be assessed in the context of sources of distress, since it may be difficult to distinguish between pain behaviors and behaviors resulting from other types of distress, such as hunger or anxiety. Observational tools rely on assessing the following items: vocalizations, facial expression, consolability, interactivity, mood, eating and sleeping, protective actions, movement, tone and posture, and physiological measures. When assessing children with severe to profound cognitive disabilities, it is important to note that they were found to have elevated scores at baseline on two pain assessment scales (Defrin, Lotan, & Pick, 2006). It is important to select a tool that is suited for an individual's ability to communicate his or her needs. Additional information on pain assessment tools are provided in chapter 20.

Evaluation

Children with IDD experience pain more frequently than the general pediatric population. Studies have reported 32%–44% of children with IDD experiencing pain on a weekly basis (Breau, Camfield, McGrath, & Finley, 2003; Houlihan, O'Donnell, Conaway, & Stevenson, 2004) and 24% on a daily basis (Stallard, Williams, Lenton, & Velleman, 2001). In contrast, 12% of healthy children experienced pain on a weekly basis (Perquin et al., 2000). Identifying the source of pain in a nonverbal individual with IDD poses a unique and significant challenge. Common, recognized pain sources in these individuals include acute causes such as fracture, urinary tract infection, or pancreatitis and chronic sources such as gastroesophageal reflux (GER), constipation, feeding difficulties from delayed gut motility, positioning, spasticity, hip pain, or dental pain. Table 6.2 outlines etiologies of acute and chronic pain to consider.

Experience shows that a pain source may not be identified, or pain may continue despite treatment of an identified source. Greco and Berde (2005) identified the category "screaming of unknown origin" to indicate children with neurologic disorders,

Table 6.2
Etiology of Pain/Irritability in Nonverbal Children with Neurological Impairment

Head, Eyes, Ears, Nose, Throat (HEENT)

- Acute otitis media, pharyngitis, sinusitis, dental abscess/gingival inflammation, corneal abrasion, glaucoma, ventriculoperitoneal shunt malfunction

Chest

- Pulmonary aspiration/pneumonia, esophagitis, pericardial effusion, supraventricular tachycardia, cardiac ischemia

Abdomen

- Gastrointestinal: gastroesophageal reflux disease, gastritis/gastric ulcer, peptic ulcer disease, food allergy, appendicitis, intussusception, constipation, delayed/impaired motility, rectal fissure, visceral hyperalgesia
- Liver/gallbladder: hepatitis, cholecystitis
- Pancreas: pancreatitis
- Renal: urinary tract infection, nephrolithiasis, neuropathic bladder, obstructive uropathy
- Genitourinary: inguinal hernia, testicular torsion, ovarian torsion/cyst, menstrual cramps

Skin

- Pressure sore/decubitus ulcer

Extremities

- Fracture, hip subluxation, osteomyelitis, hair tourniquet

Psychosocial

- Loss of caregiver, change in home environment, nonaccidental trauma

General

- Medication toxicity, sleep disturbance

severe developmental delay, neurodegeneration, or severe motor impairments with persistent agitation, distress, or screaming. Evaluation may identify a specific nociceptive cause, or painful stimulus, but in many other cases these evaluations can be frustrating for patients, families, and clinicians. In their chapter, Pain and Children with Developmental Disabilities, Oberlander and Craig note that pain in children with cognitive disabilities is typically thought to be nociceptive in origin; however, after repeated injury or surgery, neuropathic pain may also occur (Oberlander & Craig, 2003, chap. 33; Schechter, Berde, & Yaster, 2003). Neuropathic pain is caused by stimulation or abnormal functioning of damaged sensory nerves, primarily in the peripheral nervous system. Because of the confusing neurologic and clinical picture, identification of neuropathic pain is challenging. Neuropathy therefore may be another source of ongoing and poorly treated pain in such children.

Parents commonly identify the gastrointestinal tract as a source of pain in children with IDD. Breau and colleagues (Breau et al., 2003; Breau, Camfield, McGrath, & Finley, 2004) identified gastrointestinal causes as the most frequent source of all episodes of pain in children with severe cognitive disabilities. Approximately half of the children with gastrointestinal pain experienced pain classified as "bowels" (not due to constipation), and a similar number had pain characterized "digestive" due to "gas" or "gastrointestinal" problems without identification of cause or location. Pain of unknown cause was the most intense, followed by pain attributed to the bowels, gastrointestinal tract, and digestive pain. Houlihan's group (Houlihan et al., 2004) reported significantly higher rates of pain in children with a gastrostomy tube and those taking medications for feeding, gastroesophageal reflux, or gastrointestinal motility. This association between gastrointestinal symptoms and consideration of neuropathy led to the hypothesis that some children with IDD experience visceral hyperalgesia that benefits from gabapentin (Hauer, Wical, & Charnas, 2007).

Management

Management of Pain and Other Distressing Symptoms

Management of pain often varies based on the specific symptoms and circumstances (Berde & Sethna, 2002; Friedrichsdorf & Kang, 2007; Goldman, Hain, & Liben, 2006; Greco & Berde, 2005; Moryl, Coyle, & Foley, 2008; Schechter et al., 2003). However, general guidelines for pain management are presented here. Specific information will also be provided regarding use of opioids and the treatment of symptoms such as dyspnea, nausea, and delirium.

When possible, it is beneficial to determine the type or types of pain in order to prescribe the optimum treatment. Pain should be distinguished as being nociceptive and/or neuropathic. Nociceptive pain is caused by stimulation of intact nociceptors—sensory receptors that sense painful stimulus—as a result of tissue injury. Stimulation of intact nociceptors in skin, soft tissue, skeletal muscle, and bone may result in somatic pain. This type of pain is well localized and described as sharp, aching, squeezing, stabbing, or throbbing. Stimulation of intact nociceptors in internal visceral organs results in visceral pain. It is characterized as poorly localized and is often described as dull, crampy, or achy, and it is not always associated with visceral injury.

Neuropathic pain, caused by stimulation or abnormal functioning of damaged sensory nerves, may be the result of compression, transection, infiltration, ischemia, or metabolic injury to the nerves. It is often described as burning, shooting, electric, or tingling and may be underrecognized in individuals with IDD.

Once the type and severity of pain is identified, one should also determine whether a specific and treatable condition is causing the pain, since in some cases treating the underlying condition can significantly relieve the symptom. Even when specific therapy is available—and especially when it is not—it is important to provide adequate symptom management to relieve suffering.

Basic Pain Management Guided by the WHO Analgesic Ladder

The World Health Organization (WHO) analgesic ladder (Figure 6.3) provides general guidelines for choosing the drug based on the degree of pain. It is also important to understand several other issues related to analgesia. Nonopioids used for mild pain may be used along with opioids when treating moderate to severe pain. In addition, codeine is ineffective in approximately one third of individuals as a result of their inability to metabolize codeine to the active metabolite morphine (Williams, Patel, & Howard, 2002). This results in the potential for experiencing side effects with no analgesic benefit. Administration of methadone requires additional expertise given its biphasic elimination. Meperidine should be avoided if other opioids are available, as its metabolite can result in seizures especially with long term use. It is also important to identify the appropriate drug and dose in individuals with renal and hepatic failure (Dean, 2004; Murphy, 2005).

Adjuvant therapies may be used at any point on the analgesic ladder. They can enhance analgesic efficacy, treat concurrent symptoms, and/or provide independent analgesic activity for specific types of pain. They are particularly helpful for neuropathic pain but may also be helpful for bone pain and other chronic pain. Adjuvant therapy includes antidepressants such as nortriptyline and amitryptyline (neuropathic pain), anticonvulsants such as gabapentin and pregabalin (neuropathic pain), steroids (hepatic distention, bowel wall edema, cerebral edema), bisphosphonates (bone pain due to metastases), and radiation therapy (bone pain due to metastases).

Barriers to Using Opioids for Management of Pain and Respiratory Depression

Barriers to the use of opioid medications may include fear of doing harm, fear of drug addiction, and fear of giving up too soon. By identifying and discussing the misperceptions that exist, we can help alleviate these common fears.

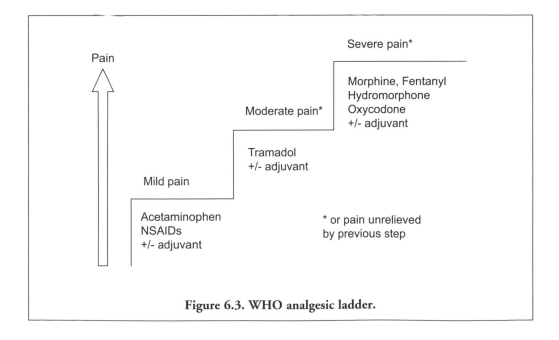

Figure 6.3. WHO analgesic ladder.

Fear over development of respiratory depression is one of the greatest barriers to the use of opioids, including at end of life. This is an unwarranted fear, as opioid-induced respiratory depression is unlikely with of a low starting dose, appropriate and standard dosing and titration, and adjustment for renal or hepatic impairment in individuals with altered mental status or compromised breathing. An exception can occur if there is a sudden change in the ability to clear opioids or a reduction in pain stimulation. The association of opioid use with end-of-life care can result in an assumption that opioids either hasten death or indicate that someone is dying when he or she is not. When used appropriately and for stated goals, opioids do not hasten death but can assure comfort throughout life.

Other Considerations for Pain Management: Dose Interval, Titration, and Breakthrough Doses

Unless pain is infrequent, an opioid dosage should be scheduled around the clock based on the duration of analgesic effect of the specific medication, typically every 4 hours. Once the opioid requirement is determined, it can be converted to a sustained release given 2 or 3 times daily with immediate release used as needed for breakthrough pain. For chronic pain, opioids should be given on a scheduled basis to maintain necessary blood levels. It is beneficial to use the same opioid for sustained release and immediate release, as it facilitates estimation of opioid requirement and better identifies the source of opioid side effects.

A general rule of thumb for determining a breakthrough dose is 20% of the sustained release dose used in 12 hours or 10% of the 24-hour opioid requirement, available as often as every 1 to 2 hours for oral dosages. Based on the patient's response, doses of analgesics may be increased by 25%–50% per day until development of adequate analgesia or intolerable and unmanageable side effects. If pain remains severe it may be necessary to increase by 50%–100%. For most opioids, there is no fixed upper limit for the effective daily dose. Occasionally, high doses of opioids are required for adequate symptom management, such as those experienced most commonly in cancer (Siden & Nalewajek, 2003). If requiring more than three or four breakthrough doses in a 24-hour period, the total scheduled and breakthrough doses are then added up and redistributed.

Equivalence of Opioid Doses

It is important to be familiar with equivalent analgesic dosing of various opioids, so that the desired analgesic effect can be achieved when switching from one opioid to another (Table 6.3). When changing opioid medications, it is important to use a dose 25%–50% lower than the calculated equivalent analgesic dose and then increase as needed, to avoid possible overmedication. This is due to the phenomena known as cross-tolerance and reflects differences in the structure of different opioids and their affinity for the various opioid receptors, which may become overstimulated due to overmedication.

Escalating Symptoms

General guidelines for management of escalating pain include the following (Moryl et al., 2008):

- Give bedside titration with IV bolus every 15 minutes until pain is relieved.
- If on opioids, set initial bolus at 10%–20% of the 24-hour opioid dose.

Table 6.3
Dosing Data for Opioid Medications (Maximum Weight for Calculation 50 kg)

Drug	Equianalgesic dose		Usual oral dose	Usual IV dose
	Oral (mg)	IV (mg)	Oral (mg)	IV (mg)
Morphine	30	10	0.3 mg/kg q 3–4 h	0.1 mg/kg q 2–4 h
Hydromorphone	7.5	1.5	0.04–0.08 mg/kg q 3–4 h	0.02 mg/kg q 2–4 h
Oxycodone	20	N/A	0.1 mg/kg q 3–4 h	N/A
Fentanyl	N/A	0.1 (100 mcg)	N/A	0.5–1 mcg/kg q 1–2 h
Methadone*	N/A	N/A	0.1 mg/kg q 6–8 h	0.1 mg/kg q 6–8 h

Doses are for individuals over 6 months of age.

* Dose dependent potency, requires expertise in use.

- Increase opioid bolus by 30%–50% every third dose if pain continues.
- Once the patient has obtained adequate pain relief, calculate the new 24-hour opioid dose including rescue doses.
- Determine route for around-the-clock dosing that is best suited to patient's ongoing analgesic needs (oral, IV, or transdermal).
- Consider adding an adjuvant or coanalgesic (e.g., a nonsteroidal anti-inflammatory drug, benzodiazepine, or corticosteroid).
- If the patient has significant opioid-adverse effects *with* adequate pain control, reduce the equianalgesic (same amount of pain relief) dose (Table 6.3) of the new opioid by 25%–50%.
- If the patient has significant opioid-adverse effects *without* adequate pain control, rotate opioids without a reduction in the equianalgesic dose.

Management of Opioid Side Effects
Anticipating and managing opioid side effects is of significant importance to assure continued use of medications for symptom management. Some side effects, such as constipation, are so common that prophylactic laxatives should be initiated when opioids are prescribed. For other side effects, management can be done in one of several ways:

- Managing symptomatic side effects (Table 6.4)
- Reducing opioid dose by 20% *if* there has been a reduction in pain
- Switching to an alternate opioid (opioid rotation) with resulting reduction in the total equivalent opioid dose as a result of incomplete cross-tolerance
- Monitoring over several days for improvement of mild symptoms such as sedation and nausea

Table 6.4
Management of Opioid Side Effects
Respiratory depression and hypersomnolence

- Breathing will become less labored once pain is controlled, but significant opioid-induced respiratory depression is unlikely with appropriate dosing
- Usually seen only with overmedication or high doses required for severe pain
- Dose reduction by 20% if analgesia is satisfactory
- Opioid rotation

Sedation

- Mild sedation is common
- Patients generally become tolerant over days to this effect of opioids

Constipation

- Opioid-induced constipation is very common, but it can be effectively prevented and treated with agents such as laxatives

Urinary retention

- Opioid rotation

Nausea and vomiting

- Patients generally become tolerant
- Can be effectively treated with one of the antidopaminergic antiemetics, such as prochlorperazine, metaclopramide, or haloperidol (Table 6.7)

Pruritis

- Antihistamines (Diphenhydramine, Hydroxyzine)

Myoclonus

- Clonazepam, Baclofen

Delirium

- Neuroleptics (Table 6.7)

Hyperalgesia

- Opioid rotation

Renal and hepatic failure can contribute to side effects through accumulation of metabolites. For patients with renal impairment, fentanyl is considered the safest, oxycodone and hydromorphone should be used with caution, and morphine sulfate should be avoided (Dean, 2004; Murphy, 2005).

SUPPORTIVE AND NONPHARMACOLOGIC INTERVENTIONS

Though not covered in this chapter, nonpharmacologic interventions are an essential part of symptom management strategies. These can include physical methods such as cuddling, massage, heat, cold, and physical and occupational therapy. Cognitive-behavioral techniques include guided imagery, distraction, storytelling, music, and art therapy.

Dyspnea

Dyspnea is the experience of shortness of breath, difficulty of breathing, or painful breathing. It is a common symptom of numerous medical disorders. Included are the diseases of the lung parenchyma and obstructions of the airway that can occur from repeated microaspiration resulting in infection, bronchiectasis, and lung scarring over time. Measures of respiratory rate, oxygen saturation, blood gas levels, and family perception do not necessarily correlate with the patient's perception of breathlessness. Instruments such as the Respiratory Distress Observational Scale (RDOS) are being evaluated for use in adults unable to report the symptoms of dyspnea (Campbell, 2008) or can be part of the Disability Distress Assessment Tool (DisDAT; Regnard et al., 2007).

Treating dyspnea is typically focused on identifying and aggressively treating the underlying cause. Evidence has been established for utilizing interventions for adults to alleviate dyspnea that persists despite maximal medical management of identified causes. These interventions include an oxygen trial, cool air from a fan or open window, repositioning, lorazepam for associated anxiety, and morphine sulfate. A recent review from the American College of Physicians identified strong evidence for treating adults with dyspnea from chronic lung disease with short-term opioids (Lorenz et al., 2008; Qaseem et al., 2008). Evidence includes demonstration of significant improvement in refractory dyspnea in participants completing a randomized, double-blind, placebo-controlled cross over study with no significant episodes of sedation (Abernethy et al., 2003). Several studies have demonstrated the safety of using morphine sulfate for management of dyspnea that occurs despite maximal treatment of the underlying cause without development of respiratory depression (Allen, Raut, Woollard, & Vassallo, 2005; Clemens & Klaschik, 2007; Mazzocato, Buclin, & Rapin, 1999). A suggested starting dose for an opioid-naïve patient is 25%–30% of the dose used for pain, with a maximum starting dose of 5 mg orally, or, if already on an opioid, increasing the dose by 30%.

Children with severe IDD have a high incidence of respiratory problems and associated distressing symptoms (Seddon & Khan, 2003). Recurrent respiratory illness leading to respiratory failure is the most common cause of mortality in children with severe cerebral palsy (Hemming, Hutton, & Pharoah, 2006; Strauss, Cable, & Shavelle, 1999). Aspiration is a frequent factor, identified in 31%–68% of children with cerebral palsy (Mirrett, Riski, Glascott, & Johnson, 1994; Taniguchi & Moyer, 1994; Wright, Wright, & Carson, 1996). Aspiration pneumonia in children with significant IDD is best understood as an acute exacerbation resulting from chronic contributing factors. Those factors include (a) ineffective cough, (b) hypoventilation from inactivity and motor impairment, (c) impaired ability to manage routine oral secretions, (d) chronic aspiration of oral bacteria resulting in a high enough inoculum over time to overcome host defenses, (e) development of inflammation, and (f) development of mucous plugs with ventilation/perfusion (V/Q) mismatch.

As the respiratory disease progresses despite maximal management of these contributing factors, respiratory distress is a frequent symptom that recurs in such children. Using the model of managing dyspnea in adults, children deserve symptom management of associated respiratory distress incorporated into chronic and acute medical management. Table 6.5 outlines chronic and acute home care strategies, based on experience and evidence, for individuals with severe IDD and associated aspiration of oral secretions. For example, the table identifies antibiotics that provide coverage of anaerobic bacteria along with other oral bacteria when treating people who chronically aspirate oral secretions (Allewelt, Schuler, Bolcskei, Mauch, & Lode, 2004; Brook, 1996; Brook & Finegold, 1980; Dreyfuss & Mier, 2001; Kadowaki et al., 2005). Table 6.5 includes morphine sulfate for consideration as goals shift from medical treatment in the early phase to treatment and comfort in the later phase as a decline in health status is observed.

In the case of DR, the option of morphine sulfate was offered for management of respiratory distress during acute respiratory exacerbations, including a lengthy review of what we know from studying its use in adults and the acknowledgment of the common worries that exist. Four months later, DR's home care nurse reluctantly utilized morphine sulfate—along with initiating one of her rotating home antibiotics as outlined in her home care plan—when DR suffered from a new respiratory illness and was very impressed with the results. It caused no respiratory or mental depression and really brought her respiratory rate and distress back to baseline.

For such reasons, we likely underutilize morphine sulfate when managing respiratory distress, instead reserving its use for comfort at the end of life. There is a need to study the integration of morphine sulfate into the care plans of patients who have chronic aspiration and recurrent, distressing respiratory exacerbations. Waiting until the goal is comfort care rather than treatment focused delays initiation of comfort strategies earlier.

Nausea, Vomiting, and Retching

Gastrointestinal symptoms are common in children with severe IDD as noted in the pain section (Breau et al., 2003, 2004; Houlihan et al., 2004). Vomiting in these children is commonly attributed to gastroesophageal reflux (GER; Del Giudice et al., 1999). Alternatively, stimulation of the emetic reflex is likely an underreported source of symptoms in these patients (Antao, Ooi, Ade-Ajayi, Stevens, & Spitz, 2005; Richards, Andrews, Spitz, & Milla, 1998; Richards, Milla, Andrews, & Spitz, 2001). Experience and limited evidence suggests the benefit of management options for GER. In addition, nausea and vomiting are commonly encountered in oncology and other disorders at end of life (Jalmsell, Kreicbergs, Onelov, Steineck, & Henter, 2006; Wolfe, Grier, et al., 2000). An understanding of the pathways and the neurotransmitters involved in generating nausea, vomiting, and retching can guide evaluation and selection of management options available (Baines, 1997; Santucci & Mack, 2007; Wood, Shega, Lynch, & Von Roenn, 2007).

SR is a 3-year-old with hydranencephaly with resulting cerebral palsy, intellectual disability, visual impairment, and seizure disorder. She eats orally with supplementation of nutrition and fluids by gastrostomy tube (G-tube). She is responsive to her family with smiles and laughter. She remained at her baseline health status until she developed vomiting and retching 3 months earlier. Persistent symptoms resulted in a switch of her feeding tube to a jejunostomy tube (J-tube) and consideration of a Nissen fundoplication.

Table 6.5
Home Management: Medical Treatment and Comfort Strategies

Chronic interventions	When needed
Suctioning	As needed for comfort
Oxygen	Assessed by appearance of patient or by oximeter
Albuterol nebulizer	Every 3–4 hours for coughing, wheezing, congestion
Ipratropium (Atrovent) nebulizer	Every 3–4 hours for coughing, wheezing, congestion
Saline or Mucomyst nebulizer	As needed for coughing, wheezing, congestion
Chest physiotherapy or vest	2 times/day, increase to 4 times/day with increased symptoms*
Nebulized budesonide (Pulmicort)	2 times/day, increase to 4 times/day with increased symptoms*
Salmeterol (Serevent)	Family history of allergies or benefit from daily albuterol

Acute Interventions **for respiratory exacerbations from chronic aspiration**

Clindamycin, Augmentin or Levofloxacin/Moxifloxacin†	10–14 days
Systemic steroids (Prednisone)‡	5 days

Additional Interventions **for symptom management and end-of-life care**

Fan on face	Relieves sensation of breathlessness
Morphine sulfate	Use for discomfort or respiratory distress; Starting dose 0.1 mg/kg/dose PO/SL/ gastrostomy tube; May increase by 30% until comfortable
Glycopyrrolate (Robinul) or Scopalamine	Might contribute to mucous plugging; Decreases oral and respiratory secretions in end-of-life care

* *Symptoms include increased coughing, secretions, congestion, respiratory rate, and breathing effort.*

† *Use in children with aspiration when symptoms persist despite an increase in chronic interventions.*

‡ *Include with third or fourth exacerbation, sooner if symptoms return within 2 months of antibiotic course.*

Reprinted with permission from the Journal of Palliative Medicine. Adapted from "Respiratory Symptom Management in a Child with Severe Neurologic Impairment," by J. M. Hauer, 2007.

The process that results in nausea and vomiting is complex. Central to the process is the vomiting center (VC) located in the medulla. The VC is the final common pathway with numerous inputs that include the chemoreceptor trigger zone, cortical inputs, meningeal and ventricular mechanoreceptors, vagal and glossopharyngeal input, and vestibular input.

The chemoreceptor trigger zone (CTZ), located in the floor of the fourth ventricle, is stimulated by toxins; medications (chemotherapy, opioids, antibiotics); and metabolic imbalance (hyponatremia, hypercalcemia, uremia, ketoacidosis). It contains significant numbers of dopamine (D2), serotonin (5HT3), and substance P (NK-1) receptors. Stimulation leads to nausea, and blockage of the receptors leads to relief of symptoms. Vestibular input is a result of disorders of the vestibular nucleus and cranial nerve VIII leading to stimulation of the VC. Nausea and vomiting brought on by position changes is a clue from history of vestibular input contributing to these symptoms.

Meningeal and ventricular mechanoreceptors are stimulated by increased intracranial pressure or directly by tumor. This leads to stimulation of the VC via cholinergic (Ach) and histamine (H1) receptors. Cortical input can provide input to both the CTZ and VC via acetylcholine and histamine receptors. Nausea can sometimes be a learned response to chemotherapy, radiotherapy, or anxiety-provoking situations. Vagal and glossopharyngeal input can result in stimulation of the VC by vagal afferents. This stimulation can be a result of mechanical (distension of a hollow viscous due to obstruction or dysmotility or direct pressure by mass or ascites) and chemical (inflammation caused by toxin, inflammation, or radiation) insults.

Opioids are a common source of nausea and vomiting. It is triggered by stimulation of the CTZ, as mediated through D2 receptors, gastroparesis (delayed gastric emptying), constipation, and labyrinth sensitization. Symptoms may peak soon after administration of the opioid. Treatment includes D2 receptor antagonists (haloperidol, metoclopramide), opioid rotation, and treatment of constipation.

Symptom management strategies based on the involved receptors are outlined in Table 6.6 in order of the origin of symptoms. As with pain, management of nausea and vomiting includes evaluating for treatable causes in addition to utilizing medications that block involved receptors. Examples include assessing for contributing medications, management of metabolic imbalance, treating identified infections, decreasing tumor burden if possible, managing mucositis, and treating constipation. It is worth noting that constipation is commonly seen in individuals with IDD (Del Giudice et al., 1999) and is known to contribute to nausea and vomiting. Treatment strategies for constipation are outlined in Table 6.7.

SR was hospitalized following an apparent life-threatening event related to an episode of vomiting. A palliative care consult was initiated. Vomiting and retching continued despite a trial of J-tube feedings and venting of the gastrostomy port. Various medication trials for medical management and comfort included cyproheptadine for its potent antihistamine (H1) and serotonin antagonist (5-HT2) properties with some limited benefit. Prokinetic medications— erythromycin and metoclopramide at prokinetic doses—were tried without improvement and with an associated increase in seizures on metoclopramide. Other treatment included an H2

Table 6.6
Treatment of Nausea and Vomiting

Central sites	Causes	Receptors/mechanisms	Therapeutic agents
Vomiting center (VC)	Final common pathway with numerous inputs	Histamine (H1)	Antihistamines (Diphenhydramine, Promethazine)
		Acetylcholine (Ach)	Anticholinergics (Scopalamine, Hyoscyamine)
Chemoreceptor trigger zone (CTZ)	*Medications* (chemotherapy, opioids, antibiotics, anticonvulsans) *Metabolic imbalance* (hyponatremia, hypercalcemia, uremia, ketoacidosis) *Toxins* (ischemic bowel)	Dopamine (D2)	Butyrophenones (Haloperidol, Droperidol); Phenothiazines (Prochlorperazine, Chlorpromazine)
		Serotonin (5-HT3)	Serotonin antagonists (Ondansetron, Granisetron)
Vestibular	Disorders of the vestibular nucleus and cranial nerve VIII	Histamine (H1)	Antihistamines (Diphenhydramine, Promethazine)
		Acetylcholine (Ach)	Anticholinergics (Scopalamine, Hyoscyamine)
Meningeal mechanoreceptors	Increased intracranial pressure, tumor, infection	Stimulation of the VC	Corticosteroids
Cortex	Anxiety	Stimulation of CTZ and VC	Relaxation techniques; Benzodiazepines, Dronabinol
Gastrointestinal sites	**Causes**	**Receptors/mechanisms**	**Therapeutic agents**
Mechanoreceptors and chemoreceptors	Stasis (anticholinergics, opioids), constipation, autonomic neuropathy, mucositis, gastritis, raciation, chemo, tumor, hepatic distention	Vagal afferents (CN X)	H2-blockers, proton pump-inhibitors (Ranitidine, Omeprazole); prokinetic agents (Metoclopramide)
		Histamine (H1)	Antihistamines (Diphenhydramine, Promethazine)
		Serotonin (5-HT3)	Serotonin antagonists (Ondansetron, Granisetron)

Table 6.7
Medications Used for Palliative Treatment of Common Symptoms
(Maximum Weight 50 kg)

Symptoms	Medications	Usual starting dose
Dyspnea	Morphine (or other opioid)	0.1 mg/kg PO or 0.05 mg/kg SQ/IV q 3–4 h prn
	Lorazepam	0.025–0.05 mg/kg PO/SQ/IV q 6 h prn (max dose 2 mg)
Respiratory secretions	Glycopyrrolate	0.04–0.1 mg/kg PO q 4–8 h
	Scopalomine	Adolescents: 1.5 mg by transdermal patch q 72 h
	Hyoscyamine	Age < 2 years: 4 gtts PO q 4 h as needed (0.125mg/ml) Age 2–12 years: 8 gtts PO q 4 h as needed (0.125mg/ml)
Fatigue	Methylphenidate	0.3 mg/kg up to 10 mg PO q AM and q noon
Anorexia/ weight loss	Megestrol acetate	Only use in children > 10 years old. 100 mg PO bid. If no effect in 2 weeks, double dose to 200 mg bid
Constipation	Polyethylene Glycol	8.5–17 gm qd
	Senna liquid	2–6 years: 2.5–3.75 ml qd 6–12 years: 5–7.5 ml qd
	Bisacodyl suppository	1 suppository PR qd
	Lactulose	15–30 ml PO bid or 5–10 ml PO q 2 h until stool
	Pediatric Fleets enema	1 PR qd as needed
Nausea/ vomiting	Metoclopramide	Prokinetic: 0.1–0.2 mg/kg PO/IV q 6 h Antiemetic: 0.5–1 mg/kg PO/IV q 6 h prn (with Diphenhydramine)
	Promethazine	0.25–0.5 mg/kg PO/IV q 4–6 h as needed
	Ondansetron	0.15 mg/kg PO/IV q 8 h as needed
	Haloperidol	0.01 mg/kg PO tid as needed
	Diphenhydramine	1 mg/kg PO/IV q 6 h as needed
	Scopolamine	Adolescents: 1.5 mg by transdermal patch q 72 h
	Lorazepam	0.025–0.05 mg/kg PO/SQ/IV q 6 h prn (max dose 2 mg)

(continued on next page)

Table 6.7
Medications Used for Palliative Treatment of Common Symptoms (Maximum Weight 50 kg) (*continued*)

Symptoms	Medications	Usual starting dose
Nausea/ vomiting	Dexamethasone (or equivalent corticosteroid)	0.1 mg/kg PO/IV TID
Fever	Acetaminophen	15 mg/kg PO/PR q 4–6 h as needed
	Ibuprofen	10 mg/kg PO q 6–8 h as needed
Insomnia	Lorazepam	0.025–0.05 mg/kg PO/SQ/IV qhs
	Trazodone	0.75–1 mg/kg (12.5–50 mg) PO qhs
Anxiety	Lorazepam	0.025–0.05 mg/kg PO/SQ/IV q 6 h prn (max dose 2 mg)
Agitation/ delirium	Haloperidol	0.01 mg/kg PO tid as needed For acute agitation: 0.025–0.05 mg/kg PO, may repeat 0.025 mg/kg in one hour as needed
Muscle spasm	Diazepam	0.05–0.2 mg/kg PO/IV q 6 h prn
	Baclofen	5 mg PO tid, increase every 3 days by 5–15 mg/day to maximum of 40 mg/day
Seizures	Lorazepam	0.1 mg/kg PO/PR, may repeat in 15 minutes
Neuropathic pain	Gabapentin	Day 1–3: 5 mg/kg/dose PO qhs Day 4–6: 5 mg/kg/dose PO bid Day 7–9: 5 mg/kg/dose PO tid Day 10–12: 5 mg/kg/dose am and midday and 10 mg/kg qhs Increase as tolerated until (1) effective analgesia occurs, (2) side effects are experienced or a total dose of 75 mg/kg/day is reached, (3) give half of the total daily dose as the evening dose, (4) titrate more rapidly for severe pain
	Nortriptyline*	Day 1–4: 0.2 mg/kg PO qhs Day 4–8: 0.4 mg/kg PO qhs Increase as tolerated until (1) effective analgesia occurs, (2) dosing reaches 1 mg/kg/day or 50 mg maximum, consider measuring plasma concentration and ECG before further dose escalation and consider twice daily dosing with 25% in the AM and 75% in the PM

Multiple sources used for table including Taketomo, Hodding, and Kraus (2007).

* *Guidelines from Pain in Infants, Children, and Adolescents (2nd ed.), edited by N. L. Schechter, C. B. Berde, and M. Yaster, 2003, Lippincott Williams and Wilkins.*

blocker, which was later switched to a proton pump inhibitor and management of constipation with polyethylene glycol, bisacodyl suppository, and enemas as needed.

Decline in nutrition was assessed as another contributing factor with total parenteral nutrition (TPN) initiated. Home TPN was arranged with plans to reinitiate J-tube feeds at home. Attempts to reinitiate enteral feeds failed. SR was later admitted with a fever and positive blood culture from a central venous line infection. The palliative care team again met with her parents to establish goals of care and to identify symptom management strategies. A team meeting occurred 1 week later.

The questions from Table 6.1 and Figure 6.2 were used to frame the palliative care discussion. This identified that for the past 3 months less than half of SR's days are quality days. She was described as "struggling," "fighting to stay alive," "uncomfortable," and needing to be held and repositioned often to be comfortable. This was in contrast to 6 months ago, when the majority of her days were good days. Her parents reported that they have "lost" part of SR, but they continue to hope for improvement in functional and health status. No improvement occurred despite treatment of the line infection, placement of a new line, and continued TPN. Discussion recognized the role of TPN as a life-sustaining medical treatment to be continued as long as it is meeting identified goals. Home TPN and home hospice were arranged with support to "hope for the best" while "preparing for the rest."

Artificial Nutrition and Hydration (ANH)

Forgoing medical nutrition and hydration remains one of the more difficult areas given the symbolic significance of nutrition, the myths about dehydration and "starvation," and underrecognition of the complications of artificial hydration and nutrition (Casarett, Kapo, & Caplan, 2005; National Conference of Catholic Bishops Committee for Pro-life Activities, 1999; Stanley, 2000). These issues are explored in further detail in chapters 10 and 11. The AAP policy statement recognizes that "life-sustaining medical treatment encompasses all interventions that may prolong the life of patients . . . [I]t also includes less technically demanding measures such as antibiotics, insulin, chemotherapy, and nutrition and hydration provided intravenously or by tube" (AAP Committee on Bioethics, 1994). Like other medical interventions, ANH should be evaluated by weighing its benefits and burdens in light of the clinical circumstances and goals of care (American Academy of Hospice and Palliative Medicine, 2006; Nelson et al., 1995). It is permissible to discontinue ANH when it is prolonging or contributing to suffering.

Forgoing artificial nutrition and hydration can lessen discomfort at the end of life as a result of decreased oral and airway secretions with reduced choking and dyspnea. The secondary effect of mouth dryness can be relieved with moistened swabs, ice chips, petroleum jelly on the lips, and careful oral hygiene. Chronically ill individuals often have no hunger when ANH is discontinued, and the resulting ketosis produces a sense of well-being, analgesia, and mild euphoria. In contrast, carbohydrate intake, even in small amounts, blocks ketone production and blunts of the positive effects of total caloric deprivation.

Individuals at the end of life without ANH often naturally take in fewer nutrients as intestinal function also slows down. Individuals at the end of life with ANH are at risk for vomiting, increase in pulmonary secretions, and development of edema when the body is no longer able to process the same quantity of nutrition or hydration. It is imperative that we monitor for unintended consequences in individuals with feeding tubes or who are receiving intravenous hydration and that we avoid the desire to act aggressively to manage these types of problems.

It is helpful to estimate for families the length of time that may pass until death occurs. The estimated time is usually 10 to 14 days after ANH has been discontinued, although it may be longer when fluids are used to flush a G-tube after medications have been given.

In the case of SR, once home, minimal J-tube feedings were introduced several times resulting in discomfort, abdominal distention, and vomiting. The follow-up discussion focused on the low likelihood of bridging back to tube feedings and SR's prior quality of life and the risk with continued TPN. SR was observed to develop peripheral edema with her current "maintenance" volume of fluids, which was assessed as a decline in the body's ability to process current artificial nutrition and fluids. A decision was made to discontinue ANH and utilize therapies for comfort. SR died peacefully at home in her mother's arms with her family feeling prepared and supported.

Delirium and Agitation

Delirium is a disturbance of consciousness with an onset of symptoms over hours to days. Associated features include fluctuating course, disordered thinking, change in cognition, inattention, an altered sleep-wake cycle, perceptual disturbances, and psychomotor disturbances (Del Fabbro, Dalal, & Bruera, 2006; Inouye, 2006). Causes for delirium include medications (opioids, anticholinergics); metabolic disturbances (infection, dehydration; renal, liver, or electrolyte imbalances; brain metastases); and psychosocial contributors (pain, emotional distress, vision or hearing impairment). In contrast, agitation is considered an unpleasant state of arousal. It may present as loud speech, crying, increased motor activity, increased autonomic arousal (diaphoresis, increased heart rate), inability to relax or concentrate, or disturbed sleep-rest pattern. Symptoms in agitation overlap with anxiety, although they are noted to have more motor, rather than psychological, manifestations.

Children and adults present with similar symptoms although at significantly different rates. Children are more frequently noted to present with an acute onset of symptoms, greater agitation, mood lability, and irritability. Adults are more likely to exhibit impaired memory and cognitive deficits (Leentjens et al., 2008; Turkel, Trzepacz, & Tavare, 2006).

Management of delirium and agitation first involves evaluation for treatable medical causes, including medications, metabolic disturbances, and sources of discomfort (pain, dyspnea, muscle spasms, position, constipation). It is also helpful to consider conditions that mimic the appearance of agitation, such as akathisia—an unpleasant state of motor restlessness—from antidopaminergic medications, myoclonus or withdrawal from opioids, and paradoxical reactions. Medications that can help manage the symptoms of delirium and agitation include benzodiazepines and neuroleptics.

Management of Escalating Symptoms at End of Life

When managing escalating symptoms at end of life, the principle of double effect is often cited (Fohr, 1998). This principle includes the following:

1. The act itself must be morally good or at least neutral.
2. The agent may not positively will the bad effect but may permit it. If one could attain the good effect without the bad effect, one should do so.

3. The good effect must flow from the action at least as immediately (in the order of causality, though not necessarily in the order of time) as the bad effect. In other words the good effect must be produced directly by the action, not by the bad effect. Otherwise the agent would be using a bad means to a good end, which is never allowed.

4. The good effect must be sufficiently desirable to compensate for the allowing of the bad effect.

All medical treatments have both intended benefit and unintended risk, including death. Examples include provision of TPN, administration of chemotherapy, and surgery. Each of these treatments or interventions is provided with the intent of doing good. However, there is the potential for harm to be done as well. When managing escalating symptoms, the interventions are ethical when the intent is to relieve suffering and not hasten death, death is a possible and not inevitable outcome of the interventions, and there is fully informed consent. When guidelines for symptom management are properly used, concerns about unintended consequences are no greater than normal and concerns about double effect rarely apply to management of escalating symptoms.

FUTURE DIRECTIONS

High-quality pediatric palliative care is considered an essential part of care for individuals with life-limiting conditions (AAP Committee on Bioethics and Committee on Hospital Care, 2000; Field, Behrman, & U.S. Institute of Medicine, Committee on Palliative and End-of-Life Care for Children and Their Families, 2003). Children and adults with IDD benefit from incorporation of this care model into the unique challenges, uncertainties, and symptom management needs faced by these individuals and their families. Attending to these needs can improve quality of life, comfort, and eventually end-of-life care. Research is needed to help guide us as to how to most effectively meet these goals.

REFERENCES

Abernethy, A. P., Currow, D. C., Frith, P., Fazekas, B. S., McHugh, A., & Bui, C. (2003). Randomised, double blind, placebo controlled crossover trial of sustained release morphine for the management of refractory dyspnoea. *British Medical Journal, 327*(7414), 523–528.

Allen, S., Raut, S., Woollard, J., & Vassallo, M. (2005). Low dose diamorphine reduces breathlessness without causing a fall in oxygen saturation in elderly patients with end-stage idiopathic pulmonary fibrosis. *Palliative Medicine, 19*(2), 128–130.

Allewelt, M., Schuler, P., Bolcskei, P. L., Mauch, H., & Lode, H. (2004). Ampicillin + sulbactam vs. clindamycin +/- cephalosporin for the treatment of aspiration pneumonia and primary lung abscess. *Clinical Microbiology & Infection, 10*(2), 163–170.

American Academy of Hospice and Palliative Medicine. (2006). *Statement on artificial nutrition and hydration near the end of life.* Retrieved Aug. 14, 2008, from http://www.aahpm.org/positions/nutrition.html

American Academy of Pediatrics (AAP) Committee on Bioethics. (1994). Guidelines on foregoing life-sustaining medical treatment. *Pediatrics, 93*(3), 532–536.

American Academy of Pediatrics (AAP) Committee on Bioethics and Committee on Hospital Care. (2000). Palliative care for children. *Pediatrics, 106*(2), 351–357.

Antao, B., Ooi, K., Ade-Ajayi, N., Stevens, B., & Spitz, L. (2005). Effectiveness of alimemazine in controlling retching after Nissen fundoplication. *Journal of Pediatric Surgery, 40*(11), 1737–1740.

Back, A. L., Arnold, R. M., & Quill, T. E. (2003). Hope for the best, and prepare for the worst. *Annals of Internal Medicine, 138*(5), 439–443.

Baines, M. J. (1997). ABC of palliative care. Nausea, vomiting, and intestinal obstruction. *British Medical Journal, 315*(7116), 1148–1150.

Berde, C. B., & Sethna, N. F. (2002). Analgesics for the treatment of pain in children. *New England Journal of Medicine, 347*(14), 1094–1103.

Beyer, J. E., & Aradine, C. R. (1986). Content validity of an instrument to measure young children's perceptions of the intensity of their pain. *Journal of Pediatric Nursing, 1*(6), 386–395.

Breau, L. M., Camfield, C. S., McGrath, P. J., & Finley, G. A. (2003). The incidence of pain in children with severe cognitive impairments. *Archives of Pediatrics & Adolescent Medicine, 157*(12), 1219–1226.

Breau, L. M., Camfield, C. S., McGrath, P. J., & Finley, G. A. (2004). Risk factors for pain in children with severe cognitive impairments. *Developmental Medicine & Child Neurology, 46*(6), 364–371.

Brook, I. (1996). Treatment of aspiration or tracheostomy-associated pneumonia in neurologically impaired children: Effect of antimicrobials effective against anaerobic bacteria. *International Journal of Pediatric Otorhinolaryngology, 35*(2), 171–177.

Brook, I., & Finegold, S. M. (1980). Bacteriology of aspiration pneumonia in children. *Pediatrics, 65*(6), 1115–1120.

Campbell, M. L. (2008). Psychometric testing of a respiratory distress observation scale. *Journal of Palliative Medicine, 11*(1), 44–50.

Casarett, D., Kapo, J., & Caplan, A. (2005). Appropriate use of artificial nutrition and hydration—fundamental principles and recommendations. *New England Journal of Medicine, 353*(24), 2607–2612.

Clemens, K. E., & Klaschik, E. (2007). Symptomatic therapy of dyspnea with strong opioids and its effect on ventilation in palliative care patients. *Journal of Pain and Symptom Management, 33*(4), 473–481.

Davies, B., Sehring, S. A., Partridge, J. C., Cooper, B. A., Hughes, A., Philp, J. C., et al. (2008). Barriers to palliative care for children: Perceptions of pediatric health care providers. *Pediatrics, 121*(2), 282–288.

Dean, M. (2004). Opioids in renal failure and dialysis patients. *Journal of Pain and Symptom Management, 28*(5), 497–504.

Defrin, R., Lotan, M., & Pick, C. G. (2006). The evaluation of acute pain in individuals with cognitive impairment: A differential effect of the level of impairment. *Pain, 124*(3), 312–320.

Del Fabbro, E., Dalal, S., & Bruera, E. (2006). Symptom control in palliative care—part III: Dyspnea and delirium. *Journal of Palliative Medicine, 9*(2), 422–436.

Del Giudice, E., Staiano, A., Capano, G., Romano, A., Florimonte, L., Miele, E., et al. (1999). Gastrointestinal manifestations in children with cerebral palsy. *Brain and Development, 21*(5), 307–311.

Dreyfuss, D., & Mier, L. (2001). Aspiration pneumonia. *New England Journal of Medicine, 344*(24), 1868–1869; author reply 1869–1870.

Dy, S., & Lynn, J. (2007). Getting services right for those sick enough to die. *British Medical Journal, 334*(7592), 511–513.

Field, M. J., Behrman, R. E., & U.S. Institute of Medicine, Committee on Palliative and End-of-Life Care for Children and Their Families. (2003). When children die: Improving palliative and end-of-life care for children and their families. Washington, DC: National Academy Press.

Fohr, S. A. (1998). The double effect of pain medication: Separating myth from reality. *Journal of Palliative Medicine, 1*(4), 315–328.

Friedrichsdorf, S. J., & Kang, T. I. (2007). The management of pain in children with life-limiting illnesses. *Pediatric Clinics of North America, 54*(5), x, 645–672.

Goldman, A., Hain, R., & Liben, S. (2006). *Oxford textbook of palliative care for children.* Oxford: Oxford University Press.

Graham, R. J., & Robinson, W. M. (2005). Integrating palliative care into chronic care for children with severe neurodevelopmental disabilities. *Journal of Developmental and Behavioral Pediatrics, 26*(5), 361–365.

Greco, C., & Berde, C. (2005). Pain management for the hospitalized pediatric patient. *Pediatric Clinics of North America, 52*(4), vii–viii, 995–1027.

Hauer, J. M. (2007). Respiratory symptom management in a child with severe neurologic impairment. *Journal of Palliative Medicine, 10*(5), 1201–1207.

Hauer, J. M., Wical, B. S., & Charnas, L. (2007). Gabapentin successfully manages chronic unexplained irritability in children with severe neurologic impairment. *Pediatrics, 119*(2), e519–e522.

Hemming, K., Hutton, J. L., & Pharoah, P. O. (2006). Long-term survival for a cohort of adults with cerebral palsy. *Developmental Medicine & Child Neurology, 48*(2), 90–95.

Himelstein, B. P., Hilden, J. M., Boldt, A. M., & Weissman, D. (2004). Pediatric palliative care. *New England Journal of Medicine, 350*(17), 1752–1762.

Houlihan, C. M., O'Donnell, M., Conaway, M., & Stevenson, R. D. (2004). Bodily pain and health-related quality of life in children with cerebral palsy. *Developmental Medicine & Child Neurology, 46*(5), 305–310.

Jalmsell, L., Kreicbergs, U., Onelov, E., Steineck, G., & Henter, J. I. (2006). Symptoms affecting children with malignancies during the last month of life: A nationwide follow-up. *Pediatrics, 117*(4), 1314–1320.

Kadowaki, M., Demura, Y., Mizuno, S., Uesaka, D., Ameshima, S., Miyamori, I., et al. (2005). Reappraisal of clindamycin IV monotherapy for treatment of mild-to-moderate aspiration pneumonia in elderly patients. *Chest, 127*(4), 1276–1282.

Klick, J. C., & Ballantine, A. (2007). Providing care in chronic disease: The ever-changing balance of integrating palliative and restorative medicine. *Pediatric Clinics of North America, 54*(5), xii, 799–812.

Leentjens, A. F., Schieveld, J. N., Leonard, M., Lousberg, R., Verhey, F. R., & Meagher, D. J. (2008). A comparison of the phenomenology of pediatric, adult, and geriatric delirium. *Journal of Psychosomatic Research, 64*(2), 219–223.

Lohiya, G. S., Tan-Figueroa, L., & Crinella, F. M. (2003). End-of-life care for a man with developmental disabilities. *Journal of the American Board of Family Practice, 16*(1), 58–62.

Lorenz, K. A., Lynn, J., Dy, S. M., Shugarman, L. R., Wilkinson, A., Mularski, R. A., et al. (2008). Evidence for improving palliative care at the end of life: A systematic review. *Annals of Internal Medicine, 148*(2), 147–159.

Mack, J. W., Hilden, J. M., Watterson, J., Moore, C., Turner, B., Grier, H. E., et al. (2005). Parent and physician perspectives on quality of care at the end of life in children with cancer. *Journal of Clinical Oncology, 23*(36), 9155–9161.

Mack, J. W., Wolfe, J., Cook, E. F., Grier, H. E., Cleary, P. D., & Weeks, J. C. (2007). Hope and prognostic disclosure. *Journal of Clinical Oncology, 25*(35), 5636–5642.

Mack, J. W., Wolfe, J., Grier, H. E., Cleary, P. D., & Weeks, J. C. (2006). Communication about prognosis between parents and physicians of children with cancer: Parent preferences and the impact of prognostic information. *Journal of Clinical Oncology, 24*(33), 5265–5270.

Mazzocato, C., Buclin, T., & Rapin, C. H. (1999). The effects of morphine on dyspnea and ventilatory function in elderly patients with advanced cancer: A randomized double-blind controlled trial. *Annals of Oncology, 10*(12), 1511–1514.

Meyer, E. C., Burns, J. P., Griffith, J. L., & Truog, R. D. (2002). Parental perspectives on end-of-life care in the pediatric intensive care unit. *Critical Care Medicine, 30*(1), 226–231.

Mirrett, P. L., Riski, J. E., Glascott, J., & Johnson, V. (1994). Videofluoroscopic assessment of dysphagia in children with severe spastic cerebral palsy. *Dysphagia, 9*(3), 174–179.

Moryl, N., Coyle, N., & Foley, K. M. (2008). Managing an acute pain crisis in a patient with advanced cancer: "This is as much of a crisis as a code." *Journal of the American Medical Association, 299*(12), 1457–1467.

Murphy, E. J. (2005). Acute pain management pharmacology for the patient with concurrent renal or hepatic disease. *Anaesth Intensive Care, 33*(3), 311–322.

National Conference of Catholic Bishops Committee for Pro-life Activities. (1999). Nutrition and hydration: Moral and pastoral reflections. *J Contemp Health Law Policy, 15*(2), 455–477.

Nelson, L. J., Rushton, C. H., Cranford, R. E., Nelson, R. M., Glover, J. J., & Truog, R. D. (1995). Forgoing medically provided nutrition and hydration in pediatric patients. *J Law Med Ethics, 23*(1), 33–46.

Oberlander, T. R., & Craig, K. D. (2003). Pain and children developmental disabilities. In N. L. Schechter, C. B. Berde, & M. Yaster (Eds.), *Pain in infants, children, and adolescents* (2nd ed., pp. 599–619). Philadelphia: Lippincott Williams & Wilkins.

Perquin, C. W., Hazebroek-Kampschreur, A. A., Hunfeld, J. A., Bohnen, A. M., van Suijlekom-Smit, L. W., Passchier, J., et al. (2000). Pain in children and adolescents: A common experience. *Pain, 87*(1), 51–58.

Qaseem, A., Snow, V., Shekelle, P., Casey, D. E., Jr., Cross, J. T., Jr., Owens, D. K., et al. (2008). Evidence-based interventions to improve the palliative care of pain, dyspnea, and depression at the end of life: A clinical practice guideline from the American College of Physicians. *Annals of Internal Medicine, 148*(2), 141–146.

Regnard, C., Reynolds, J., Watson, B., Matthews, D., Gibson, L., & Clarke, C. (2007). Understanding distress in people with severe communication difficulties: Developing and assessing the Disability Distress Assessment Tool (DisDAT). *Journal of Intellectual Disability Research, 51*(Part 4), 277–292.

Richards, C. A., Andrews, P. L., Spitz, L., & Milla, P. J. (1998). Nissen fundoplication may induce gastric myoelectrical disturbance in children. *Journal of Pediatric Surgery, 33*(12), 1801–1805.

Richards, C. A., Milla, P. J., Andrews, P. L., & Spitz, L. (2001). Retching and vomiting in neurologically impaired children after fundoplication: Predictive preoperative factors. *Journal of Pediatric Surgery, 36*(9), 1401–1404.

Santucci, G., & Mack, J. W. (2007). Common gastrointestinal symptoms in pediatric palliative care: Nausea, vomiting, constipation, anorexia, cachexia. *Pediatric Clinics of North America, 54*(5), x, 673–689.

Schechter, N. L., Berde, C. B., & Yaster, M. (Eds.). (2007). *Pain in infants, children, and adolescents* (2nd ed.). Philadelphia: Lippincott Williams & Wilkins.

Scornaienchi, J. M. (2003). Chronic sorrow: One mother's experience with two children with lissencephaly. *Journal of Pediatric Health Care, 17*(6), 290–294.

Seddon, P. C., & Khan, Y. (2003). Respiratory problems in children with neurological impairment. *Archives of Disease in Childhood, 88*(1), 75–78.

Sharman, M., Meert, K. L., & Sarnaik, A. P. (2005). What influences parents' decisions to limit or withdraw life support? *Pediatric Critical Care Medicine, 6*(5), 513–518.

Siden, H., & Nalewajek. (2003). High dose opioids in pediatric palliative care. *Journal of Pain and Symptom Management, 25*(5), 397–399.

Stallard, P., Williams, L., Lenton, S., & Velleman, R. (2001). Pain in cognitively impaired, noncommunicating children. *Archives of Disease in Childhood, 85*(6), 460–462.

Stanley, A. L. (2000). Withholding artificially provided nutrition and hydration from disabled children—assessing their quality of life. *Clinical Pediatrics (Phila), 39*(10), 575–579.

Steele, R. (2005a). Navigating uncharted territory: Experiences of families when a child is dying. *Journal of Palliative Care, 21*(1), 35–43.

Steele, R. (2005b). Strategies used by families to navigate uncharted territory when a child is dying. *Journal of Palliative Care, 21*(2), 103–110.

Strauss, D., Cable, W., & Shavelle, R. (1999). Causes of excess mortality in cerebral palsy. *Developmental Medicine & Child Neurology, 41*(9), 580–585.

Taketomo, C., Hodding, J., Kraus, D. (Eds.). (2007). *Lexi-Comp's pediatric dosage handbook* (14th ed.). Hudson, OH: Lexi-Comp.

Taniguchi, M. H., & Moyer, R. S. (1994). Assessment of risk factors for pneumonia in dysphagic children: Significance of videofluoroscopic swallowing evaluation. *Developmental Medicine & Child Neurology, 36*(6), 495–502.

Tuffrey-Wijne, I. (2003). The palliative care needs of people with intellectual disabilities: A literature review. *Palliative Medicine, 17*(1), 55–62.

Tuffrey-Wijne, I., McEnhill, L., Curfs, L., & Hollins, S. (2007). Palliative care provision for people with intellectual disabilities: Interviews with specialist palliative care professionals in London. *Palliative Medicine, 21*(6), 493–499.

Turkel, S. B., Trzepacz, P. T., & Tavare, C. J. (2006). Comparing symptoms of delirium in adults and children. *Psychosomatics, 47*(4), 320–324.

Valdimarsdottir, U., Kreicbergs, U., Hauksdottir, A., Hunt, H., Onelov, E., Henter, J. I., et al. (2007). Parents' intellectual and emotional awareness of their child's impending death to cancer: A population-based long-term follow-up study. *Lancet Oncology, 8*(8), 706–714.

Williams, D. G., Patel, A., & Howard, R. F. (2002). Pharmacogenetics of codeine metabolism in an urban population of children and its implications for analgesic reliability. *British Journal of Anesthesia, 89*(6), 839–845.

Wolfe, J., Grier, H. E., Klar, N., Levin, S. B., Ellenbogen, J. M., Salem-Schatz, S., et al. (2000). Symptoms and suffering at the end of life in children with cancer. *New England Journal of Medicine, 342*(5), 326–333.

Wolfe, J., Klar, N., Grier, H. E., Duncan, J., Salem-Schatz, S., Emanuel, E. J., et al. (2000). Understanding of prognosis among parents of children who died of cancer: Impact on treatment goals and integration of palliative care. *Journal of the American Medical Association, 284*(19), 2469–2475.

Wong, D. L., Wilson, D., Hockenberry-Eaton, M. J., Winklestein, M. L., & Schwartz, P. (2000). *Wong's essentials of pediatric nursing* (6th ed.). St. Louis, MO: Mosby/Elsevier.

Wood, G. J., Shega, J. W., Lynch, B., & Von Roenn, J. H. (2007). Management of intractable nausea and vomiting in patients at the end of life: "I was feeling nauseous all of the time . . . nothing was working." *Journal of the American Medical Association, 298*(10), 1196–1207.

Working Party of Association for Children's Palliative Care (ACT) and Royal College of Paediatrics and Child Health (RCPCH). (2003). *A guide to the development of children's palliative care services* (2nd ed.). Bristol, UK: Doveton Press.

World Health Organization. (1998). *Cancer pain relief and palliative care in children*. Geneva: World Health Organization.

Wright, R. E., Wright, F. R., & Carson, C. A. (1996). Videofluoroscopic assessment in children with severe cerebral palsy presenting with dysphagia. *Pediatric Radiology, 26*(10), 720–722.

ADDITIONAL RESOURCES

Association for Children's Palliative Care, http://www.act.org.uk

Doyle. D., Hanks, G. W. C., Cherny, N., Calman, K. (Eds.). (2005). *Oxford textbook of palliative medicine* (3rd ed.). Oxford: Oxford University Press.

End-of-Life Physician Education Resource Center, http://www.eperc.mcw.edu

Initiative for Pediatric Palliative Care, http://www.ippcweb.org

Innovations in End-of-Life-Care, http://www2.edc.org/lastacts

Last Passages End-of-life care for Persons with Disabilities, http://www.albany.edu/aging/lastpassages

CHAPTER 7

Nutrition Issues in End-of-Life Care

SARI EDELSTEIN, SHARON WESTON, AND VANESSA LUDLOW

INTRODUCTION

Nutrition for people facing end-of-life care may provide many challenges for the patient, caregiver, and medical team. The provision of nutrition not only offers sustenance with potential comfort and sensory pleasure but also may cause discomfort at the end of life. In the best of circumstances, the patient, caregiver, and medical team can face these challenges together and come to a consensus on the nutrition support method (Biedrzycki, 2005). For some people with intellectual and developmental disabilities (IDD), however, communication may not always be optimal. During these times, the caregiver and the medical team must make decisions based on the presumed wishes and the best interest of the patient in terms of nutrition support versus burden/discomfort in end-of-life care (Buiting et al., 2007; Dorner, Gallagher-Allred, Deering, & Posthauer, 1997).

The registered dietitian—an allied medical associate who has completed at least an accredited bachelors program in nutrition or dietetics, dietetic internship, and national examination—is the medical team member who can assist with providing a nutrition assessment for patients at end of life (American Dietetic Association, 2002; Teitelbaum et al., 2005). A nutrition assessment will help determine if food and nutrition can add to the patient's quality of life. This assessment is a complex gathering of information. The Nutrition Care Process presented by the American Dietetic Association represents the "best practice" for evaluating nutrition options that can be utilized for end-of-life care. The Nutrition Care Process contains four phases for nutrition assessment and diagnosis, with a plan for treatment and ongoing evaluation (Lacey & Pritchett, 2003). These four phases are nutrition assessment, nutrition diagnosis, nutrition intervention, and nutrition monitoring and evaluation.

Step One: "Nutrition Assessment"

"Nutrition Assessment" is the first of four steps of the Nutrition Care Process. Its purpose is to obtain adequate information in order to identify nutrition-related problems. It is initiated by referral and/or screening of individuals or groups for nutritional risk factors. Nutrition assessment is a systematic process of obtaining, verifying, and interpreting data in order to make decisions about the nature and cause of nutrition-related problems. The specific types of data gathered in the assessment will vary depending on a) practice settings, b) individual/groups' present health status, c) how data are related to outcomes to be measured, d) recommended practices such as ADA's Evidence Based Guides for Practice and e) whether it is an initial assessment or a reassessment. Nutrition assessment requires making comparisons between the information obtained and reliable standards (ideal goals). It is an on-going, dynamic process that involves not only initial data collection, but also continual reassessment and analysis of patient/client/group needs. Assessment provides the foundation for the nutrition diagnosis at the next step of the Nutrition Care Process. (Lacey & Pritchett, 2003)*

The use of selected nutritional assessment tools will vary and should be used with consideration of the information reported by the child, adult, or caregiver. Examples of nutritional references and assessment tools include the Dietary Reference Intakes, the CDC Growth Charts, Nutrition Analysis Tools and System (http://nat.uiuc.edu/), and National Cancer Institute's Dietary Questionnaire (http://riskfactor.cancer.gov/DHQ/forms/).

Considerations for End-of-Life Care

The nutrition assessment will help confirm the extent of nutritional support that is required for maintenance. In many end-of-life situations, the collective medical team may or may not elect to provide full nutritional support depending on the discomfort level this support may induce. Instead, a realistic portion of total nutrients may be provided by the route found most comfortable to the patient, whether that be oral, nonoral, or a combination of the two modalities. The health professional should note that guidelines, standard references, and tools are designed for the provision of optimal nutrition, which needs to be interpreted by the dietitian for the goal of providing comfort for the patient at end of life.

Step Two: "Nutrition Diagnosis"

"Nutrition Diagnosis" is the second step of the Nutrition Care Process, and is the identification and labeling of the specific nutrition problem that dietetics professionals are responsible for treating independently. Unlike the medical diagnosis, which may or may not resolve with nutrition intervention, the goal of the nutrition care process is to resolve the nutrition diagnosis.

At the end of the assessment step, data are clustered, analyzed, and synthesized. This will reveal a nutrition diagnostic category from which to formulate a specific diagnostic statement. Analyzing assessment data and naming the nutrition diagnoses provide a link to setting realistic and measurable expected outcomes, selecting appropriate interventions and tracking progress in attaining those expected outcomes.

The nutrition diagnosis is summarized into a structured sentence named the nutrition diagnosis statement. This statement, also called a PES statement, is written in a format that states the Problem (P), the Etiology (E), and the Signs &

---

* Reprinted with permission from Elsevier: "Nutrition Care Process and Model: ADA adopts road map to quality care and outcomes management," by K. Lacey and E. Pritchett, 2003, *Journal of the American Dietetic Association*, 103(8), p. 1061(12).

Symptoms (S). The etiology and signs and symptoms are found in the nutrition assessment and the problem is the specific nutrition diagnosis derived from the nutrition diagnosis reference sheets. A well-written nutrition diagnostic statement should be clear and concise, specific, related to one client problem, and be based on reliable and accurate assessment data. (Lacey & Pritchett, 2003)

Considerations for End-of-Life Care

The nutrition diagnosis identified by the registered dietitian will take into consideration the needs and goals identified from the assessment, as well as those from the health care team, patient, and caregiver, in order to implement appropriate interventions. Common problems that affect which interventions are chosen may include refusal of nutrition, inability to make independent decisions, and withholding or withdrawal of nutritional support.

Step Three: "Nutrition Intervention"

"Nutrition Intervention" is the third step of the Nutrition Care Process. An intervention is a specific set of activities and associated materials used to address the identified nutrition problem (or nutrition diagnosis). Nutrition interventions are purposefully planned actions designed with the intent of changing a nutrition-related behavior, risk factor, environmental condition, or aspect of health status for an individual, target group, or the community at large. This step involves a) selecting, b) planning, and c) implementing appropriate actions to meet patient/client/groups' nutrition needs. The selection of nutrition interventions is driven by the nutrition diagnosis and provides the basis upon which outcomes are measured and evaluated. Dietetics professionals may actually do the interventions, may include delegating or coordinating the nutrition care that others provide. All interventions must be based on scientific principles and rationale and, when available, grounded in a high level of quality research (evidence-based interventions).

Dietetics professionals work collaboratively with the patient/client/group, family, or caregiver to create a realistic plan that has a good probability of positively influencing the nutrition diagnosis or problem. This client-driven process is a key element in the success of this step, distinguishing it from previous planning steps that may or may not have involved the patient/client/group to this degree of participation. (Lacey & Pritchett, 2003)

Considerations for End-of-Life Care

The nutrition interventions are unique for each case and as such must be handled individually. The expressed desires of the child, adult, family, and/or caregiver regarding the extent of medical care provided must be known in order to determine the level of nutritional intervention (Biedrzycki, 2005). The expected benefits, in contrast to the potential burdens, of nonoral feeding must be evaluated by the health care team and discussed with the patient, family, and/or caregiver. The focus of care should emphasize the patient's physical and psychological comfort (Maillet et al., 2002). For example, if a patient cannot eat by mouth, the dietitian may discuss the use of artificial nutrition.

Step Four: "Nutrition Monitoring and Evaluation"

"Nutrition Monitoring and Evaluation" is the fourth step of the Nutrition Care Process. The purpose of monitoring and evaluation is to determine the degree to which progress is being made and goals or desired outcomes of nutrition care are being met. It is more than just "watching" what is happening; it requires an active commitment to measuring and recording the appropriate outcome indicators (markers) relevant to the nutrition diagnosis and intervention strategies. Data from this step are used to create an outcomes management system. Progress should be monitored, measured, and evaluated on a planned schedule until discharge from care. Short inpatient stays and lack of return for ambulatory visits do not preclude monitoring, measuring, and evaluation. Innovative methods can be used to contact patients/clients to monitor progress and outcomes. Patient confidential self- (or caregiver) report via mailings and telephone follow-up are some possibilities. (Lacey & Pritchett, 2003)

Considerations for End-of-Life Care

A systematic review and measurement should be taken of the individual's nutritional status. The ongoing evaluation of nutritional support for the patient receiving end-of-life care should continually be monitored for the goals set forth by the patient (when possible), caregiver, and medical team. The team will need to address any changes in patient comfort, which may require alterations in the treatment plan.

CHALLENGE OF PROVIDING NUTRITIONAL SUPPORT AT THE END OF LIFE

The difficulty of providing adequate nutrition support of malnourished patients has been well documented (Kochevar, Guenter, Holcombe, Malone, & Mirtallo, 2007). Nutrition support may be achieved in a variety of ways, with the medical team evaluating the risks and benefits to the patient. Nutrition may be provided directly into the gastrointestinal tract (enteral) or intravenously (parenteral). Enteral nutrition may be appropriate for patients whose gastrointestinal tract is still working and continues to utilize the stomach and/or intestines to digest food. Nutrition may be delivered via nasogastric, nasojejunal, gastrostomy, or jejunostomy tubes. Enteral nutrition may not be appropriate or well tolerated in certain situations.

There are times when a patient is quite ill and has a poorly functioning stomach and/or intestine, interfering with the absorption of nutrients by the gastrointestinal tract. Enteral nutrition also may not be appropriate in situations in which significant portions of the gastrointestinal tract have been removed. Similarly, a bowel obstruction precludes the provision of enteral nutrition. There are also some instances in which severe gastrointestinal symptoms, such as severe nausea, vomiting, and/or diarrhea, interferes with providing feeds through the gut. In addition, significant abnormalities in clotting mechanisms of the blood or severe hematologic issues at times may also interfere with safe provision of enteral feeds (*National* Cancer Institute, 2008).

Parenteral nutrition provides another modality to deliver nutrition to the patient. It is used when the patient is not able take food by mouth or by enteral feeding. Parenteral feeding bypasses the normal digestive system. Nutrients are delivered to the patient directly into the blood, through a catheter inserted into a vein. If a person is not able to eat orally or has the conditions that preclude enteral feedings, then parental nutrition may be indicated. In addition, severe ulcerations or fistulas in the mouth and/or esophagus may also be indications to provide parenteral nutrition (National Cancer Institute, 2008).

It is important that experienced medical staff manage the administration of, as well as the removal from, parenteral nutrition support. The weaning of parenteral nutrition support needs to be done gradually and under medical supervision. The parenteral feedings are reduced in small increments over time as the patient is transitioned to enteral or oral feeding.

Refusal of Nutrition

Refusal to eat is a significant problem to providing nourishment (Shah, 2006). In this instance, consideration may be given to insertion of nasogastric or gastric tube feed for parenteral nutrition and hydration. However, the patient or surrogate decision maker needs to provide permission to do so. There are instances in which a patient does not want to receive nutrition via any route, which presents both medical and ethical challenges that must be dealt with knowledgably, with systematic care, and sensitivity.

Addressing Nutrition Care Issues for Patients at the End of Life

When a patient is dying there are many questions that need to addressed and answered when considering what type of nutrition should be provided to the patient (Monturo & Strumpf, 2007). Physicians, nurses, and others on the care team will have an ongoing obligation to weigh the benefits of nutrition support in relation to the patient's burden to accept the nutrition. It is also important that the patient and/or the family be part of the discussion and decision making. In many cases, the medical team may provide less than optimal nutrition support to provide benefit without discomfort.

Inability to Independently Make Health Care Decisions

There are situations in which a patient may not be able to provide information about his or her wishes for feeding or nutrition support (McCarron & McCallion, 2007). In those situations, it is important to work with family members, loved ones, or surrogate decision makers. There are instances in which no one is available to function in that role. In those instances, a guardian may be appointed by the courts to determine what should be done to meets the patient's needs and to act in his or her best interest.

Withdrawing or Withholding Nutrition Support

There are situations in which the decision is made to withhold or withdraw feeding at the end of life (Ferrell, 2006). These are decisions that take into account the patient's medical condition, nearness of death, and/or the discomfort that may be caused by providing nutrition through the gastrointestinal system. These decisions are complex and involve the medical team in concert with the patient, family, and/or other surrogate decision makers. At times, consultation is obtained from the bioethics committee to be able to consider the issues from varying perspectives, while supporting the rights and dignity of the patient.

BIOETHICS COMMITTEES AND THE ROLE OF THE DIETITIAN

The registered dietitian has a well-defined and consistent role concerning the ethical issues and dilemmas of nutrition care for patients. The dietitian is the link between the patient and the medical team or physician in assisting difficult decision making about nutrition care. A description of the dietitian's role in terms of managing the nutrition support of a patient may be as follows.

When patients choose to forgo artificial nutrition and hydration or when patients lack decision-making capacity and others must decide whether to provide artificial nutrition and hydration, the registered dietitian has an active and responsible professional role in the ethical deliberation around that decision (American Dietetic Association, 2002).

As early as 1988, Schiller pointed out that the dietitian's practice involves difficult decisions about feeding patients in both the right-to-live and right-to-die situations. These decisions may include refusal of feeding by a competent individual, benefit versus burden of nutrition care, and the issue of assigning a surrogate decision maker. Usually, the dietitian's role in feeding dilemmas is as a consultant, while the physician is charged with managing the medical plan and treatment. In reality, the dietitian is an important link in the chain of care decisions, often serving as consultant or fact gatherer for the physician and/or as a member of the medical team. Ethics or bioethics committees have been established due to the growing expansion of complex ethical choices for patients, families of patients, physicians, and other health care professionals. Their goal is to identify the ethical implications of medical problems and attain resolutions. Dietitians serve as committee members in many areas of the country, providing relevant input as to feeding benefits and burdens.

THE NUTRITION CARE PROCESS AT THE END OF LIFE

The following case study depicts nutrition issues that were involved in the case of a young child with a neurodegenerative disorder and developmental disabilities.

Initial Nutrition Assessment

Presenting History

Eddie was a 2-year, 10-month-old boy with a complex medical history and multiple medical problems including spinal muscular atrophy, cystic fibrosis, gastroesophageal reflux, chronic constipation, and failure to thrive. He was nonambulatory and received multiple medical treatments. A nutrition referral was made by the Early Intervention team because of their concerns for his poor weight gain and his difficulty with oral-feeding skills. There was also the concern of feeding safety due to a risk of aspiration, as Eddie had chronic upper respiratory tract infections He was initially evaluated in his home by a community-based Nutrition, Feeding, and Swallowing team, consisting of a registered dietitian, speech pathologist, and occupational therapist in the presence of his Early Intervention coordinator and mother. Socially, Eddie lived with his mother and 4-year-old sister in a low-income housing development; his father was not involved.

Food- and Nutrition-Related History

His mother was asked to provide a 24-hour recall of his diet, which consisted of a combination of table foods and 24 ounces of Pediasure per day by mouth. Intake provided 104 kilocalorie per kilogram per day, 3.1 grams of protein per kilogram per day, and 700 milliliters of free water per day. He was fed 3 meals and 3 snacks per day, with each meal taking up to an hour to finish. Eddie was described as having difficulty with eating and swallowing, especially with thin liquids. His mother regularly provided him with appropriate amounts of enzymes with all meals and snacks as prescribed to manage digestive issues related to cystic fibrosis.

Eddie's medications included Prevacid, Reglan, ADEK, Ultrase, Glycolax, Pulmicort, and Albuterol.

Anthropometric Measurements

Eddie's presenting measurements were as follows:

- *Weight: 10.6 kg (< 3rd percentile weight/age, CDC Growth Chart)*
- *Length: 91.4 cm (18th percentile length/age, CDC Growth Chart)*
- *BMI: 12.7 kg/m2 (< 3rd percentile/age, CDC Growth Chart)*
- *Ideal Body Weight: 13.3 kg*
- *Eddie was at 79.7% of his standard weight for height, indicating a moderate degree of wasting (Waterlow Criteria)*

Comparative Standards

- *Estimated Energy Needs: 102 kcals/kg/day*
- *Estimated Catch-up Growth Needs: 128 kcals/kg/day*
- *Protein Needs: 1.2 g/kg/day*
- *Maintenance Fluid Needs: 1,030 ml/day*

Nutrition Diagnosis

Inadequate oral food and beverage intake related to increased nutrient needs, as well as food and nutrition-related knowledge deficit of the mother as to a high calorie diet, as evidenced by insufficient growth and a BMI significantly below the 3rd percentile.

Nutrition Intervention

1. *Nutrition Prescription: 128 kcals/kg/day, 1.2 g protein/kg/day, 1,030 ml fluid/day.*
2. *Medical food supplement: Increase to 1.5 cal/ml formula by mouth and continue to promote 24 ounce per day consumption.*
3. *Comprehensive nutritional education: Provide information and instruction to family and caretakers on appropriate high-calorie diet, appropriate use of enzymes, and fluid-rich food. Established goals to increase fluid by 10 additional ounces per day. After calling the child's pediatrician to discuss the issues, it was agreed to provide samples of a 1.5 cal/cc formula for the child to try.*
4. *Coordination of other care during nutritional care: Videofluoroscopy swallow study scheduled for the following week.*

Nutritional Monitoring and Evaluation

1. *Total energy intake: will monitor and evaluate if intakes meet his nutritional prescription as above per 24-hour dietary recall*
2. *Oral fluid intake: will monitor and evaluate if intakes meet maintenance needs above per 24-hour recall*
3. *BMI: will monitor and evaluate if BMI is increased to the 3rd percentile for age*

First Follow-Up Nutrition Assessment
Food- and Nutrition-Related History

Following the initial visit, Eddie began accepting the new, higher calorie formula, but he continued to have difficulty with lengthy feeding times and meeting fluid goals. Recommendations from the videofluoroscopy swallow study (described later) concerned the mother, as feeding this child was a source of comfort and nurturing. However, she also realized that the liquid aspiration likely contributed to his recurrent respiratory infections. Intake provided 118 kcals/kg/day, 3.5 grams protein/kg/day, and 750 ml free water/day.

Biochemical Test and Procedures

Results of a videofluoroscopy swallow study confirmed that the child was aspirating on all liquids. All other consistencies were deemed safe, but fatigue was noted as a concern for safe feeding. Because meals were taking up to 60 minutes per session, and he was not able to meet fluid needs orally, it was recommended that a feeding tube be placed.

Anthropometric Measurements

Eddie's follow-up measurements were as follows:

- *Weight: 10.8 kg (< 3rd percentile weight/age, CDC Growth Chart)*
- *Length: 91.8 cm (21st percentile length/age, CDC Growth Chart)*
- *BMI: 13.2 kg/m^2 (< 3rd percentile/age, CDC Growth Chart)*

Nutrition Diagnosis

Inadequate oral food and beverage intake related to increased nutrient needs, as well as food and nutrition-related knowledge deficit of the mother of a high calorie diet, as evidenced by insufficient growth and a BMI significantly below the 3rd percentile.

Nutrition Intervention

1. *Nutrition prescription: 128 kcals/kg/day, 1.2g protein /kg/day, 1,030 ml fluid/day*
2. *Initiate enteral nutrition: 24 ounces/day of 1.5 kcal/ml pediatric formula and additional 10 ounces free water to be provided by gastrostomy tube (G-tube)*
3. *Comprehensive nutritional education: continue to offer table foods, limit feeding times to 20 minutes*
4. *Coordination of other care during nutrition care: G-tube placement*

Nutrition Monitoring and Evaluation

1. *Total energy intake: monitor and evaluate if intakes meet nutritional prescription as above per 24-hour dietary recall*
2. *Total fluid intake: monitor and evaluate if intakes meet maintenance needs above per 24-hour recall*
3. *BMI: monitor and evaluate if BMI is increased to the 3rd percentile for age*

Follow-Up Nutrition Assessment: Summary of the Next 6 Months
Food- and Nutrition-Related History

Oral feeding became more of a challenge as Eddie's strength diminished, and he required tube feedings to meet the majority of his nutritional needs. His mother felt that if the tube feedings were decreased, he may eat more food. However, because of his weakening strength, his ability to eat adequate quantities was significantly impaired.

The decision to change from intermittent bolus feeds to use of a feeding pump to provide slow, continuous feedings was made because Eddie was no longer able to tolerate large amounts of fluid in order to meet his nutritional requirements. This change required additional medical supply instruction for the mother and also added limitations on how mobile the child and family could be, since he required being connected to his feeding pump throughout the day. A portable pump was used so that they could leave home without discontinuing the pump feeds.

Eddie was meeting 100% of his estimated nutritional needs, and he was maintaining fluid requirements. He was tolerating continuous feeds for 16 hours a day without difficulty, but he was eating minimally by mouth. Constipation was resolved with extra fluid intake, as well as using a formula that had additional fiber. Following his hospitalizations, he was followed monthly in the home.

His mother was able to get home nursing to assist with some of Eddie's medical care. This was helpful, but it infringed on some the family's privacy.

Anthropometric Measurements

Eddie exhibited improvements in growth parameters, although his BMI continued to be below the 3rd percentile.

Client History

Nutrition visits occurred initially every 2 to 3 weeks. His respiratory system continued to be compromised due to liquid aspiration, and he required lengthy hospitalizations over the winter months. Following his hospitalizations, he was followed monthly in the home. However, medically, his condition was progressively deteriorating, and after 3 months at home, his health deteriorated to the point that he passed away.

CONCLUSION

This chapter provides an overview of the roles and responsibilities of the registered dietitian in the care of individuals, specifically for those with IDD, at the end of life. The nutritional care process is complex, and the relationship between the patient and his or her family members and the dietitian forms the center around which different interactions and actions revolve. The elements of nutrition assessment, diagnosis, intervention, and monitoring reflect the dietitian's knowledge base, skills, and competencies. The dietitian must be able to apply critical thinking and collaborate and communicate with other team members in addition to the patient and his or her family. The dietitian's practice should be evidence based and follow high ethical standards. All of this is performed within the context of the health care system, social and practice settings, and economic milieu.

End-of-life care from a nutritional standpoint adds another level of medical and emotional complexity. The processes outlined within this chapter require careful consideration of individual needs based on the person's nutritional, medical, and psychosocial situation. Ethical dilemmas occur and should be carefully addressed, with the registered dietitian serving as a source of information and support to the bioethical team, medical staff, and the patient and his or her family.

References

American Dietetic Association. (2002). Position of the American Dietetic Association: Ethical and legal issues in nutrition, hydration, and feeding. *Journal of the American Dietetic Association, 102*(5), 716–727.

Biedrzycki, B. A. (2005). Artificial nutrition and hydration at the end of life: Whose decision is it? *Oncology Nursing Society News, 20*(12), 8.

Buiting, H. M., van Delden, J. J. M., Rietjens, J. A. C., Onwuteaka-Philipsen, B. D., Bilsen, J., Fischer, S., et al. (2007). Forgoing artificial nutrition or hydration in patients nearing death in six European countries. *Journal of Pain and Symptom Management, 34*(3), 305–314.

Dorner, B., Gallagher-Allred, C., Deering, C. P., & Posthauer, M. E. (1997). The "to feed or not to feed" dilemma. *Journal of the American Dietetic Association, 97*(10), S172–S176.

Ferrell, B. R. (2006). Understanding the moral distress of nurses witnessing medically futile care. *Oncology Nursing Forum, 33*(5), 922–930.

Kochevar, M., Guenter, P., Holcombe, B., Malone, A., & Mirtallo, J. (2007). ASPEN statement on parenteral nutrition standardization. *Journal of Parenteral and Enteral Nutrition, 31*(5), 441–448.

Lacey, K., & Pritchett, E. (2003). Nutrition care process and model: ADA adopts road map to quality care and outcomes management. *Journal of the American Dietetic Association, 103*(8), 1061–1072.

Maillet, J. O. (2002). Position of the American Dietetic Association: Ethical and legal issues in nutrition, hydration and feeding. *Journal of the American Dietetic Association, 102*(5), 716–726.

McCarron, M., & McCallion, P. (2007). End-of-life care challenges for persons with intellectual disability and dementia: Making decisions about tube feeding. *Intellectual and Developmental Disabilities, 45*(2), 128–131.

Monturo, C. A., & Strumpf, N. E. (2007). Advance directives at end-of-life: Nursing home resident preferences for artificial nutrition. *Journal of the American Medical Directors Association, 8*(4), 224–228.

National Cancer Institute. (2008). *Nutritional screening and assessment.* Retrieved April 23, 2008, from http://www.cancer.gov/cancertopics/pdq/supportivecare/nutrition/Patient/page4

Schiller, M. R. (1988). Ethical issues in nutrition care. *Journal of the American Dietetic Association, 88*, 13–15.

Shah, S. H. (2006). A patient with dementia and cancer: To feed via percutaneous endoscopic gastrostomy tube or not? *Palliative Medicine, 20*(7), 711–714.

Teitelbaum, D., Guenter, P., Howell, W. H., Kochevar, M. E., Roth, J., & Seidner, D. L. (2005). Definition of terms, style, and conventions used in A.S.P.E.N. guidelines and standards. *Nutrition in Clinical Practice: Official Publication of the American Society for Parenteral and Enteral Nutrition, 20*(2), 281–285.

Part III

Current Controversies and Ethical Dilemmas

CHAPTER 8

Practical Guide to Health Care Decision Making

Betsy B. Johnson

INTRODUCTION

This chapter focuses on making important and often difficult health care decisions within the context of end-of-life care for and with children and adults with intellectual and developmental disabilities (IDD). Topics include understanding key principles used in health care decision making, recognizing and addressing areas of potential conflict, and developing guidelines for addressing many of these conflicts. Explanations of often used treatment abbreviations are also provided. These principles are applied and interpreted based on individual and family needs. Case studies will be used to exemplify how these ideas may be put into practice. In addition, values, areas of potential bias, and specific issues faced by children and adults with IDD will be explored.

PRINCIPLES

When facing difficult medical decisions, some key ethical principles are often used to provide guidance. These principles include *autonomy, beneficence, nonmaleficence,* and *justice*.

Autonomy refers to the ability to make one's own decisions. It stems from Greek meaning "self rule." An adult can accept or refuse medical treatment based on his or her "autonomous" wishes. One may agree or disagree with a person's choice, but if the individual understands the potential benefits and burdens of a treatment, he or she has the right to accept or refuse any proposed medical treatment. A key factor needed to make these decisions is that of informed consent. An individual requires adequate and appropriate information in order to make an informed decision to accept or refuse suggested treatments. In their book *Clinical Ethics*, Jonsen, Siegler, and Winslade (2006, p. 7) outline four components that are considered imperative for disclosure and informed decision making:

1. The patient's current medical status, including the likely course if no treatment is provided
2. The interventions that might improve prognosis, including a description and the risks and benefits of those procedures, as well as some estimation of probabilities and uncertainties associated with the interventions
3. A professional opinion provided to the patient about alternative choices
4. A recommendation based on the physician's best clinical judgment

These four tenets need to be closely considered when caring for a person who may be unable to provide informed consent or informed refusal for a treatment. In addition, a key question to consider is whether the person has the *capacity* to make a specific decision. Capacity refers to a person's ability to understand, even with extra help, a proposed procedure and to give informed consent or informed refusal (Table 8.1). For example, does the individual understand he or she is sick or needs a medical test or procedure? Can the person understand the risks or benefits of a procedure? Individuals may need explanations in particular formats depending on how they receive or process information. For people with IDD, it is imperative not to underestimate a person's capacity simply because they may need additional time to process information or need additional explanations. Often, medical professionals provide perfunctory information regarding procedures and even people without IDD have difficulty comprehending medical information. This does not necessarily mean a person lacks capacity; he or she may simply need more education about a procedure. It is critical to remember that a person with IDD may typically need extra information regarding names and functions of the organs of the body. For instance, a doctor concerned about kidney function may assume a person knows what a kidney is and how it functions. One cannot make this assumption with a person with IDD because it is reasonable to assume that person may not have had the benefit of science or anatomy classes. Hence, it is important to take the time to explain what a kidney is and what it does. This need for more assistance to understand something is not necessarily a sign of lack of capacity. Many adults, with or without IDD, have difficulty understanding complex medical issues, especially when they are under stress.

Table 8.1

Key Points Regarding Capacity in People With Intellectual and Developmental Disabilities

- Do not underestimate a person's ability based solely on a diagnosis of IDD.
- The individual may need extra information based on lack of education, not lack of capacity.
- Consider how the person receives and expresses information. Does communication from the medical professional reflect specific communication needs?
- Are any communication aids needed to ensure understanding?
- Just because someone may require extra assistance to understand information or needs additional time to think about a procedure does not mean he or she lacks capacity.

Capacity is very different from the legal term *competency*. Any individual 18 years of age and older is generally considered as being legally competent under the law and typically makes his or her own medical decisions. An individual who is legally competent and has capacity to make decisions may still require extra assistance, particularly for treatment decisions that are very complex. He or she may therefore require additional explanations in order to provide informed consent or informed refusal.

In addition, an adult has the option of assigning someone as a health care surrogate for decision making in case of a loss of capacity. The terminology for this documented decision maker may vary between states, such as health care proxy, health care power of attorney, or health care surrogate. Any adult not adjudicated in a court of law as incompetent may choose to select a health care surrogate of his or her choosing, which can be very useful. Adults with IDD have the same opportunity as anyone else to exercise this option. It is important, however, to provide explanations and education about the intent of this type of representation and the power it can potentially give to another person. A health care surrogate, assigned by the individual, will have the power to authorize any medical treatment the surrogate believes the individual would authorize if he or she would be able to understand the proposed treatment. Unless otherwise designated, a surrogate has full authority to accept or refuse any medical treatment on behalf of the individual. This authority includes removal of life support, should that be the choice they believe the individual would make in a particular circumstance. A surrogate acts when a treating physician states that the principle—that is, the person who assigned the surrogate—has lost capacity. Simply put, a surrogate acts in place of the principle who assigned him or her to make decisions. The surrogate is responsible for making medical decisions that best reflect the choices the individual would make, if he or she had not lost capacity.

In emergency situations where there is no surrogate, any needed treatment will be initiated. Additionally, in the absence of other documents or legal decrees in a hospital setting, next of kin may be allowed to make health care decisions for adults who have lost capacity. In cases involving children, parents or legal guardians usually make medical decisions, as the child has not reached the age of majority. In circumstances when a child understands a treatment, it is desirable to obtain his or her "assent" or refusal to "assent" to a proposed treatment. The parents or guardians still retain legal decision-making power due to the child's age. However, it is important to listen to the child's concerns and give weight to his or her potential refusal, especially if he or she has experience with a treatment.

If a person's wishes are unknown and the individual lacks the capacity to make medical decisions, the principles of beneficence and nonmaleficence can provide guidance to the decision-making process.

Beneficence has its roots in the Hippocratic oath and means the promotion of good for another person or persons. In medical decision making, beneficence is represented by the decision that promotes the most good for the individual patient. Conversely, *nonmaleficence*, which also has its roots in the Hippocratic oath, promotes the treatment option that does the least harm. Promoting good and doing no harm appear to work well together. However, at times these two principles may actually come into conflict.

A simplistic example may be illustrated in a situation in which a person presents with appendicitis. Surgery is typically the best option, and it promotes good for the patient.

However, nonmaleficence states that medical professionals must do no harm. Surgery will require administering anesthesia and making an incision in the individual, both treatments that carry potential risks. How does one reconcile these two important principles? Weighing benefits and burdens becomes paramount. In the example of appendicitis, operating quickly will save the person's life. It is true there will be burdens and potential harms. However, in this straightforward case, the benefits of surgery clearly outweigh the burdens of the surgical intervention and do not generally give one pause in terms of whether or not to proceed with surgery. However, there are situations in which the benefits and risks are not as clearly evident.

The benefits and burdens may not be as clear when considering the recommendation to insert a gastrostomy tube (G-tube) for feeding. For instance, a G-tube may be recommended as the safest way for someone to receive nutrition due to swallowing difficulties. This may appear straightforward when considering issues regarding the safety of receiving nutrition. However, the burdens may be overwhelming for an individual who loves to eat and savors his or her food. One must individually consider the person and his or her quality of life. Might one consider a shorter life span that includes no G-tube? One must acknowledge and discuss the risks of aspiration and/or choking. The key is discussion of benefits and burdens from the perspective or the values of the individual for whom the G-tube is being considered. Many people may experience little or no burden from a G-tube. From another person's perspective, a G-tube may offer little actual benefit and a host of burdens.

It is very important to take each situation individually and weigh burdens and benefits of treatment options with and on behalf of individuals who lack capacity to make an informed decision, even with extra assistance. A person with IDD should be presented with the same medical options to treat a medical condition as any other person, as intellectual functioning is a separate issue from treatment of an acute medical problem. In these types of situations, other relevant prognostic issues may need to be considered; however, the disability itself should not be the focus of offering or denying treatment.

Thus far, treatment decisions have focused primarily on adults with IDD. Age is certainly one key factor when medical decisions must be made, with decisions typically being made by parents for children. Decisions made for an infant or young child may be difficult, as the child has not had a chance to live a full life and does not have the ability to provide preferences. Parents of all children generally reach health care decisions after conferring with medical professionals as well as other significant people in their lives, such as family members, friends, and clergy, when needed. Is there a difference in decision making when caring for a child with IDD?

When one considers potential bias regarding disability, decision making for an individual with IDD has unique components. Parents of medically fragile infants may have spent time in a neonatal intensive care unit (NICU) worried their infant would not survive. In intensive care settings, the physicians and nurses go to great lengths to save their baby. It is a time of hope as well as stress. Will their baby fully recover? Will he or she have an ongoing disability? What are the hopes and dreams for this baby? In the NICU setting, it is often too early to provide a definitive diagnosis about long-term disability.

If the infant survives, a child with disabilities may subsequently require multiple hospitalizations and medical appointments, admissions to intensive care settings, or to a children's specialty hospital. It is true that parents of children without IDD may also face difficult treatment dilemmas. However, parents of a child with disabilities should not bear the additional burden of wondering if medical professionals provide different treatment options than they would for typically developing children.

This issue of parity is important because for many parents of children with IDD, hospital admissions to intensive care settings may well be the beginning of making complex and ongoing medical decisions for their child. In interviews this author has conducted with parents of children with IDD, one of the most mentioned concerns was the tendency of medical professionals to focus primarily on the child's problems rather than their abilities. Well-meaning medical staff may not appreciate living a life with significant disabilities and may wonder aloud whether this child's life is a life worth living. This attitude may have the potential of setting up some very difficult dilemmas and conflicts for both parents and medical professionals.

Medical professionals may wonder why parents of children with IDD are not able to see the degree to which their child is suffering. Parents may question why these doctors do not seem to understand how much this child means to them or how capable the child may be. Are there assumptions being made about the value of this child's life? For infants, children, and individuals whose wishes are unknown, the "best interest" standard has been used when faced with difficult medical decisions. The use of this standard, however, is not simple as it also takes into account value judgments of the stakeholders.

The main components of this standard include the amount of suffering and potential relief of suffering, the severity of impairment and likelihood of restoration of function, life expectancy, and the potential for personal satisfaction and enjoyment (President's Commission, 1983).

Justice will be used in this chapter in the context of medical decision making with and for people with IDD. A primary concern for people with disabilities is treating "equal" diagnoses "equally." For example, if a person has end-stage renal disease, the typical course of treatment is dialysis and kidney transplant. If the medical facts are the same for two individuals, one with an intellectual disability and one without, *justice* requires offering the same "gold standard" treatment to both individuals, regardless of disability. A person, or his or her surrogate, may refuse a treatment option. However, the refusing of treatment differs significantly from receiving no offer of treatment based on perceived judgments about an individual's quality of life.

These principles offer parties guidance when facing difficult medical decisions. It is important to consider additional safeguards for individuals with IDD, particularly to guard against potential bias or misunderstanding. Caution needs to surround key "buzzwords" such as quality of life, suffering, or pain.

Additional Terminology and Concepts

Quality of life is a subjective term and is defined from the perspective of the individual. The phrase "quality of life" refers to the experience of life as viewed by the patient, that is, how the patient—and not the parents or health care providers—perceives or evaluates his or her experience (American Academy of Pediatrics, 1994).

It is also important to consider whether a decision to offer or deny treatments is based on a bias against a disability. It is essential to determine whether bias against a person's disability exists. One should consider the perspective of the individual in question in regards to his or her quality of life. What is important to him or her? The questions regarding treatment are not what others want for the person but what that person might want for himself or herself. A treatment may be medically appropriate but what about the individual's other quality of life considerations? Is a G-tube a consideration for a person who loves food? Many factors may need to be considered. One needs to weigh specific burdens and potential benefits for this specific person. One may choose a potentially shortened *quantity* of life for this individual so he or she could enjoy food, with the thought that a G-tube could extend the person's life but the burdens may outweigh this benefit. However, without a G-tube a person may experience more illnesses and discomfort due to aspiration of food or swallowing problems. Again, one must consider what is important to the individual—not just what is medically recommended—as well as the consequences of the decision. An individual, whether legally competent or not, still has the right to accept or refuse any medical treatment.

When considering issues related to quality of life, it is important to ask whether a proposed treatment will improve, maintain, or actually permanently reduce the person's quality of life. For example, one could argue chemotherapy might be very burdensome. However, if the treatment has a good chance of offering cure or remission, one would consider accepting it by weighing burdens and benefits. However, if a proposed treatment is not going to offer an overall improved quality of life—or at least maintain current quality—it is very reasonable to refuse such treatment.

In decision making for others, it is also important to look at one's own value system. One may hear a medical professional state, "If this were my brother/sister/mother/father (etc.) I would do the following . . ." Alternatively, families may ask a physician, what would you do if this were your family member? These statements or questions are not as helpful as they may seem. People have their own set of values and they may differ from those of the individual who is considering treatment. Just because one person might accept a particular treatment, does not mean another individual will choose the same. It is important for individuals who are recommending treatment options to be aware of their own value system and actually try to avoid superimposing those values on others. The values of the individual for whom treatment is considered are the only values that truly count in discussions of treatment options. This does not imply that a medical professional may not provide this type of insight, but he or she should be able to acknowledge the potential differences in value systems. It is important, however, to ascertain what the individual would ask of those charged with making difficult medical decisions.

At times, significant *suffering* that cannot be adequately eased or reversed may justify forgoing certain treatment options. However, one needs to use extreme caution regarding the use of this word. Even though people may be well meaning, assumptions about poor quality of life based on disability can lead to assumptions about a treatment being too burdensome. Additionally, others may perceive a person with a disability as living a life of suffering when, in fact, the individual is quite happy and has a positive quality of life.

When contemplating a difficult medical decision, one needs to look for the generally accepted "gold standard" for a specific condition. For example, if a person were in respiratory failure, a typical treatment may be the use of a ventilator. It is true that mechanical ventilation is burdensome and may actually cause some suffering. It is important to consider the specifics of the situation that could influence the decision to be placed on a ventilator. One may want to consider whether the use of the ventilator is temporary or long term, the likelihood that the condition will improve or change, the expected course of the illness, and/or whether the person would want to be live with ventilator support if the condition is felt to be longstanding. It is crucial to be able to understand the facts, the potential courses of illness, and the options of care in these types of highly charged situations.

Another crucial consideration for anyone is *pain management*, which is further discussed in chapters 6 and 20. People with disabilities are particularly vulnerable in situations that require management of pain. The Joint Commission on Accreditation of Health Care Organizations (Dahl, Pasero, & Patterson, 2000; JACHO, 1999) approved new pain assessment and management standards. The commission developed these standards because of the "reality that under treatment of pain is a major public health problem in the United States." People with disabilities, especially anyone with a history of behavioral difficulties, are at risk of receiving inadequate pain medication. The individual also is at risk for treatment with sedatives or antipsychotic medications rather than adequate treatment with pain medications. It is imperative to rule out a potentially painful medical condition when a person with IDD presents with any unexplained behavioral change.

Sam was placed on a psychiatric unit for increased negative behaviors. Over a period of two months, Sam had demonstrated an increase in behaviors such as head banging, slapping at staff that came near him, and increased agitation at mealtimes, including sometimes throwing food at staff. Sam has a history of behavioral and psychological issues and had four past admissions to a psychiatric unit. He therefore was readmitted to the psychiatric unit for evaluation of his increased behavioral concerns. Rather than initially ruling out a medical cause, staff at the unit assumed Sam needed a medication adjustment, since this intervention worked in the past. Multiple psychotropic medication changes failed to affect his behavior. On week three of this admission, a medical work-up was ordered, including a CT scan of his abdomen. Only then was stomach cancer discovered.

Issues of quality of life, potential suffering, and pain management need to be considered in any situation that involves a person with IDD. It is also important to consider how best to address conflicts and decisions. The following provides some guidelines when addressing complex and difficult issues, as well as a template for decision making.

Decision Making

Issues that may potentially be a source of conflict with and for people with IDD include differing value systems, assumptions about quality of life, and inclusion of many stakeholders in the decision-making process with potentially varying opinions. Difficult medical decisions, especially ones involving end-of-life care, are emotionally highly charged. Facts help dissipate some of the negative issues arising from assumptions or misunderstandings.

Assumptions and misunderstandings often occur with the use of confusing medical terminology when communicating with stakeholders without medical backgrounds. It is important to ensure adequate understanding of key terms or abbreviations often encountered, especially when discussing issues pertaining to end-of-life care. This terminology is also reviewed in chapters 9 and 10.

The following are terms and abbreviations that may be used when referring to patients' resuscitation status. Some of the abbreviations have not been universally adopted but are included here because of their widespread use in different settings.

A hospitalized patient may have an order written by his or her physician for Do Not Resuscitate (DNR). This order typically means the person will not receive cardiopulmonary resuscitation (CPR) in the event his or her heart stops. A physician writes this order based on the wishes of the decision maker(s) and taking into consideration the medical condition of the patient. This is usually used when someone has a condition in which death is imminent or there is little likelihood of surviving CPR. The individual therefore will not receive artificial means to promote breathing or resume his or her heartbeat. A person may have a DNR order yet continue to receive treatment for acute illnesses, such as pneumonia, urinary tract infections, fractures, and other acute conditions. Generally, a DNR order assumes that a patient will not be intubated—with a tube placed in the trachea to which oxygen and artificial respiratory support is delivered—or be on a ventilator or other mechanical means of breathing. However, there may be situations in which a person or the surrogate wants to include intubation with the DNR order. Desire for intubation would then be noted in the actual DNR order. If a person wishes to explicitly exclude intubation with a DNR order, a specific Do Not Intubate (DNI) order would be written by the physician.

Health care providers sometimes refer to a person's "code status," referring to what type of resuscitation measures are provided or withheld. A person's code status may be "full code" meaning all means of resuscitation and treatment will be used to restart beating of the heart and breathing. "No code" or DNR means that artificial means to augment cardiac and pulmonary function will not be used; however, comfort measures will continue to be provided.

There are other orders that may be written by the physician, often in the context of DNR orders. A person who is being cared for outside of an acute care facility may have a Do Not Hospitalize (DNH) order. Typically the person would be able to receive the level of care consistent with the setting in which they reside, but would not return to an acute care facility like a hospital. A Do Not Transfer (DNT) order may be similarly written to indicate that a patient should remain in the current setting in which they reside. In this situation a patient should be transferred neither to a hospital for admission nor to an emergency room for evaluation. Treatment, therefore, would continue to be provided consistent with the level of care at the person's current setting, as specified in his or her medical orders. Typically, a DNT order indicates a decision not to transfer from an existing facility to a hospital, similar to the DNH.

A patient should always receive adequate pain management in order to be made comfortable, regardless of his or her resuscitation status. However, there also comes a time in which curative treatment is no longer desired or appropriate, and care is directed to provision of "comfort measures only." The individual receives pain medication and other treatment to ensure the person is comfortable at the end of life but does not receive active treatments of illness or medical conditions.

There is concern that assumptions about poor quality of life may lead to premature treatment limitations. Therefore, it is imperative to rule out any bias toward an individual due to his or her disability (or disability type) when considering any of the aforementioned treatment limitations. As noted throughout this chapter, difficult health care decisions with and for people with intellectual disabilities require unique considerations. At its most basic, any medical decision with and for a person with IDD needs to take into consideration the question, "What would this person ask of us?" When facing difficult medical decisions, the following guidelines, template for decision making (Table 8.2), and case examples offer some support for this process.

Table 8.2
Template for Medical Decision Making

Diagnosis	• What is the diagnosis? Is there a desire or need for a second opinion?
Prognosis	• What is the prognosis? What will happen without the proposed treatment? What will happen with the proposed treatment? Will the proposed treatment improve the person's quality of life or only maintain it? Alternatively, will the proposed treatment significantly diminish the individual's quality of life?
Stakeholders	• Typically, these are the family, staff (day and residential), and medical professionals such as doctors and nurses. Does the individual have capacity to make his or her own medical decisions? Has he or she expressed a preference? Is there a surrogate decision maker? Is he or she in attendance?
Options	• What are the proposed options? Consider all possible treatment options. It is critical not to prematurely rule out any option.
"Gold standard"	• Rule out bias before ruling out options. Is there a standard, typical treatment option for this particular diagnosis? Is there an offer of this treatment? If not, why not? Refusal of an option is very different from not offering an option based on disability bias.
Recommendations	• After fact gathering, confirmation of diagnosis and prognosis, identification of stakeholders, and option exploration, recommendations are given. Even the best recommendations, based on all available information, can cause disagreement among parties. The most important aspect of any deliberation is making a recommendation that best reflects the values of the individual for whom treatment is being proposed.

Guidelines for Conflict Resolution

Obtain a facilitator. A need may exist for a neutral and experienced facilitator. Good facilitators ensure everyone stays on track and focused. These skills are critical during highly charged discussions, and mediation skills may offer needed assistance. The goal of involving someone with mediation skills is not one of finding compromise but rather of offering ways of dealing with anger and extreme emotion that may accompany difficult discussions.

Understand all stakeholders' frames of reference. Often a number of people have roles in the life and care of the person for whom the decisions are being made, and these stakeholders are also impacted by these decisions. It is important to check the assumptions and perceptions of everyone involved.

Determine the facts of the situation rather than go on assumptions. This may require private interviews with individual stakeholders when clarifying or correcting assumptions.

Focus on the person directly impacted by the medical treatment. Issues related to the needs, wishes, and the value system of the person making decisions or for whom decisions are being made are critical to the decision making process.

Involve the key decision makers and stakeholders. These individuals need to be actively involved in the process of decision making.

Seek input from others who are participating in the person's care. This input is especially important if day and residential services are involved.

Grace: Transplant or Hospice?

Grace is a 42-year-old adult with IDD who is dying of end-stage liver disease. She is on a transplant list, but her primary care physician, Dr. Curran, thinks the best option for Grace is to die at home. Dr. Curran strongly believes that Grace has suffered enough. From his perspective, Grace's quality of life has plummeted, and she no longer enjoys many of her favorite activities. Grace used to have her own apartment and now resides in a nursing home. Dr. Curran believes Grace should return home to die with hospice services in place. He has spoken with her residential staff and they are very willing to have Grace return with hospice services in place.

Grace's sisters are very close to her and believe she ought to remain on the transplant list, as this is her only hope of living. They go with her to every appointment to offer support to Grace during this difficult time of hoping and waiting for a liver. Grace's support staff and her physician do not agree with Grace's sisters. Communication has become very strained and the sisters now refuse to talk with Grace's residential support staff. Additionally, they will not consider hospice or her removal from the transplant list.

How does one address this conflict? A nurse involved with Grace sought an ethics consultation.

Facilitation of discussion. All parties were able to express their concerns. Initially, there were private interviews due to strong emotions and conflict among the stakeholders.

Perception and assumptions by Dr. Curran and staff. They believed that Grace's quality of life was so poor that active treatment should be discontinued. They felt the best option for her would be hospice care. Hospice services that would provide treatment to Grace would focus on comfort. Staff expressed their own emotional discomfort watching her suffer.

Perceptions and assumptions of Grace's sisters. Grace's sisters do not want her to die. She is their little sister, and they have always protected her. Grace assigned both sisters as health care surrogates, with one having primary decision-making authority, if needed.

Key discovery. When interviewing Grace privately, it was clear that she actually had capacity to make her own decisions. Grace needed education regarding the technicalities of actual liver transplantation. Once she understood the issues, she wanted to wait for a liver and remain on the transplant list.

Review of Case

Diagnosis: Liver failure.

Prognosis: Death without transplant.

Stakeholders: Grace, her sisters, her doctors, and health care staff.

Options: Transplant or hospice.

Recommendations: Grace has capacity to make her own decisions. Once she was educated more thoroughly about liver transplantation, Grace made her own decision to remain on the list rather than opt for hospice. Either option was reasonable to consider but Grace's autonomous choice was to continue waiting. A few months after the meeting, Grace was fortunate enough to receive a needed liver and is doing well.

This case illustrates that the key stakeholder, Grace, was absent from the initial discussions about her treatment options. Conflict arose in discussions between a primary care doctor, residential staff, and Grace's sisters. This entrenched conflict could have been avoided had anyone talked to Grace about her preferences. However, of noted importance is the presumption by others about Grace's quality of life. Grace, however, did not agree with the assumptions made by the staff and her physician. It is true her quality of life had declined during her illness. However, from Grace's perspective, it was important to seek treatment that offered her the only possibility of a return to function.

Would the outcome have been different if Grace lacked the capacity to make her own decisions? In this case, Grace previously assigned her sisters as her health care surrogates. Hence, they were charged with making the medical decisions that best reflected Grace's values. Had she not had the capacity, her sisters would have considered Grace's past decisions and any expressed wishes regarding a transplant. In essence, Grace protected herself by assigning people she knew would express her wishes, even if she could not. Had Grace been adjudicated in a court of law as incompetent and had a guardian, the guardian would have legal decision-making authority regarding the choice of transplant or hospice. Grace's guardian would consider any of Grace's expressed wishes and would ultimately make the choice that reflected, in the guardian's opinion, what was in Grace's best interest. Note the distinction: A court chooses a guardian for the person. Grace, being legally competent, chose her surrogate for herself. Even if she lost capacity later, she would not have needed a guardian, because she previously assigned a health care surrogate to act for her if she could no longer communicate her wishes.

Susan

Susan is 9-years-old and has been in the hospital for 3 weeks with an overwhelming sepsis (infection throughout the bloodstream) and pneumonia. She has significant lung damage and needs a ventilator to breathe. The doctors in the pediatric intensive care unit (PICU) do not believe Susan is able to recover. She has failed multiple trials of weaning her from ventilator support. Despite their best efforts, she continues to decline, cannot breathe on her own, and has little likelihood coming off the ventilator.

Susan's family is very involved in her life and advocates tirelessly on her behalf. Many times, through her short life, doctors told the family she would die. However, her parents characterize her as being a fighter, as she has outlived everyone's expectations. Susan's parents are familiar with dire predictions from doctors, and Susan repeatedly has proven them wrong. According to Susan's parents, medical professionals have always underestimated her abilities to recover and function. It is true Susan now has a tracheotomy (airway tube) and is on a ventilator, which is new for her. However, the family finds it difficult to believe what the PICU doctors are telling them. Is Susan really dying? It has never been true before during past hospitalizations. Why would it be true now?

Susan is a child and unable to make her own decisions. Her parents, as decision makers, are in conflict with the treating physicians. Communication between PICU staff and the family is at a stalemate. Susan's parents no longer trust the treating doctors, and the medical staff are frustrated. From the perspective of the medical team, the parents do not seem to understand or want to accept the gravity of her illness.

The doctors are recommending removal of life support because of her overwhelming organ failure. Her kidneys and lungs have failed and her liver is failing, despite all the medical teams' interventions provided to her. Susan continues to require the use of a ventilator. She also requires medications in order to maintain her blood pressure. The infectious disease doctors indicate that her chances of survival are very slim because of the fulminate infection that is not adequately responding to intravenous antibiotic treatment.

The family is initially unable to understand or hear this information because they are defending against the assumption that Susan has had a generally poor quality of life. They want the doctors to understand that Susan has fought back before and lived, why is this so different? In reality, this is different because Susan previously has not had sepsis or multiorgan failure. However, the doctors needed to demonstrate an understanding that Susan was a valued member of her family before the family was able to listen to the medical professionals' poor prognosis for Susan.

Facilitation: Initially, interviews with Susan's parents took place separately from the PICU staff. From the parents' perspective, they were in the position of defending Susan's right to treatment. Susan has IDD, and her parents previously faced insensitive comments about her quality of life. To her parents, she is a joy. They do not want her to suffer, but they are concerned PICU staff may be giving up on her because they are judging her based on disability.

The PICU staff indicates that Susan is very sick and has a poor chance of recovery. The doctors indicate they are not judging her quality of life; rather, they are clinically assessing her medical condition. During the course of the meeting, the medical staff indicate they will assure the parents that Susan is very much valued. However, her physical condition is critical. In the very slim likelihood she would survive, she would require ongoing use of a ventilator.

Review of Case

Diagnosis: Susan has an overwhelming infection, which has spread throughout her bloodstream, as well as pneumonia. She is beginning to have multisystem organ failure.

Prognosis: Susan's prognosis is very poor with or without continued treatment. Her lungs have failed and now her liver and kidneys are failing.

Stakeholders: Susan, her parents, her siblings, the medical staff in the PICU.

Options: Keep her on ventilator or remove her from life support, institute comfort measures, and allow her to die.

Recommendation: Facts in this case were critical in seeking resolution. It was key to have an in-depth discussion about Susan's prognosis in a manner that did not discuss her disability. The medical staff were respectful of her parents' concerns about potential bias toward their child. The PICU staff showed sensitivity toward Susan's parents and did not push for an immediate decision. Rather, they asked questions about what gave meaning to Susan's life. What would it mean to Susan to live life on a ventilator? There was careful consideration of all options without focus on her disability.

While the other doctors had been wrong previously, this was a different diagnosis. Only when trust and mutual respect were established could both parties understand each other. The doctors needed to understand that Susan was not just the patient in bed three. Rather, she was a beloved daughter and a valued family member. In the end, Susan's parents made the extremely painful decision to remove her from life support. The critical factor in making this difficult decision was the medical team's display of respect for Susan and her needs. They did not put focus on her as a child with a disability but rather centered their discussions on what gave meaning to her life.

Difficult decisions are less daunting when there is a cohesive way to address accompanying issues. When discussions best reflect the values of an individual and what gives meaning to his or her life, recommendations and decisions will come forth that respect the dignity of the person. Respecting the dignity of a person with an intellectual disability is, in essence, not radically different from respecting any person's dignity, as also noted in chapter 13. Is the process of decision making respectful? Does it take into consideration all the important aspects of the person? Does it give voice to the person, even when clear wishes are unknown? These are critical factors for anyone. The biggest difference in dealing with medical decision making with and for people with IDD is the need for increased diligence to eliminate decisions based on disability bias.

REFERENCES

American Academy of Pediatrics. (1994). Guidelines for forgoing life sustaining medical treatment. *Pediatrics, 93*, 532–536.

Dahl, J., Pasero, C., & Patterson, C. (2000, November). Institutionalizing effective pain management practices: The implications of the new JCAHO Pain Assessment and Management Standards (No. 302) [Abstract]. Program and Abstracts of the 19th Annual Scientific Meeting of the American Pain Society, Atlanta, GA.

JACHO Standards for Pain Management. (1999). Comprehensive accreditation manual for hospitals, Update 3.

Jonsen, A. R., Siegler, M., & Winslade, W. J. (2006). *Clinical ethics* (6th ed.). New York: McGraw-Hill.

President's Commission for the Study of Ethical Problems in Medicine and Biomedical and Behavioral Research, Final Report. (1983, March 31).

CHAPTER 9

Do-Not-Resuscitate Orders and Redirection of Treatment

JEFFREY P. BURNS AND CHRISTINE MITCHELL

Decision making about life-sustaining treatments for children and adults with intellectual and developmental disabilities (IDD) requires careful reflection on a range of issues. At its essence it must be founded on a sound understanding of the conceptual framework for these decisions that has evolved over the past 30 years in the United States. While children and adults with disabilities usually cannot make their own health care decisions, a few can be involved and almost all have parents or other legally authorized surrogate decision makers. The practices associated with the right of competent adult patients to choose whether they want cardiopulmonary resuscitation (CPR) in the event of a cardiopulmonary emergency are generally transferable to parents or others authorized to make decisions for children and adults who are not able to make their own choices—with a few cautionary notes. In this chapter we therefore trace the development of the core principles related to Do-Not-Resuscitate (DNR) orders and decisions to redirect the priorities of treatment and highlight areas of ongoing controversy, attending to special circumstances involved in making ethical and clinical decisions about CPR for children and adults with disabilities.

HISTORICAL PERSPECTIVE: ORIGINS AND PURPOSE OF THE DNR MEDICAL ORDER

Cardiac resuscitation after cardiac arrest or ventricular fibrillation has been limited by the need for open thoracotomy and direct cardiac massage. As a result of exhaustive animal experimentation a method of external transthoracic cardiac massage has been developed. Immediate resuscitative measures can now be initiated to give not only mouth-to-nose artificial respiration but also adequate cardiac massage without thoracotomy. The use of this technique on 20 patients has given an over-all permanent survival rate of 70%. Anyone, anywhere, can now initiate cardiac resuscitative procedures. All that is needed are two hands.

—Kouwenhoven, Jude, and Knickerbocker (1984)

This first description of CPR by closed-chest message coupled with artificial respiration in 1960 by Kouwenhoven and colleagues was a landmark article describing a revolutionary breakthrough in resuscitation procedures that was miraculous for its effectiveness and simplicity. For the first time, anyone, anywhere, could use the simple technique of external chest massage to sustain life long enough to bring a defibrillator to the patient. Yet it was not for another 16 years that the first description of formal hospital polices establishing procedures for determining when not to attempt to resuscitate a patient were published in the medical literature (Clinical Care Committee, 1976; Rabkin, 1976).

Notably, CPR as originally described was intended for patients experiencing a witnessed cardiac arrest from an etiology thought to be easily reversible. Indeed, this first description of CPR concerned its application on a case series of 20 patients experiencing a witnessed cardiac arrest either upon the induction of anesthesia or upon emergence from anesthesia at Johns Hopkins Hospital in the late 1950s.

Yet the simplicity of its application soon led to widespread and indiscriminate attempts at CPR on a wide range of patients, some of whom were revived to transient physiologic stability only to suffer and die again. Reports in the medical literature described repeated resuscitation attempts on terminally ill patients that appeared only to prolong suffering and delay death (Russell, 1968). Medical evaluation of the efficacy of CPR—or even expert consensus about its efficacy in a context other than witnessed, anesthesia-induced cardiac arrest—remained absent throughout the 1960s, and thus there was no open decision-making framework about decisions for the use of CPR with patients and their families.

Decisions about who would, or would not, receive a resuscitation attempt became increasing ad hoc by medical staff when it was not discussed with the patient and his or her family. Hospital culture soon developed new terms, such as "chemical code," "show code," "Hollywood code," and "slow code," to describe situations where the staff employed less than a full resuscitation attempt in the belief that CPR was not "beneficial." In addition, many institutions developed somewhat surreptitious means of communication among the staff—such as placing purple dots on the patient's chart—to quickly convey their decisions about whether to attempt a full resuscitation in the event of cardiopulmonary arrest (Burns, 2004).

The absence of an established and transparent framework for informed consent around resuscitation decisions in the event of cardiac arrest was an increasing concern to many in medicine in the 1960s and early 1970s. In 1974 the American Medical Association (AMA) became the first professional organization to propose that decisions not to resuscitate be formally documented in progress notes and communicated to all clinical staff. Moreover, the AMA stated that "CPR is not indicated in certain situations, such as in cases of terminal irreversible illness where death is not unexpected" (AMA, 1991). This recommendation was followed in 1976 by reports from two Boston teaching hospitals describing their policies on the process for implementing decisions about resuscitation status. This movement toward explicit DNR policies rapidly spread to other hospitals with the result that medical staff now had a framework to deliberate with the patient, or patient's surrogate, on the rationale for attempting, or withholding, CPR in the event of cardiac arrest well before the actual event. Transparent decision making around resuscitation attempts was in turn openly communicated to potential rescuers, many of whom could have only limited personal knowledge of each patient's case but who could now feel more confident about the process through which decisions had been made.

Legal Perspectives on DNR Decisions

The first reported legal case regarding entry of a DNR medical order occurred in Massachusetts in 1978 and focused on two questions: (a) could a DNR order be entered in the medical record of a terminally ill patient? and (b) must the physician first obtain court authorization? The Massachusetts Appeals Court in this case based its ruling on a determination that appropriate measures in the treatment of a terminally ill patient are a matter that is peculiarly within the competence of the medical profession. Therefore, with the concurrence of the family, the physician can enter a DNR order without prior court approval (*Superintendent of Belchertown v Saikewicz*, 1977). Subsequent cases in other states confirmed that patients have the right, based on common law and on the federal (or state) constitution, to refuse medical treatment, including CPR. While the right to refuse treatment was most clearly established for competent patients, almost all courts have also held that incompetent patients hold this "right" (at least theoretically), which can be implemented in appropriate circumstances through surrogate decision makers and most typically without prior court approval. Chapter 8 provides further explanation of competency.

Parents as Decision Makers

In general, cognitively competent persons now have a well-established right to make their own decisions about health care that includes both informed consent for hospitalization, transfer, treatments, procedures, and surgeries they want to have—including CPR—and informed refusal of those they do not, including DNR. By extension, persons with IDD have the same right, though it must be exercised by a surrogate decision maker, usually, in the case of children, his or her parent(s), who is presumed to be responsible for determining either what their child or ward would want if they could choose for themselves (substituted judgment) or what would be best for them (best interests, Tibbalis, 2006). Deference to parents' decisions for their children is based on the fact that most parents have a profound love and commitment to their child's welfare—the child will likely grow up to espouse many of the same values and cultural attitudes as the parents, and the parents are usually the ones who will have to deal with the consequences of whatever decisions are made (American Academy of Pediatrics [AAP] Committee on Bioethics, 1996). One notable exception is children in state custody for whom parents are no longer the child's surrogate decision makers. Depending on state law, decisions about whether to limit life-sustaining treatments such as CPR may be made by responsible persons in the state department of health and human services, by the court, or by a court-appointed guardian.

Health care professionals—especially those in pediatrics and those caring for adults who cannot make their own decisions—also have a responsibility to consider and advocate for what they believe to be best for their patients. Indeed, health care professionals have a legal responsibility to report cases of alleged neglect or abuse when they believe a parent or guardian is failing to take proper care, including in cases of consent for medical care for a person who cannot care for himself or herself.

One of the more common problems leading to ethics consultation is disagreements between health professionals and parents or guardians about whether a child is being over treated or under treated. Studies of children with Trisomy 21, or Down syndrome, show significant gains in survival and life expectancy over the years due to improved medical care to address health problems and less than 25% of individuals needed assistance with personal care (Schieve, Boulet, Boyle, Rasmussen, & Schendel, 2009). Sometimes, however, parents may refuse to consent for their child with Down syndrome to have surgical repair of a gastrointestinal anomaly or heart defect, preferring instead to allow the child to die. As a result of some cases publicly discussed in the media (e.g., Baby Doe in Bloomington, Indiana), research about physicians' and parents' attitudes regarding medical care for such children, congressional hearings, and new disability laws, there is now widespread consensus among health professionals that children with Trisomy 21 should not be allowed to die simply because of their disability and should receive needed medical interventions. Usually, but not always, this includes CPR (AAP Committee on Fetus and Newborn, 2008)

When there is disagreement between the parents and health professionals, an ethics consult is often requested, sometimes leading to parental consent for needed medical treatment or a decision by the parent(s) to allow their child to be placed in state custody for foster care or adoption. In clearer cases of what has come to be called "medical neglect" (Section 504 of the Rehabilitation Act; Federal Register, 1985), parents who do not consent for needed medical treatment may have their rights temporarily or permanently withdrawn as health care providers turn to the court for treatment authorization. In ambiguous cases, an ethics consult team would talk with parents, physicians, nurses, and others about why and whether disputed medical treatments—including CPR—are believed to be beneficial or harmful, with the aim of coming to a common understanding by gathering relevant factual information and engaging in respectful discussion of parental and professional values and perspectives. Similarly, when the parents insist on CPR for a child that the clinical team believes is irreversibly dying and should not have to endure efforts at resuscitation, an ethics consult may also be requested.

In both types of disagreement, the ethical question of who should decide is not as simply answered as it is in cases involving a competent adult who has a nearly absolute right to make his or her own decision, even when it may result in their own death. Although, by social agreement and with legal protections, parents are generally expected to make decisions for their children, this practice must be legally authorized when children with IDD reach adulthood and when parents' decision-making authority is no longer absolute. Parents who do not appear to understand essential medical information, who are unable to make a decision about CPR when one is needed, who seem to act with untoward preference for their own interests and neglect their child's or ward's interests, or who are persistently unavailable to be with their child and talk with clinician's about their child's needs may be disqualified as decision makers. In such rare circumstances, health professionals should seek legal counsel and petition the department of social services or the court for an alternate decision maker.

Outcome Studies on Resuscitation Decisions

Advances in medical knowledge and therapies have allowed more children with neurodevelopmental disabilities and complex medical conditions to survive infancy. Children and young adults with neurodevelopmental disabilities are a growing segment of the general population. Many do remarkably well despite their higher incidence of health problems and their increased utilization of health and education services (Boulet, Boyle, & Schieve, 2009). Yet, outcome data remain limited on decisions regarding resuscitation for children and adults with IDD.

Graham and colleagues recently examined the experience of children with congenitally or perinatally acquired neurodevelopmental diagnoses at a large, tertiary, academic, pediatric medical center and found that this population represented nearly one quarter of approximately 2,000 annual admissions to the pediatric intensive care unit (ICU; Graham, Dumas, O'Brien, & Burns, 2004). Of these children, 85% were cared for at home before hospitalization. The majority of admissions were for scheduled surgery (45%) or for management of acute respiratory illness (26%). Of the patients with preexisting tracheostomy, nonrespiratory conditions accounted for 70% of acute admitting diagnoses. Of all admissions, 223 (52%) required noninvasive or transtracheal ventilatory support, yet the length of stay and mortality rate were consistent with those reported in other general pediatric intensive care unit populations. However, use of life-sustaining medical technology increased significantly for some—for example, enterostomy (feeding tube) support increased from 181 patients on admission to 191 patients upon discharge and mechanical ventilation increased from 103 patients on admission to 120 patients upon discharge.

The stability of DNR orders after admission to a pediatric rehabilitation facility for patients with IDD has recently been examined. Friedman (2006) studied the relationship of providing explanatory information regarding resuscitation to DNR status for parents and guardians of patients aged 2 to 32 years residing in a pediatric-skilled nursing facility. At the outset, families of 11 (18%) of 60 patients had requested DNR orders for their child in the event of cardiopulmonary arrest. After provision of informative material regarding the meaning of resuscitation and its implications, there was an increase to 26 patients (43%) who had DNR orders written for them. In this study, there was no significant difference in characteristics between the groups that changed to DNR and those that remained full resuscitation, although there was a marginal trend that the parents of children in the group with an acquired etiology for their developmental disabilities were more apt to change their child's resuscitation status than those with children who had congenital diagnoses. In a follow-up to this study, Friedman and Gilmore (2007) examined the resuscitation decisions and factors that impact these choices on the same cohort. They found that interpersonal relationships—such as those with family members, a religious leader, or physician—were more influential for families who chose full resuscitation compared to those with DNR preferences. Factors such as the perception of quality of life and medical condition of the individuals with developmental disabilities were not significantly different between these two groups.

Taken together, these limited data dispel conventional wisdom that children with IDD have markedly different outcomes in the ICU setting. These data reveal that children and adolescents with IDD have more comorbidities and technology dependence on readmission to the hospital but a similar mortality rate and length of stay in the ICU when compared to the general population. Moreover, these data reveal that when families are provided with explanatory information regarding resuscitation in a nonacute, pediatric, skilled nursing home setting, there is a significant increase in request for DNR in some 25% of the population under study, but this rate is similar to changes in resuscitation preference found among adults in the general population on readmission to the hospital (Heyland et al., 2006).

DNR Order as Threshold for Discussion of the Goals of Therapy

Discussion about the resuscitation status of the patient is often the opening to discussion of more fundamental issues around the dying process (Sulmasy, Sood, & Ury, 2008). As an order that focuses strictly on what will not be done in specific circumstances of cardiopulmonary arrest, discussion about DNR status would seem to be an illogical starting point for the inherently important discussion of what is important to parents in the last few months of their child's life. In part, talking about CPR creates the need, and becomes the opportunity, to discuss dying and death openly because end of life is an inevitable point in the future that can no longer be ignored. This fact provides a reason for even the most reluctant parent, guardian, or clinician to prepare for death or at least have a talk about dying, an uncomfortable topic in our culture. In part, resuscitation decisions—absent previous discussion around life-sustaining treatments and what will be done for the patient regardless of physiologic stability—reflect an artificial decision node driven by a mistaken notion by the lay public and medical professionals alike that there is something distinctly different about resuscitation procedures.

Integrating Family Values With Medically Indicated Treatment Plans

Discussion about the resuscitation status of the patient is often too narrowly focused and misses the opportunity to explore and clarify more fundamental decisions that will form the basis for guiding all treatment decisions given the unique life context for each patient. To begin, a broad consensus among ethicists in the United States holds that there is no morally relevant or logically valid distinction among life-sustaining treatments, including various resuscitation treatments that can potentially be administered at the time of cardiac arrest. In other words, it may be justifiable to refuse CPR, just as it may be ethically justifiable to refuse medically administered hydration, nutrition, antibiotics, renal dialysis, Extra Corporeal Membrane Oxygenation (ECMO), and so on. Ethical justifiability rests on the reasons, not on the type of medical treatment. Similarly, some aspects of CPR may be warranted in selected circumstances while others may not. For example, the parent who wants CPR for their child in the context of respiratory arrest for an easily reversible mucous plug or a seizure might also decline CPR when the child has lung failure that cannot be corrected, and the parent feels the child would not be able to enjoy life dependent upon mechanical ventilation. The essential framework that should guide such treatment decisions is not whether a treatment can be administered but whether the proposed treatment furthers the goals, interests, and values of the patient as expressed by their appropriate surrogate. Resuscitation decisions sometimes place misdirected focus on whether patients will receive medications if the heart stops. However, what is morally and medically relevant and most important to the patient may not be just dramatic medical procedures only when the heart stops but also the full range of possible medical treatments as they relate to the patient's goals and what the patient's clinicians believe to be medically indicated under the circumstances (Heyland et al., 2006; Tibballs, 2006).

Comparative and Noncomparative Quality-of-Life Considerations

Perhaps no variable in making decisions about life-sustaining treatments, especially life-sustaining treatments for individuals with IDD, is as controversial as quality-of-life assessments. At one extreme, bias enters when the decision makers apply their own subjective assessment of the quality of life experienced by the patient. At the other extreme is the view that one cannot make *any* quality-of-life assessments because one can never know accurately or fully the quality of another person's life. Between these two extremes, it is helpful to distinguish comparative quality-of-life assessments from noncomparative ones. A comparative quality-of-life assessment is generally ethically suspect because it compares the quality of life of a person with a disability to the quality of life experienced by those without the disability in a way that unfairly disadvantages the former person, typically based on the false belief that only those without disabilities can experience full enjoyment in life.

Historically, discrimination, abuse, and even killing of people with IDD have been erroneously based on such comparisons. Yet, failure to weigh the impact of an advancing illness and the possibility that life-sustaining treatment might be more burdensome than beneficial upon a person's quality of life can be unethical, too. While it is right to protect individuals with intellectual, developmental, and other disabilities from discriminatory comparisons that deprive them of important rights and benefits—including the same respect for their lives and right to beneficial health care resources that other persons have—it is possible to leave people with disabilities in the paradoxical state of being unfairly marooned on nonbeneficial life support by refusing to make any assessment of its effect on their quality of life. Noncomparative quality-of-life assessments weigh the impact of advancing disease and escalating dependence on life-sustaining treatment against the prior quality of life only as experienced by that patient. In essence, the reference standard is not some ideal type, nor other patients without a disability; rather, it is the patient serving as his or her own control.

Procedure-Specific Versus Goal-Specific DNR Orders

Reframing the DNR discussion away from a checklist about specific therapies and toward a more focused discussion of the patient's goals and values puts the patient in a position to speak authoritatively on issues about which they alone are the expert and to define what is important to them (Sulmasy, Sood, & Ury, 2008). Such an approach also appropriately frames the role of the physician in these discussions as the medical expert on treatment alternatives who recommends treatment plans that align with the expressed goals and values of the patient. This deductive, rather than inductive, approach allows treatment choices to flow more coherently from the patient's goals. Treatments that promote the patient's values are medically indicated, and any treatment that does not promote the patient's values is not indicated.

These concepts serve as the basis for better understanding of procedure-specific versus goal-specific DNR orders. Procedure-specific orders delineate which procedures will and will not be attempted, typically as a list that is checked on a DNR form in a hospital setting. The greatest advantage of the procedure-directed DNR order is its clarity. This type of order should be supplemented with a detailed note in the chart explaining the justifications for the order and documenting the discussions between the clinicians and the patient or surrogate. By focusing on procedures, the form addresses in very concrete terms exactly what will or will not be done in the event of a cardiac or respiratory arrest; it is especially useful in a hospital setting where various clinicians care for the patient around the clock but cannot, practically, be privy to intimate discussions with the patient about their values and goals of care.

Goal-directed DNR orders emphasize the patient's goals, values, and preferences, rather than specific individual clinical procedures. Because patients or their surrogate decision makers are not medical experts on the technical details of resuscitation, proponents of the goal-directed approach believe the focus should be on what patients know best—their goals, values, and preferences (Truog, Waisel, & Burns, 1999). Discussion focuses on learning what the patient or their surrogate values most and what goals they are trying to achieve in selecting whether CPR or a DNR order is best for their child. For example, some parents choose CPR because it might enable their child to live longer, and life in any condition is preferable to death. Alternatively, some parents choose CPR for their child because they want to be present when the child dies and CPR might enable the child to live long enough for the parents to arrive. Or parents might believe that CPR will cure their child's underlying problem, which may or may not be the case. Knowing the parents' goals enables the clinicians to correct any erroneous beliefs and choose with the parents whether CPR can reasonably meet their goals. When patients or their surrogates ask questions as to the efficacy of CPR and other resuscitation measures—questions such as "Will my child suffer severe neurological damage if he survives? Will resuscitation be painful? Will my child be left in a worse state after CPR than she is in now?"—the physician is able to provide medical information and focus on learning what is most important to the decision maker, leaving medical decisions about which specific procedures should be performed aside until they can be chosen in light of the parents' values and goals.

This approach has been advocated to guide clinicians in caring for patients who have a DNR order suspended during an operative or interventional procedure (AMA Council on Ethical and Judicial Affairs, 1991). If the patient experiences profound hypotension or an arrhythmia after receiving a medication required to induce anesthesia, for example, then several moments of "resuscitation" (vasoactive agents, chest compressions, etc.) may be indicated while the disturbance is corrected. On the other hand, if the patient suffers a cardiac arrest from a massive intraoperative myocardial infarction, then chest compressions may not be indicated in light of the patient's or parent's goals. By this approach, decision making is left to the anesthesiologist and surgeon, based upon a clear understanding of the context of the medical situation as well as the patient's values and goals in undergoing the procedure.

Revisiting DNR Orders During the Perioperative Period

Controversy remains around automatically suspending all DNR orders during the perioperative period because, in essence, general anesthesia involves the deliberate depression of vital systems followed by their resuscitation (Truog, Waisel, Burns, 2005). Since the induction of anesthesia necessarily involves using medications that may produce respiratory or circulatory instability, which can usually be readily corrected, anesthesiologists generally feel responsible for resuscitating the anesthetized patient with cardiovascular medications, assisted ventilation, and tracheal intubation (if the patient is not already intubated). Separating resuscitation from anesthesia by leaving a DNR order in place during surgery is therefore somewhat artificial. Nevertheless, some patients or their surrogates may prefer dying during surgery to being resuscitated with the possibility of being worse off or dying during the resuscitation itself. For example, the parents of a child with a severe disability may decide that surgery, such as a palliative procedure to place a cardiac stent, is in the child's interest because it may reduce apnea and make him more comfortable. However, if the child's cardiopulmonary condition became so unstable during the procedure that it could not be easily corrected and the parents believe that cardiac defibrillation and other CPR procedures carry too high a risk of leaving the child worse off than before surgery, they might both want to have the procedure attempted and want to have the DNR order apply during it. For this reason, the American Society of Anesthesiologists (ASA) and the American College of Surgeons have adopted formal positions that state that the automatic suspension of DNR orders is not appropriate, and that all decisions about resuscitation status should be based on the goals of the informed patient undergoing surgery (or their surrogate decision maker) or a procedure requiring anesthesia, using the goal-directed approach outlined earlier (Waisel, Burns, Johnson, Hardart, & Truog, 2002).

DNR in the Home and School

First-responders and emergency medical services (EMS) personnel were traditionally expected to initiate CPR on all persons found in cardiopulmonary arrest. As it became clear that CPR is not always a beneficial intervention for all patients and as hospitals and other health care facilities developed policies permitting decisions not to resuscitate it was necessary to figure out how to deal with persons who had DNR orders once they were no longer in a health care institution. Professional organizations have, therefore, developed policies allowing EMS personnel to be guided by out-of-hospital DNR orders. These assert that first-responders should not attempt to resuscitate terminally or irreversibly ill persons who wish to forego such interventions and who have legal out-of-hospital DNR orders stating that transport to a hospital and care directed toward comfort should still be provided. Further, all these states have some form of unique identification procedure to certify the authenticity of the DNR order. These range from single page forms kept in the home, to wallet cards, bracelets, or necklaces kept on the patient (Burns, Edwards, Johnson, Cassem, & Truog, 2003).

The validity of DNR orders in the school setting has recently been the focus of more attention. The Americans With Disabilities Act of 1990, the Education for All Handicapped Children Act, and advances in health care have allowed minors with disabilities greater access to public education. As a result, some chronically ill or technology-dependent children are at risk for having a cardiopulmonary arrest while at school. The AAP, the National Education Association, and the National Association of School Nurses all have statements affirming the inclusion of students with DNR orders in the school setting. Despite this, only a few state protocols for EMS personnel explicitly extend out-of-hospital DNR orders to cover minors, and even fewer encompass the school setting (Burns et al., 2003). Even for states that legally authorize DNR orders for children outside a health care facility, problems arise in determining exactly what should be done if a child suffers a cardiopulmonary arrest (AAP Committee on School Health and Committee on Bioethics, 2000). We have found that thoughtful planning and coordination with school and home care staff are essential to insuring that a child's care is carried out with respect for the decisions the parents or legally authorized surrogate has made. Even for a child with a DNR order, calling emergency services for transport to a health care facility is often the first step in their end-of-life care. Emergency personnel may assess, stabilize, and provide medical treatments other than CPR and bring the child to a hospital as quickly as possible. However, if the child has died, many emergency service personnel will not transport a dead body, which state laws often prohibit. Clarification with the state's department of emergency services about how to handle such circumstances may be helpful. Even though the child may appear dead, it is often the case that he has not been pronounced dead by a legally authorized physician or nurse practitioner and may be transported to a hospital where such a determination may be formally made. Otherwise, it may be necessary to call the parent(s) and make arrangements for a funeral home to pick up the child. Clearly, foreseeing and planning for such a possibility, while difficult, should be done. An example of these types of issues in the school setting may be illustrated in the case of *ABC School and DEF School, Plaintiffs vs. Mr. and Mrs. M., individually and in their capacity as parents of their minor child, Minor M, Defendants*. In this situation, the school made a motion for injunctive and declaratory relief allowing it to refuse to honor the child's DNR order, which the court denied (Commonwealth of Massachusetts, 1997).

THE MEDICAL FUTILITY DEBATE: HOW DOES IT IMPACT CHILDREN WITH IDD?

From the earliest days of CPR, few issues have been more contentious than determining who ultimately decides whether a resuscitation attempt is indicated (Annas, 1982).

Most medical institutions in the United States require the informed consent of the patient (or their legally authorized surrogate) to withhold CPR. Some hospitals have adopted a "don't ask, don't tell" approach to this question by allowing "unilateral" or "futility-based" DNR orders without asking or informing the patient of the decision. Still other policies employ a "don't ask, do tell" approach where unilateral DNR orders can be written at the discretion of the attending physician who then informs the patient or patient's family of the decision, allowing them (at least theoretically) the option to transfer the patient to other caregivers. One state has adopted a public policy consistent with this approach. The Texas Advance Directives Act legally authorizes clinicians to unilaterally withdraw life-sustaining treatments if (a) the patient's physician determines that continuing life support is medically futile, (b) a second opinion from another physician is in agreement, and (c) an ethics committee reviews the case and concurs. The hospital is then required to give the family 10 days notice, during which time attempts may be made to transfer the patient to another health care provider or institution willing to continue caring for the patient on life support. If transfer is not possible, life support may be withdrawn (Smith, Gremillion, Slomka, & Warneke, 2007).

The concept of futility remains highly contentious. In a recent review of the topic, Burns and Truog (2007) have argued that the futility concept can be understood by viewing its three generations of evolution. The first generation was characterized by attempts to define futility in terms of certain clinical criteria. These attempts to define futility failed because they proposed limitations to care that were inherently and inevitability based on value judgments for which there is no consensus in our society. The second generation was defined by a procedural approach that empowered hospitals, through their ethics committees, to decide whether interventions demanded by families were futile. Many hospitals have adopted such policies, and some states incorporated this approach into legislation. This approach has also failed because it gives hospitals authority to decide whether or not to accede to demands that the clinicians regard as unreasonable, because there remains no local or national public policy on what defines "beneficial treatment." Absent such a consensus, procedural mechanisms to resolve futility disputes inevitably confront the same insurmountable barriers as the initial attempts to define futility. These authors therefore predict emergence of a third generation that is focused on communication and negotiation at the bedside, similar to paradigm that has proven successful in business and law.

Children and adults with IDD especially may be caught in so-called futility debates because of the inherent value judgments that so often underpin the real meaning of those who invoke the term "futility." On the other hand, cases where surrogates are demanding care that the clinicians believe is not indicated (if "not indicated" is simply restricted to demanding treatment that cannot maintain biologic life, let alone a broader definition) remain a source of real concern for all in our society for the number of times it arises in a modern hospital. Such cases seriously undercut public trust in the medical profession, and they equally undermine the integrity of the foundation of the medical and nursing profession to provide care that is beneficial.

Future Directions

The development of so-called DNR orders marked a pivotal change in health care. Up to that time all other orders in a hospital setting described what therapies would be provided for the patient. However, the DNR order established a fundamental change in this conceptual framework as it was the first specific order to direct the withholding of a potential treatment—what would not be done for the patient. The DNR order has since become commonplace in the delivery of health care, and yet it remains symbolic of the ongoing controversy in our society about decisions around life-sustaining treatments. For the individual patient, whether in the hospital or at home, a DNR order— or the absence of a DNR order—likely determines whether emergency personnel will be summoned and what procedures will occur around the time of death. At a societal level, the decision whether to perform CPR is emblematic of the ongoing debate over fundamental questions about foregoing medical treatment at the end of life: When is it appropriate, and who is to decide?

The conceptual foundation of a DNR order has inherent limitations. First, discussions about whether to perform CPR necessarily focus on the final event in the dying process— cardiopulmonary arrest—while many other important aspects of the process of dying are often not discussed. Second, the DNR order describes what will not be done for the patient, as opposed to what should be done for the patient. Yet the problems inherent in the current concept of DNR orders also point the way toward alternative frameworks. These insights are not new. Accompanying the first publication of hospital DNR policies in the New England Journal of Medicine in 1976 was a third article promoting the need for advance directives on all aspects of end-of-life care (Bok, 1976). This article, like many others at the time, was a harbinger of the development of more comprehensive palliative care—not simply for the dying but as an integral part of all treatment plans regardless of the trajectory of illness. Such an approach recognizes that good care at the end of life depends much more on what we provide than upon what we forego. We may withhold or withdraw treatments in accordance with the patient's or parent's values, but we should never withhold or withdraw caring for the patient.

REFERENCES

American Academy of Pediatrics Committee on Bioethics. (1996). Ethics and the care of critically ill infants and children. *Pediatrics, 98*(1), 149–152.

American Academy of Pediatrics Committee on Fetus and Newborn. (2008). Hospital discharge of the high-risk neonate. *Pediatrics, 122*(5), 1119–1126.

American Academy of Pediatrics Committee on School Health and Committee on Bioethics. (2000). Do not resuscitate orders in schools. *Pediatrics, 105*(4, Part I), 878–879.

American Medical Association Council on Ethical and Judicial Affairs. (1991). Guidelines for the appropriate use of do-not-resuscitate orders. *Journal of the American Medical Association, 265*(14), 1868–1871.

Annas, G. J. (1982). CPR: When the beat should stop. *Hastings Center Report, 12*(5), 30–31.

Bok, S. (1976). Personal directions for care at the end of life. *New England Journal of Medicine, 295*(7), 367–369.

Boulet, S. L., Boyle, C. A., & Schieve, L. A. (2009). Health care use and health and functional impact of developmental disabilities among U.S. children, 1997–2005. *Archives of Pediatric and Adolescent Medicine, 163*(1), 19–26.

Burns, J. P. (2004). DNR (Do Not Resuscitate). In S. G. Post (Ed.), *Encyclopedia of bioethics* (3rd ed., pp. 683–685). New York: Macmillan.

Burns, J. P., Edwards, J., Johnson, J., Cassem, N. H., & Truog, R. D. (2003). Do-not-resuscitate order after 25 years. *Critical Care Medicine, 31*(5), 1543–1550.

Burns, J. P., & Truog, R. D. (2007). Futility: A concept in evolution. *Chest, 132*(6), 1987–1993.

Clinical Care Committee of the Massachusetts General Hospital. (1976). Optimum care for hopelessly ill patients. *New England Journal of Medicine, 295*(7), 362–364.

Commonwealth of Massachusetts, Superior Court Civil Action No. 97–518 (1997).

Federal Register. (1985). Nondiscrimination on the basis of handicap; procedures and guidelines relating to health care for handicapped infants—HHS. Final Rules, 50, 14879–14892.

Friedman, S. L. (2006). Parent resuscitation preferences for young people with severe developmental disabilities. *Journal of the American Medical Directors Association, 7*(2), 67–72.

Friedman, S. L., & Gilmore, D. (2007). Factors that impact resuscitation preferences for young people with severe developmental disabilities. *Intellectual and Developmental Disabilities, 45*(2), 90–97.

Graham, R. J., Dumas, H. M., O'Brien, J. E., & Burns, J. P. (2004). Congenital neurodevelopmental diagnoses and an intensive care unit: Defining a population. *Pediatric Critical Care Medicine, 5*(4), 321–328.

Heyland, D. K., Cook, D. J., Gafni, A., Giacomini, M. K., Kuhl, D. R., & Tranmeret, J. E. (2006). Understanding cardiopulmonary resuscitation decision making: Perspectives of seriously ill hospitalized patients and family members. *Chest, 130*(2), 419–428.

Kouwenhoven, W. B., Jude, J. R., & Knickerbocker, G. G. (1984). Landmark article July 9, 1960: Closed-chest cardiac massage. *Journal of the American Medical Association, 251*(23), 3133–3136.

Rabkin, M. T., Gillerman, G., & Rice, N. R. (1976). Orders not to resuscitate. *New England Journal of Medicine, 295*(7), 364–366.

Russell, W. R. (1968). Not allowed to die. *British Medical Journal, 1*(5591), 576.

Schieve, L. A., Boulet, S. L., Boyle, C., Rasmussen, S. A., & Schendel, D. (2009). Health of children 3 to 17 years of age with Down syndrome in the 1997–2005: National Health Interview survey. *Pediatrics, 123*(2), 253–260.

Smith, M. L., Gremillion, G., Slomka, J., & Warneke, C. (2007). Texas' hospitals' experience with the Texas Advance Directives Act. *Critical Care Medicine, 35*(5), 1271–1276.

Sulmasy, D. P., Sood, J. R., & Ury, W. A. (2008). Physicians' confidence in discussing do not resuscitate orders with patients and surrogates. *Journal of Medical Ethics, 34*(2), 96–101.

Superintendent of Belchertown v. Saikewicz. North East Rep Second Ser, 370, 417–435 (1977).

Tibballs, J. (2006). The legal basis for ethical withholding and withdrawing of life-sustaining medical treatment in children. *Journal of Law and Medicine, 4*(2), 244–261.

Truog, R. D., Waisel, D. B., & Burns, J. P. (1999). DNR in the OR: A goal-directed approach. *Anesthesiology, 90*(1), 289–295.

Truog, R. D., Waisel, D. B., & Burns, J. P. (2005). Do-not-resuscitate orders in the surgical setting. *Lancet, 365*(9461), 733–735.

Waisel, D. B., Burns, J. P., Johnson, J. A., Hardart, G. E., & Truog, R. D. (2002). Guidelines for perioperative do-not-resuscitate policies. *Journal of Clinical Anesthesia, 14*(6), 467–473.

Chapter 10

Ethical Issues in the Withdrawal of Support

Charting a Course Between Scylla and Charybdis

Peter J. Smith and John J. Hardt

Introduction

During this first decade of the 21st century, individuals with intellectual and developmental disabilities (IDD), their families, and the medical professionals who serve them have confronted dilemmas that must be considered within the context of current medical, ethical, practical, and theoretical contingencies. It is an understatement to suggest that the current historic moment is more complex than any that have preceded it—both when considering the increased number of options relating to withdrawal of support at the end of life for individuals with intellectual disabilities and when considering the weight of moral decisions in our increasingly morally plural culture. In this chapter, the authors will propose a framework based upon the conviction that decision making for individuals with IDD must chart a "middle way" between a vitalistic inclination to preserve life at all costs and a utilitarian impulse to undervalue the personhood of individuals with IDD. Such a course requires that those involved be familiar with not only the opposing risks mentioned earlier but also medical technologies that bear upon such difficult work. This chapter will first review the medical and technological aspects of the withdrawal of supports including a consideration of what constitutes support, how support is maintained, and what medical considerations bear upon such decisions. It will then consider the broader, theoretical aspects of these difficult decisions. The authors do not consider this chapter to be complete in its treatment of this complex subject. They also recognize that their viewpoint is limited by their perspectives, which are predominantly shaped by Western medicine and the Christian tradition of moral reflection. The authors hope that despite these limitations, the information presented will nonetheless be helpful for a diverse population of professionals, families, and individuals.

What Constitutes Treatment and Support?

It is a truism that medical technology has expanded tremendously in the past 50 to 100 years. This expansion has had many profound results both inside and outside of health

161

care centers. Three examples serve both to demonstrate this point and set the stage for later considerations. First, there are an increasing number of conditions that, while previously considered "lethal," are currently treated "successfully" insofar as they lengthen the life span of these affected individuals. Second, there are an increasing number of conditions that require long-term treatments or therapies, changing them from "acute" to "chronic" conditions. Finally, there are an increasing number of treatment options that extend life with variable "costs" and "benefits." For the sake of this chapter, the authors will consider *any* action by a licensed clinician to be a treatment. This includes the use of medications, whether prescription controlled, over the counter, or "alternative"; surgical interventions; diagnostic procedures; ongoing and invasive medical technologies including mechanical ventilators; nutritional supplementation; and coordinated actions by groups of clinicians including efforts aimed at attempting to resuscitate those whose hearts have stopped beating in a regular fashion. All of these actions, by this definition, require advanced training and an institutional setting to initiate their use. Moreover, these kinds of treatments and supports are becoming increasingly common in the contemporary health care context, increasingly effective in maintaining various life processes such as circulation or respiration, and increasingly present in the day-to-day lives of those persons affected not only within the institutional setting but also, it is worth noting, outside of the institutional location.

All of these treatments have a life cycle of their own. For example, mechanical ventilators were initially rare and restricted to a small population of individuals, namely, persons undergoing surgery in a hospital operating room. Now, they are widely used across multiple settings including homes and schools as well as intensive care units (ICUs) to support a wide variety of individuals from the youngest to the oldest among us. Because treatments themselves are so rapidly changing, it is crucial that any discussion of particular individuals is grounded both in the particularities of their current conditions and the current accepted applications of various treatment options. For this reason, all historical positions regarding the use of any treatment are subject to change as the treatments change. The current treatments that are most often involved in decisions to withdraw support at the end of life can be broken into three main categories: medicines, devices, and professional actions.

Medicines

The list of medications that are involved with the end of life is not easily limited. Main categories include medications to diminish pain; medications to support heart functionality; medications to help maintain chemical balances; medications to fight infections; medications that impact body fluids, including those in the lungs, urine, and gastrointestinal (GI) tract; and medications used to decrease or prevent seizures. All of these have individual costs and benefits, and most have a potentially significant effect on other medications. Therefore, those who are discussing withdrawal of supports for any individual who is on any medications will need to calculate not only each one individually but also their collective impact. However, simple maxims such as "do everything" or "stop them all" are rarely clinically useful because of the complexity of the pharmacological options currently available. For example, most individuals who do not want to extend life do not, when pushed, have difficulty imagining that they would accept medications that fight infections or inflammation even if they declined other therapies. Likewise, treatment options for most cancers are limited by their usefulness and toxicity. It does little good to "kill the cancer" if, by doing so, one kills the patient.

Devices

Devices that support life include mechanical ventilators as well as systems to deliver oxygen other than ventilators, devices to assist circulation for extended periods, devices to clean the body of toxins, and devices to deliver nutritional support. Each one of these treatment interventions, which substitute for major organ systems of the human body, requires significant clinical and technical expertise to initiate, but some require considerably less expertise to maintain. This discrepancy in required expertise between initiation and maintenance of treatment interventions has caused decisions around the foregoing or withdrawing of such supports to be an ethically contentious arena of health care in which families and clinicians may disagree. In the past, the limited effectiveness of treatments for serious medical problems (e.g., organ system failure), combined with a limited number of treatment options, left few treatment decisions to be made as certain physiological conditions were incompatible with life. Now, however, individuals and families can choose from a wider range of increasingly effective treatment interventions that can extend life spans considerably—although often at great effort and expense. A variety of treatment options that are both increasingly effective and able to be maintained outside of an institutional setting has placed upon families and surrogates wider decisional latitude, authority, and responsibility in treatment decisions for persons with IDD.

Professional Actions

Finally, there are a set of treatments that are themselves the actions of professionals. Most well known in this category is cardiopulmonary resuscitation (CPR). This procedure holds a special status within Western medicine because it is the one medical procedure that is usually considered an intrinsic part of care that cannot be withheld absent the directly stated consent of the individual who is in possible need of it. Therefore, it is has become a symbolic representative of the whole of the interventions, decisions, and actions associated with the health care team. Both families and clinicians recognize the privileged status of resuscitation among treatment interventions and the symbolism involved in our society's current approach to this issue. This creates an especially sensitive atmosphere around discussions of the future use of CPR and related interventions. These discussions have been labeled as discussions around Do-Not-Resuscitate (DNR) orders: strictly speaking they are actually about "attempting to resuscitate." Unfortunately, they are often too limited in scope such that they do not adequately consider the larger question concerning long-term goals of care, hope of meaningful recovery, and they frequently occur too late in the course of the individual's life and care. All parties who have examined this issue have concluded that everyone is better served by having a thoughtful discussion of the goals of care between the clinicians and the individual and families. Consideration of future situations that may lead to attempting to resuscitate is one part of these discussions. In this respect, individuals with IDD are not unlike other individuals: Like all persons who are not medically trained, persons with IDD need help with communication in the clinical encounter in order to discern how their general life patterns are best represented by the practical choices at hand. Such assistance should include advocating for these choices throughout their care program, which spans up to and potentially including the withdrawal of care.

Special Features of Care for Individuals With Intellectual Disabilities

There are several features of the care of individuals with IDD that are unique to their situation. They include an incongruence of values between patients, families, and the care team due to the historic undervaluing of the lives of persons with IDD, complications due to prior lack of communication of personal desires for care, and the increased frequency of "outside" forces weighing in upon decisions, including representatives of the state, residential institutions, and oversight organizations.

The readers of this text need not be reminded that individuals with disabilities have too often been undervalued. This has certainly been true within health care institutions. Therapies have been withheld or discontinued simply because the individuals have been deemed to have less value than others due to their real—or perceived—intellectual disability. This terrible legacy is not relegated to the distant past; rather, it is recent and even ongoing and unfortunately has many current implications. For example, it is only recently that individuals with Down syndrome were even considered "worthy" of transplantation, and therefore there are many clinicians who still have not had the experience of caring for this type of patient in that situation. This dearth of experience in care can lead to a lack of understanding when confronted with questions of life-sustaining therapies. This is especially true for questions that hinge upon the use of limited resources such as transplanted organs or kidney dialysis. Among many well-meaning clinicians, there is an unspoken—and clinically unwarranted—sense of hopelessness for such patients that creates an undertow for individuals with IDD, pulling them out of the realm of possible intervention. Many clinicians have had experiences confronting clinical scenarios similar to those with typically developing individuals whose sole differentiating feature is that in one the person in question has an intellectual disability—albeit mild—that entirely changed the consideration of options offered. The destructive assumptions that lead to undervaluing persons with IDD are still too often present in decision-making meetings; they must be monitored, discovered, and addressed forcefully if they are to be ended. In decisions concerning withdrawal of care for individuals with intellectual disabilities, the undervaluing of persons with IDD is likely to be one of—if not the—most important special consideration in such cases.

Regarding the second special feature, individuals with IDD can be divided into two groups for this portion of the discussion. First, there are those who at some point have been able to indicate their life preferences in ways that those around them have been able to meaningfully interpret. Second, there are those who have not been able to do so whether due to features intrinsic to themselves or due to features of the situations within which they find themselves. For those who have had the opportunity to express themselves in a way that has been heard and recorded, the most important resulting obligation for decision makers is to seek them out if possible for further discussion about the particular decision at hand. If that is not possible, decision makers should seriously consider how prior communication might bear upon the decision at hand. This is not easy due to the fact that prior communications are usually difficult to apply in new and potentially unconsidered circumstances. Furthermore, because of the undervaluing mentioned in the prior section, the expressed wishes of individuals with disabilities are often undervalued or discounted. For individuals without prior meaningfully understood communications, the burden on those shaping decisions on their behalf is to rely on a standard of "best interest" when weighing potential options. This standard is different than the "substituted judgment," which is possible when individuals have prior communications on which to formulate decisions regarding what their wishes would be.

The third feature that makes the decisions regarding withdrawal of treatments for individuals with intellectual disabilities special is the involvement of persons or groups outside of the traditional cohort of decision makers consisting of clinicians, family members, and the individuals themselves. The involvement of these "outsiders" stems from several factors. First, as has been noted earlier, individuals with IDD have been historically undervalued. Procedural safeguards have been instituted in an attempt to combat this phenomenon. These procedures are most often institutional—for example, mandatory involvement by a hospital ethics committee—but can be mandated by legislation or judicial ruling.

Second, individuals with IDD, when considered with other populations, are more often supported within residential programs that involve nonfamily care providers. Therefore, it is not uncommon that these individuals, who have no mandated or explicitly recognized role to play within the decision-making process, either voluntarily step forward with opinions or are solicited to offer their views.

Finally, numerous organizations have been created around and for individuals with intellectual disabilities, not unlike many other identifiable groups within the population. Because these organizations are formed explicitly to advocate for this population, they can become involved in actual clinical cases and in health care policy formation. These groups often play a vital role in empowering persons with IDD. Such groups are often not perceived as helpful by institutions given that their involvement can frequently be seen by the institutions as disruptive. They certainly serve as a special feature in this process.

MIGUEL'S STORY

Miguel was a baby born with an anterior encephalocele, which meant that a large portion of his brain was wrapped in a sac that grew outside his forehead. This sac had to be surgically removed in the first days of life to prevent an infection and subsequent death. After surgery, his medical difficulties were many, and he required both a gastrostomy tube for feeding and a tracheostomy to protect his airway. His brain was not only smaller than average, but it showed signs of significant abnormalities resulting in profound cognitive impairments. The abnormalities of his brain made even the basic function of maintaining a stable body temperature frequently difficult for him. Most of the nurses and doctors taking care of him thought he should be allowed to die peacefully. They recommended that a DNR order be placed in Miguel's chart.

However, Miguel's parents disagreed. They loved him and wanted him to live. His parents were a young, unmarried, immigrant couple. Given his parents' stated wishes, every available medical technology was used to keep him alive and as comfortable as possible. It was not easy. Many people involved in his care voiced strong opposition to working with him. Not only was he medically fragile and technologically dependent, but his body—especially his face—had been physically transformed by his congenital malformation and the subsequent surgeries.

In addition, relationships with the family were difficult. His parents had very different lives and perspectives than his medical care team: They did not speak English as their first language, they were devoutly religious, and his father was often disruptive and unpleasant to the hospital staff. Some staff suspected him of illicit drug use. Finally, it was reported that Miguel's mother had been told by her mother that Miguel's problems were "God's punishment" for her out-of-wedlock pregnancy and his suffering was a "cross to bear" for his mother. According to Miguel's grandmother, to try to fight "God's will" would further compound her sin. Eventually, Miguel became so sick that he was admitted to the pediatric intensive care unit (PICU), where he was placed on a mechanical ventilator and required multiple medications to stay alive. Eventually, many of the staff wanted not only to place a DNR order in the chart but also to withdraw the life-sustaining medical interventions that were keeping Miguel alive.

Many questions are raised by this story, which may be summarized into two basic questions that are common to most moral deliberation: What ought to be done? and, Who decides? It is important to note that the assumptions that are brought into the struggle to answer these questions will usually shape the inquiry. Thus, the "facts" or "truths" offered to justify a particular decision will not symmetrically counter the arguments of another opinion. Due to the different ways in which the questions at hand were framed, arguments between opposing opinions often appeared to speak past each other. For example, some within a natural law tradition of moral reasoning may suggest that the crucial issue is whether the care offered to Miguel beyond feeding him is "morally extraordinary" and therefore not obligatory. Others, arguing from the principle of "beneficence," might suggest that a determination of Miguel's "best interests" is important. Virtue ethicists might see the need for caregivers to learn to serve this type of patient and family, precisely because of the difficulty of the task, as part of the formation of virtuous clinicians. The answers to what ought to be done hinge upon who is designated—whether actively, by default or accident—as the person or group who "gets to decide." Therefore, often times, such conversations eventually devolve into a power struggle over decision making given the lack of common ground from which arguments are made.

Modern Society and Modern Ethics

The first step in understanding the current state of medical ethics is to examine the underlying assumptions and predispositions of the larger society. Simply stated, the current consensus in Western countries is that culture and society ought to be structured upon the foundations of "life, liberty, and the pursuit of happiness." Because of this orientation, it is important to point out that the conception of "liberty" implies a freedom "from" oppressive restrictions. It is critical to note that this framework is based upon the definition that personhood is determined by an ability to choose. Over time, liberal society has responded to these criticisms regarding membership and has greatly expanded its definition of citizen. However, it has not been able to expand this definition beyond the strict limits that are inherent in its conception of citizens as competent choice makers and therefore sees any who do not fit into this rubric as, by definition, "defective" and "needing to be fixed." In addition, the modern American bioethics movement, starting with the Nuremberg Trials at the end of World War II, was born within a worldview that not only mistrusted previous systems but also saw the need to safeguard individuals from the domination of larger entities (Rothman, 1991).

Although concerns for liberty and individual human rights are clearly good influences upon society and the practice of ethics, they have steadily come to dominate in a manner that is less than desirable in many cases. Exclusive focus upon the individual when attempting to wrestle with complicated clinical conditions can result in too narrowly conceiving of the ethical problem at hand, especially when one is attempting to advocate for individuals with intellectual disabilities. Exclusive focus on the individual can often times fail to adequately consider the morally relevant contextual details of a case and marginalize values beyond the language of liberty and rights. Ironically, the exclusive focus on the individual as the locus of the ethical dilemma often leads to decisions that do not best protect and respect the individual. This is especially true for those with strong relational ties to families, friends, and communities such as individuals with intellectual disabilities.

Modern Society and Modern Medicine

The 20th century witnessed both the birth of modern medical ethics and the rise of a modern medical system. Some of the most notable of the scientific and technological innovations of the last century include the rise and expanded use of antibiotics; the advent and increasing sophistication of mechanical ventilation supports; multiple surgical innovations across all surgical specialties, patient groups, and disease processes; and the creation and ongoing expansion of the modern intensive care units.

For this discussion, it is important to highlight two points that are common across all of these developments. First, the individuals who are sickest have benefited the most from these developments. Second, because of the nature of associations between illness and cognitive impairments, individuals with IDD are significantly overrepresented in the group of people who utilize and benefit from these developing technologies.

Modern Society and Our Modern Dilemma

Individuals with IDD are more frequently receiving life-sustaining therapies than members of other identifiable populations. Therefore, family members and care providers for these individuals are more frequently in the position of weighing decisions regarding foregoing and withdrawing these therapies. Because of the complexity of these situations, family members and care providers often do not agree about these decisions. It is in the attempt to frame arguments in these contentious disagreements that participants often mistakenly narrow the consideration of the values and principles that shape their decision by focusing on the individual patient. As was noted before, an exclusive focus upon the individual will frequently end with impasse. Seemingly intractable disagreements about facts ensue, insurmountable differences between judgments regarding "best interest" block agreement, and increasing hostility and conflict eventually dominate discussion. The most common pattern in these impasses is that two "sides" emerge in a struggle between avoiding "vitalism" on one hand or "futility" on the other.

AN UNSATISFACTORY DICHOTOMY: "VITALISM" VERSUS "FUTILITY"

The drive toward "vitalism" starts with the noble motive of protecting life, especially the lives of vulnerable individuals. This appropriate concern for the protection of life at all costs has been pointedly demonstrated in the dramatic historical examples documenting when such a moral impulse was blatantly ignored. The inherent value of all persons, whether impaired or not, remains a question for social debate. This ongoing debate makes necessary an ongoing vigilance by all advocates for individuals with any type of intellectual and developmental disability. The risk that is inherent in this advocacy is that the individual will, as a secondary consequence, be forced to endure increased suffering and burden such that it may become disproportionate to the benefit of pursuing life-sustaining interventions. Ultimately, the danger of vitalism-based arguments is that the only moral end that carries weight is the end of maintaining life, which leads to the loss of all other values, a position that can ultimately diminish the moral meaning of the life being "saved."

On the other hand, attempts to avoid engaging in futile interventions begin with the equally noble motive of recognizing the limits of human interventions, including medical interventions. Simply put, all humans will die, and there seems to be some consensus that medicine as a practice should recognize this. One of the great fears becoming increasingly relevant in our contemporary context is that life will be extended "too long," and those who advocate for limitations in care are often directly motivated by clear statements from individuals that they "do not want to live on a machine." However, there are also inherent risks in this movement as well. First, errors of discernment occur both because of the diverse clinical and personal variations between individuals regarding "living on machines" as well as the unpredictable, but not unrecognized, pattern of individuals changing their minds regarding how they feel about invasive life-sustaining technologies as prognoses change—whether for the better or worse. Those who propose futility as a key feature in any dilemma are at risk of making quality of life judgments prematurely and thereby limiting interventions too soon. Of particular importance to people with IDD is the possibility that such judgments could be incorrectly made in the case of particularly vulnerable patient populations because of an inaccurate perception of the patient's burden. The ultimate danger of futility-based arguments is that decision makers will "give up too soon" due to inaccurate information or personal biases that, when repeated across communities, can lead to systematic discrimination.

SCYLLA AND CHARYBDIS

In Greek mythology, there were stories about two deadly monsters that were situated on opposite sides of the Strait of Messina between Sicily and Italy. They were located in close proximity to each other and posed an inescapable threat to passing sailors: avoiding Charybdis meant passing too closely to Scylla and vice versa. The phrase "between Scylla and Charybdis" has come to mean being in a state where one is between two dangers: moving away from one will cause you to be at risk from the other. That is precisely the description of the dangers that lurk when attempting to navigate the difficult ethical dilemmas related to withdrawal of support from individuals with IDD. Charting a course between the Scylla of vitalism and the Charybdis of futility is an apt metaphor for the difficulty inherent in end-of-life decision making. Participants in these morally profound decisions generally agree that they desire to avoid both the unnecessary suffering of patients and the unwarranted prolongation of death that can sometimes accompany decisions for life-sustaining treatment options. Similarly, participants in these decisions share a desire to avoid bias and discrimination against those with IDD and seek to resolve conflicts among parties involved. The disagreements lie in their interpretations of the course that they need to plot to navigate between these menacing dangers.

THE IMPORTANCE OF PROCESS

Moral philosopher Alasdair MacIntyre makes the following observation about the process of forming one's moral judgments. He writes,

> We are always liable to error in making particular moral judgments, sometimes intellectual errors such as going beyond the evidence or relying upon some unsubstantiated generalization, sometimes moral errors such as being over-influenced by our liking and disliking of particular individuals or projecting on to a situation some unrecognized fantasy. And our intellectual errors are often rooted in moral errors. We need therefore to have tested our capacity for moral deliberation and judgment in this and that type of situation by subjecting our arguments and judgments systematically to the critical scrutiny of reliable others, of co-workers, family, friends. Such others, of course, are not always reliable and some may influence us in ways that strengthen the propensity to error. So to have confidence in our deliberations and judgments we need social relationships of a certain kind, forms of social association in and through which our deliberations and practical judgments are subjected to extended and systematic critical questioning that will teach us how to make judgments in which both we and others may have confidence. (MacIntyre, 1999)

As MacIntyre observes, because we, as human beings, are liable to making errors in moral judgment, especially when the course is difficult—as is the case in modern medical care for individuals with intellectual disability—we need to engage in discussions of ethical deliberation with our peers as part of our professional routine and not simply in an "ad hoc" method. We should also engage in discussions with individuals who do not agree with us in order to critically test our thinking and conclusions. Finally, we should engage in discussions with individuals who are simply different from us in order that the professional and cultural biases that congregate among like-minded and similarly skilled persons can be tested by a moral vantage point that is wholly different from our own.

CONTEXT AND CONVERSATIONS MATTER

Clinicians need to avoid a failure of moral perspective. This failure is a real possibility given that professionals spend so much of their lives working alongside individuals who share a similar perspective and set of concerns. New moral perspectives must be found through honest engagement with a wider circle of concern than those of only like-minded colleagues. Such a circle would include the perspective of families and other "outsiders" who bring a new perspective to clinical moral dilemmas. These types of conversations necessarily take time, a fact that poses a challenge to the time-sensitive nature of clinical practice. Beyond the necessity of time, it is important to foster and maintain a professional culture that values the building of consensus through the protection of moral values and the exploration of alternative moral vantage points when considering questions of foregoing or withdrawing support; this culture of moral deliberation would then be increasingly tolerant of moral ambiguity and the possibility that multiple decisions could prove to be "right."

REFERENCES

MacIntyre, A. (1999). Social structures and their threats to moral agency. *Philosophy, 74*, 316.

Rothman, D. J. (1991). *Strangers at the bedside*. New York: Basic Books.

CHAPTER 11

Forgoing Nutrition in Infants and Children With Intellectual Disabilities

ROBERT M. VEATCH

There was a day, up until the end of the 20th century, when many people believed that infants with intellectual and developmental disabilities (IDD) were not worth saving (Duff & Campbell, 1973; Gustafson, 1973; Indiana Supreme Ct., 1982; President's Commission, 1983, p. 467). Especially in cases in which infants and children suffered concomitant medical problems, physicians, parents, and others sometimes decided to forgo medical interventions necessary to save the lives of these patients. Beginning in the 1980s, the interventions that were omitted sometimes included the provision of nutrition and hydration by medical means such as of nasogastric feeding tube, intravenous feeding, or gastrostomy (a direct opening into the stomach).

Today that attitude seems horribly cruel and insensitive. These decisions were challenged morally and legally, leading to a substantial consensus that intellectual disability was not a justifiable reason for withholding life support, including medically supplied nutrition and hydration. Nevertheless, certain patients have such severe medical problems that continuing life support inflicts grave burden on them or is useless in helping them. This chapter explores the moral and legal issues of forgoing nutrition and hydration in infants and children with intellectual disabilities. It presents the thesis that life support may be foregone in those with intellectual disabilities in those cases (and only those cases) in which it would be omitted or withdrawn in a person without intellectual impairment.

An infant I have called Jimmy McCarthy (names and other details are changed to protect anonymity) was born 4 weeks prematurely. At birth he did not do well. He required immediate life support, including resuscitation. He was soon diagnosed as suffering from a combination of complex genetic and anatomical anomalies including a ventricular septal defect of the heart, a duodenal atresia (blockage of the intestine) that did not allow for feeding by mouth, and liver abnormalities that may or may not have been correctable. His genetic problems included monosomy 18, a chromosomal abnormality that would cause severe intellectual and physical impairments and would eventually lead to Jimmy's death within months or a few years.

The most immediate problem was the intestinal blockage that prevented normal feeding. The pediatric surgeon indicated that eventually he could correct the blockage, but Jimmy's prematurity prevented operating until he had grown for a few weeks. He recommended intravenous feeding in the interim. The cardiac septal defect would require one or more heart operations when the child had matured for a few months. The liver problems might be self-correcting but could require a liver transplant. All agreed that the intellectual disabilities could not be corrected and that Jimmy would, in any case, deteriorate and die within a few years, perhaps sooner.

At a hospital ethics committee meeting attended by Jimmy's parents, the treatment options were explored. Jimmy would require temporary intravenous feeding, intestinal surgery in a few weeks, heart operations, and perhaps corrective interventions for his liver problems. Nevertheless, he would remain severely impaired mentally and would die within a few years.

After these treatments were described to Jimmy's parents, they presented their views. They arrived at the meeting with Bibles in hand and were later described by one of the committee members as "fundamentalist Catholic." Deeply religious people, they had consulted with their parish priest as well as medical specialists at a local research center. They had also contacted one of the leading attorneys in the area dealing with medical consent and treatment refusal issues. They told the committee that they had prayed about the decision and had concluded that "God's place for Jimmy is in heaven." They insisted that no intravenous feeding be provided. They acknowledged that they understood that Jimmy would die soon from lack of nutrition and fluids.

The ethics committee, initially shocked by the parents' decision, faced many issues. Most critically, some members of the committee felt it was unethical to withhold nutrition and hydration even if it would be morally acceptable to forgo the anticipated surgeries. Other committee members were aware of legal requirements that infants must always be provided "appropriate nutrition," even if other means of life support were being withheld. The remainder of this chapter will explore these issues.

THE MORALITY OF FORGOING NUTRITION AND HYDRATION

The Argument That Nutrition and Hydration Are Always Required

Many people hold that nutrition and hydration are special—that even if other life supports can be withdrawn, nutrition and hydration still should be provided. These arguments usually come in three forms.

The Basic Care Argument

Gilbert Meilaender, a leading conservative, Protestant commentator on this subject and a member of the national President's Council on Bioethics, argues that providing food and fluids is not medical treatment but rather is "basic human care" (Meilaender, 1984). He suggests that basic care is required for all human beings even if they are beyond benefit from medical treatments.

Many moral theologians and philosophers recognize that some medical treatments are sometimes gravely burdensome or useless in treating patients' medical problems (Pope Pius XII, 1984). It has long been acknowledged that such treatments that offer no benefit, or offer only benefits offset by the burdens of the treatment, are morally expendable. They were traditionally called "extraordinary means" of life support but now are often simply referred to as "disproportional" or simply morally expendable treatments (President's Commission, 1984).

Meilaender and others who are generally critical of withholding or withdrawing nutrition and hydration acknowledge that some treatments offer no proportional benefit and are morally expendable but insist that nutrition and hydration are fundamentally different. They are not so much medical treatments as they are basic care, and therefore they must be provided even if other interventions, such as the surgeries in Jimmy McCarthy's case, can be omitted.

The Symbolic Care Argument

Daniel Callahan (1983) offered a somewhat different claim. He argued that nutrition and hydration are symbolic of our concern for the hungry and thirsty, and that society should show its commitment to the most needy of the community by always providing nutrition and hydration even if other means of life support can be omitted.

The Omission-Commission Argument

A third concern behind the view that nutrition and hydration are special and should be provided to everyone focuses on a somewhat different problem. Some have claimed that, if it is acceptable to withhold nutrition and hydration from the critically ill, this will become a substitute for active mercy killing. It is claimed that what is called the "omission-commission" distinction protects most people from having their lives ended prematurely, but that including forgoing of nutrition and hydration will radically expand the number of people who can end up dead from mere omission of treatment.

This argument is complex, and the explanation is lengthy. It holds that one reason to accept what is called the "omission-commission distinction" (the idea that there is a moral difference between actively killing the terminally ill and merely letting them die) is that interventions that actively kill can potentially kill many more people than the mere decision to let someone die. The reasoning is that if decisions related to the end of life are limited to omission of life support, most people will simply not die. Most of us, most of the time, are not in need of medical life support and will, therefore, continue to live if the only permissible decisions related to end of life are decisions to withhold or withdraw life support. Thus, restricting decisions to omissions will pose at most a limited threat to continued existence.

By contrast (so the argument goes), if we open the door to active interventions to end life, literally every person could be made dead soon with such a choice. Those following this reasoning conclude that normally we should maintain the omission-commission distinction (the position that it is acceptable to forgo life support, but that it is not acceptable to actively, intentionally intervene to terminate life) because as a practical matter this significantly limits the number of people who are at risk of being made dead by such decisions.

This is a kind of "rule-utilitarian" defense of the omission-commission distinction (Lyons, 1965; Rawls, 1955). A "rule-utilitarian" position is one that holds that instead of evaluating every action based on its consequences, we should evaluate alternative rules and choose the rule that has the best consequences. It is held that the consequences of the rule that would merely tolerate omissions of life support are much better than the consequences of a rule that would permit active interventions to kill. If this is the basis for supporting the omission-commission distinction (and there are other reasons that may be offered), then proposals to omit medically supplied nutrition and hydration introduce a special problem. While most people will not die because of decisions to omit most forms of life support, omission of nutrition and hydration escalates the consequences of omission dramatically. Literally everyone would die if a decision were made to omit nutrition and hydration for a significant time (days or weeks). Hence, there is something special about nutrition and hydration. For those who defend the omission-commission distinction on the grounds that the consequences of omission are normally much less severe than the consequences of active intervention designed to terminate life, the normal rule cannot be supported in the case of nutrition and hydration. In this special case, the consequences of omission are just like active killing. Literally everyone could die from this particular kind of omission.

For those who rest their support of the omission-commission distinction on these consequence-based arguments, it may make sense to make an exception for nutrition and hydration and to insist that they never be omitted. This view holds that withholding nutrition and hydration is morally like active killing because the consequences are similar. Even though most people most of the time could not die from decisions to omit medical treatments, everyone could die from omitting nutrition and hydration just like everyone could die from decisions to actively kill them. This is a third reason why some people have concluded that nutrition and hydration are morally unique and must always be provided even if other means of life support can justifiably be withheld in cases of critical and terminal illness. If acceptance of omission-commission distinction was rule utilitarian, then withholding nutrition and hydration should be treated like commission.

The Defense of Forgoing Nutrition and Hydration

The three versions of arguments in favor of treating nutrition and hydration as special and always morally required have generated persuasive responses.

Nutrition and Hydration Are No More Basic Than Other Life Supports

First, in response to Meilaender's claim that nutrition and hydration are different because they represent basic caring, defenders of withholding nutrition and hydration respond that these interventions are no more basic than other means of life support. Ventilators, for example, are now often withheld in the case of certain terminally ill patients when the ventilator is deemed not to provide any benefit. That was the conclusion in the famous case of Karen Quinlan, for example. Ventilators provide a very basic bodily function; they oxygenate the blood when normal respiration is not possible. The defenders of omission of nutrition and hydration claim that medical means of supplying food and fluid are no more basic than medical means of supplying oxygen. If omission of a ventilator is—under certain conditions—moral and legal, then omission of medically supplied nutrition and hydration should be as well.

Similarly, antibiotics are now routine for fighting bacterial infections. They are safe, simple, and a reasonably sure treatment that has become quite standard. Nevertheless, antibiotics may be omitted legally, and many would consider such omission moral if the antibiotic merely prolongs an inevitable dying process. Once again, medical means to supply nutrition do not seem any more "basic."

This may lead to a slightly different version of the claim that nutrition and hydration are basic. It may be claimed that they are different because they are not so much medical interventions as merely the caring of the sort we provide for all human beings. This seems to suggest, however, that useless medical means are expendable while useless, nonmedical means are required—a position that seems hard to defend.

Treating Those Who Are Not Hungry and Thirsty

The argument that nutrition and hydration should always be provided because providing food and fluid is symbolic of our pervasive social commitment to the hungry and thirsty also faces problems. Some dying patients are not hungry and thirsty. In fact there is some evidence that providing food and fluid to some critically or terminally ill patients may make them more uncomfortable (Lynn & Childress, 1983). In the cases in which food and fluids make patients uncomfortable or have no effect whatsoever, they surely should not be required. It makes no sense to provide extra burdens to the dying by providing nutrition or hydration when it offers no benefit to them and may actually make them more uncomfortable. They cannot be made the victims of our symbolic actions, no matter how important it is for a society to maintain its commitment to feed those who really are hungry. We should be respectful when discontinuing food and fluids (just as we are when we discontinue a respirator), but it is truly disrespectful to continue useless and burdensome food and fluids when we accept the idea that other treatments that are useless and burdensome and therefore could be refused.

Thus, many conclude that no logical reason exists to limit this to medically administered food and fluids. In fact, if normal oral food and fluids are useless or burdensome, they should be discontinued as well. In fact, that is standard policy. If someone is made extremely uncomfortable when fed orally, he or she is given nothing by mouth. The same policy should apply to the terminally or critically ill.

Problems With the Rule-Utilitarian Defense of the Duty to Provide Food and Fluids

This brings us to the third and final argument for providing nutrition and hydration, the rule-utilitarian defense. It holds that, while normally the consequences of forgoing a treatment are necessarily limited, in the case of nutrition and hydration literally every human being could die simply by omission. If the consequences are that substantial (so the argument goes), we should treat this particular kind of forgoing like we treat active interventions intended to kill. We should prohibit them because of the vast and potentially horrendous consequences.

First, it should be noted that forgoing nutrition and hydration is not the only potential omission with vast consequences. Withholding many other medical treatments could also have very extensive consequences. Withholding oxygen or antibiotics or insulin or CPR would, at various times, lead to many unnecessary deaths.

More fundamentally, it is questionable whether the omission-commission distinction really should rest on the rule-utilitarian claim that the consequences are potentially much more serious with commissions than with omissions. Many would defend the distinction on grounds unrelated to consequences. The debate over whether there is a principled difference between active killing and merely letting someone die is a convoluted and lengthy one. This is not the place to rehearse it in detail. Suffice it to say, many people who defend the difference do so on grounds that are not utilitarian. They hold to the doctrine of "double effect," which relies, in part, on the claim that the intention is different in the case of omissions when compared with active interventions intended to kill (Graber, 1979; Marquis, 1991; Pellegrino, 1995). If the omission-commission distinction can be sustained, it probably is not on the basis of a significant difference in consequences. In fact, in many cases the consequences of letting someone die are similar to those of actively killing. The real difference, if it exists at all, must lie in some other theoretical distinction, such as the double effect doctrine. It cannot be that the mere fact that many people could potentially die from forgoing nutrition and hydration changes our duty to be compassionate to those who will actually be harmed by receiving them. It cannot be that showing compassion to small numbers is morally acceptable, but showing similar compassion to larger numbers in itself would make it immoral.

If that is true, then the claim that nutrition and hydration must always be provided because the potential bad consequences of permitting their omission will not stand up. We are left with the conclusion that there is nothing intrinsically unique or different about nutrition and hydration. Since almost all human beings benefit from receiving food and fluid, the duty to provide them to those who cannot otherwise obtain them is quite stringent. Normally, we should feed and hydrate those who are dependent on the care of others including critically and terminally ill patients, especially infants. However, in the special case in which providing them offers no benefit and may actually cause net harm, they should be foregone. Just like any other intervention that is not proportionally beneficial, nutrition and hydration should only be provided when there is an expected net benefit to the person receiving them. If an intervention offers no benefit, or will do more harm than good, it is expendable. In fact, it should not be provided.

That is the conclusion not only of those who are more liberal defenders of forgoing life support but also of those who have clear track records with more conservative, prolife inclinations. For example, a large group of leading conservative bioethicists published a statement on the topic of withholding nutrition and hydration. The group was made up of a who's who of religious and secular leaders—Catholic, Protestant, Jewish, and religiously unaffiliated. They said the obvious: Normally, almost all human beings benefit from nutrition and hydration. Those in society with responsibility have a duty to see that these people receive food and fluid. Occasionally, however, there are special cases— normally involving critically or terminally ill patients, including newborns and other infants—for whom provision of nutrition and hydration does more harm than good. In these special cases, the providing of food and fluid is not required. It is excluded by our duty to avoid harming. Their conclusion is

> when specific objective conditions are met, the withholding and withdrawing of various forms of treatment, including the provision of food and fluids by artificial means, do not necessarily carry out a proposal to end life. One may rightly choose to withhold or withdraw a means of preserving life if the means employed is judged either useless or excessively burdensome. (May et al., 1987)

In the light of the controversial case of Terri Schiavo, Dan Sulmasy, a physician and a member of a Catholic religious order as well as a holder of a doctorate in bioethics, showed that the Catholic tradition is in agreement with the conclusion of this group of bioethicists. He showed that the idea of burdensome or useless means of life support— including nutrition and hydration—goes back as far as the 4th century in Catholic thinking and has been endorsed regularly since the 16th century. In discussing tube feedings for critically and terminally ill patients, he concludes that "tube feeding in these types of patients will often result in great burden, no net benefit, and multiple complications and will in many, many cases meet criteria by which the treatment could be considered extraordinary or morally optional" (Sulmasy, 2005).

Our conclusion seems inescapable: Nutrition and hydration should always be initially presumed to be beneficial, but there are special exceptions. This applies to competent patients who normally should be able to express in their own words whether they are receiving benefit from nutrition and hydration that are offered. It also applies to the case of incompetent patients for whom the responsible surrogate decision maker must decide. This is likely to be the parents in the case of newborns, infants, and small children. As long as that decision maker is within the limits of reason, society should accept that person's judgment. The hospital ethics committee responsible for Jimmy McCarthy's medical treatment accepted the parents' judgment as well within reason and honored their wish to withhold intravenous feeding. That decision meant that the infant died somewhat sooner than he otherwise would have, but he was spared the weeks or months of suffering that would have accompanied the long string of surgeries and other medical interventions that would have had to take place before his eventual, inevitable death.

Special Public Policy Problems in Forgoing Nutrition and Hydration

These moral conclusions about forgoing nutrition and hydration apply to all human beings—adults, children, and infants, the mentally competent as well as the incompetent (including those with intellectual disabilities). In general, if a treatment such as medically supplied nutrition and hydration can be withheld from those without intellectual disabilities who have medical problems, then it can be withheld from those who have such disabilities and who have similar medical problems. Only in special situations, which will be discussed later in this chapter, might the presence of a disability be relevant in deciding about forgoing treatment.

While that is a conclusion that represents a widespread consensus of both conservative and liberal thinkers, when we examine public policies about forgoing life support, we discover some odd and complicated restrictions that need to be addressed. In particular, some state laws treat the act of forgoing nutrition and hydration as unique and have strange and controversial implications—especially for patients who are not mentally competent to make their own decisions. Also, the federal government promulgated regulations often called the "Baby Doe Regulations" that have important legal implications for babies for whom nutrition and hydration might be withheld. The babies who were the focus of the controversy that generated these regulations were babies with intellectual disabilities. We need to examine this legal situation to see if it is justified.

State Laws Requiring Nutrition and Hydration

In the 1980s, when the issues of nutrition and hydration first surfaced, many states were actively adopting laws that governed advance directives and related decisions to forgo life support. These laws were designed to clarify the legal status of documents (generically called "advance directives") in which people stated their wishes about terminal care. These laws began to be adopted in 1976 (California, 1976). At that time, the presumption was that people would use their advance directives to refuse major technological interventions such as organ transplants, hemodialysis, and mechanical ventilators. Eventually, however, people realized they might also want to refuse more common and simple interventions such as antibiotics, routine medications, and even medically supplied nutrition and hydration.

By the 1980s, many states were active in passing such legislation. Since cases had occurred in which competent persons or surrogates on behalf of incompetent persons were refusing nutrition and hydration (Cruzan, 1988, p. 8; New Jersey, 1983), state legislation sometimes explicitly addressed decisions to forgo these treatment modalities. The result has been that the right of patients to refuse nutrition and hydration varies from state to state.

Some states presume that nutrition and hydration will be administered even for patients who have written an advance directive refusing life support unless the directive specifically directs the withholding or withdrawal of food and fluids (see Table 11.1). Other states create no presumption about the withholding or withdrawing of nutrition and hydration.

In addition to state policies regarding the interpretation of advance directives of competent patients, states also vary in whether they will let a surrogate make a decision to forgo nutrition or hydration for their wards. Some explicitly authorize such decisions. Others limit surrogate decisions to cases in which the patient, while competent, previously and explicitly addressed nutrition and hydration.

Thus, even if a person with IDD is mentally competent to make his or her own medical decisions and is legally capable of exercising an advance directive, it is critical that the individual clearly states whether nutrition and hydration are included in any statements refusing life support.

Of course, many persons with such disability may not be legally competent and, in fact, may never have been so. Surely, this would be true of all infants and children. Laws that address only the right of competent persons to accept or refuse nutrition and hydration leave such persons exposed. One plausible interpretation is that the presumption in favor of providing these supports applies in the case of these individuals. A significant number of states authorize surrogates to withhold or withdraw so-called artificial nutrition and hydration if it is consistent with the patient's wishes in an advance directive, but this only would be relevant in cases in which the patient was at one time capable of writing such a directive. A few states authorize surrogates to withhold or withdraw if the patient's wishes are unknown and/or an advance directive does not exist (or such wishes are not explicitly stated in the directive).

The net result is that in many states a person with IDD who has never been in a position to exercise a valid advance directive may have no one who can determine that nutrition and hydration may ever be withheld. If Jimmy McCarthy were in one of these many states, he would be left with an imperative to be supplied as long as he lives even if his parents concluded it was not in his interest and even if his health care delivery team and the family's church advisors concurred. Persons with IDD who have never been able to express their own views may not have the same rights as competent persons to avoid such treatment no matter how painful or burdensome the result may be. On the other hand, they may be aggressively protected against surrogates who attempt to make treatment-forgoing decisions on their behalf.

Table 11.1

State Policies Regarding Forgoing Nutrition and Hydration

States banning withdrawal of artificial nutrition and hydration in all cases	Missouri
States presuming the administration of nutrition and hydration unless an advance directive directs withholding or withdrawal	Arizona, Florida, Georgia, Kentucky, Iowa, Michigan, Minnesota, New Hampshire, New Jersey, North Carolina, North Dakota, Oklahoma, Oregon, Pennsylvania, South Carolina, Tennessee
States that create no presumption about the withholding or withdrawal of artificial nutrition and hydration	Alabama, Arkansas, Louisiana, Montana, New Mexico, New York, Ohio, Texas, Utah, Virginia
States where surrogates may authorize withholding or withdrawal of artificial nutrition and hydration if it is consistent with patient's wishes in advance directive	Alabama, Arizona, Arkansas, Colorado, Connecticut, Delaware, Florida, Georgia, Idaho, Iowa, Kentucky, Louisiana, Maine, Maryland, Massachusetts, Mississippi, Nevada, New Hampshire, New Mexico, New York, North Dakota, Ohio, Oklahoma, Oregon, South Carolina, South Dakota, Utah, Vermont, Virginia, West Virginia, Wyoming
States where surrogates may authorize withholding or withdrawal of artificial nutrient and hydration if patient's wishes are unknown and/or an advance directive does not exist and/or instructions are not explicitly stated in the advance directive	Louisiana, Maine, New Mexico, New York, South Dakota, Vermont, West Virginia, Wyoming
States with no mention of surrogates	Illinois, Montana, Indiana, Rhode Island

Note. Adapted from "Terminating Artificial Nutrition and Hydration in Persistent Vegetative State patients: Current and Proposed State Laws," by D. Larriviere and R. J. Bonnie, 2006, American Academy of Neurology, 66, pp. 1624–1628; and "Refusing Artificial Nutrition and Hydration: Does Statutory Law Send the Wrong Message?" by C. E. Sieger, J. F. Arnold, and J. C. Ahronheim, 2002, Journal of the American Geriatrics Society, 50, pp. 544–550.

Baby Doe Regulations Requirement of "Appropriate Nutrition"

Thus, the legal status of persons with IDD when it comes to state law governing decisions to forgo nutrition and hydration is confusing. All of this is embedded, however, in an even more confusing set of federal regulations that apply to what the government calls "infants."

In 1982, a baby born in Indiana with Down syndrome and a cardiac septal defect was left to die on the basis of his parents' decision not to provide treatment (Indiana Supreme Ct., 1982). The records were sealed, so little is known about the case. According to some interpretations, the cardiac defect was severe and had only a 50% chance of being corrected with surgery, even with repeated operations. In the minds of some people, the burdens related to the surgeries and the bleak prognosis might justify the parental decision. In the minds of others, the parental decision was not justified.

Regardless of the interpretation of that case, it stimulated considerable public debate and led to the Reagan administration's development of legislation calling for regulations called the "Baby Doe Regulations." After several false starts, a set of regulations was promulgated that requires every state receiving federal funds for activities to protect against child abuse to have in place regulations conforming with federal standards (U.S. Department of Health and Human Services, 1985). Under these standards no infant can be allowed to die by the forgoing of life support unless one of three conditions is met:

1. The infant is chronically and irreversibly comatose.
2. The provision of such treatment would merely prolong dying, not be effective in ameliorating or correcting all of the infant's life-threatening conditions, or otherwise be futile in terms of the survival of the infant.
3. The provision of such treatment would be virtually futile in terms of the survival of the infant and the treatment itself under such circumstances would be inhumane.

Even if one of these conditions is met, the decision makers for the infant's medical care must provide "appropriate nutrition, hydration, and medication." This raises the question of exactly what is meant by "appropriate" in these circumstances.

Two interpretations of what would be "inappropriate nutrition" have been suggested. The more obvious meaning would permit omission only of nutrition that would cause explicit medical harm (e.g., oral feeding of a baby with a tracheoesophageal fistula, an opening between the trachea and the esophagus that would permit food particles to pass into the lungs, a potentially lethal development). Under this more conservative interpretation, oral feeding in such a case would be excluded, but intravenous or nasogastric feeding would be required since food could then not enter the lungs. Likewise, under this more conservative interpretation, a food to which a baby was allergic would be excluded, as would purines for a baby with phenylketonuria. The requirement of "appropriate feeding" has been widely assumed to permit exclusion only of those kinds of feeding that would produce direct medical harm to the baby.

Since the days of the writing of the regulations, there has also existed a second interpretation of "inappropriate nutrition." One might claim that any feeding that fails to satisfy the proportionality criterion could plausibly be called inappropriate. This suggests that any food that produced no benefit or did more harm than good for a baby could be excluded as inappropriate. Recalling the rich discussion of what counts as disproportional means of providing nutrition and hydration, this interpretation could permit exclusion of some feeding that did not produce direct medical harm (such as in the case of the tracheoesophageal fistula or allergy). It could permit excluding any feeding that leaves the child with additional burdens. It could conceivably permit excluding intravenous feeding in the case of Jimmy McCarthy on the grounds that the feeding would preserve his life so that he survives to experience the significant burdens of repeated surgery. Some decision makers, such as Jimmy's parents, could argue that the benefits of the feeding are exceeded by the burdens of the surgeries (especially since he is inevitably going to die fairly soon anyway).

These two interpretations are substantially different. In the decades since the promulgation of these Baby Doe Regulations, no litigation or regulatory action has ever clarified which interpretation is correct. Since most of the infants who are plausible candidates for forgoing nutrition and hydration have IDD, the interests of, indeed the lives of, this group of patients hangs in the balance.

INFANTS VERSUS OTHER PERSONS WITH PERMANENT DISABILITIES

There is a final puzzle in the Baby Doe Regulations. It is clear that they apply only to "infants," not to other persons who are permanently impaired and have never been able to express their views about nutrition and hydration. Hence, if the more obvious, conservative interpretation of "appropriate feeding" is assumed, parents are restricted from refusing nutrition and hydration for their infants even though, at least in some states, they would be permitted to refuse the same feeding for their small children who had exactly the same medical conditions. Since the small children are not "infants," the Baby Doe Regulations would not apply. This is surely a serious flaw in the Baby Doe Regulations. There is no relevant difference between an infant and a small child in terms of their ability to make their own rational, autonomous decisions about life support, including nutrition and hydration. Whether one holds that no permanently impaired person should ever have nutrition and hydration withheld or holds the more plausible position, endorsed by Catholic theologians and most other reasonable people, that in rare instances medically supplied nutrition and hydration may present greater harm than benefit, there seems no justifiable reason to have one federal rule apply to infants and another to other people who have never been able to express their own views.

The problem is made more difficult by the ambiguity in the federal regulations about how "infant" is defined. The Baby Doe Regulations define an "infant" as "an infant of less than one year of age." In defining "infant," the regulations use the word "infant," which provides little information. The regulations state that "in addition to their applicability to infants less than one year of age, the standards set forth in paragraph (b)(2) of this section should be consulted thoroughly in the evaluation of any issue of medical neglect involving an *infant older than one year of age* who has been continuously hospitalized since birth, who was born extremely prematurely, or who has a long-term disability" (emphasis added). The term "infant" is used in such a way as to lead one to believe that an "infant" could be older than one year of age, but the regulation establishes no point at which an individual is no longer an infant.

A FINAL WORD

The central theme of this chapter is that persons with IDD deserve the same treatment as those without such impairments. This therefore means recognizing the rare instances in cases for individuals with IDD in which medically supplied nutrition and hydration do more harm than good and therefore can be withheld or withdrawn. There is, however, a special qualification. It could be that intellectual disability itself impacts the judgment about the extent of benefit and burden that a patient can experience.

Consider the case of a child who faces the prospect of repeated surgery with nevertheless a very bleak prognosis. For example, a very bright 12-year-old girl who had experienced many cardiac surgeries was now facing the prospect of a heart transplant even though that transplant had little chance of solving her total medical problems (Kuehl, Shapiro, & Sivasubramanian, 1992). She and her parents faced the question of whether to refuse the transplant on the grounds that the burdens of this and future surgeries exceeded the benefits. It was considered relevant in that decision that, since she was very bright and mature, a significant part of her agony was the mental anguish of realizing that she was facing repeated painful and difficult surgeries. Most people consider it legitimate to take this mental suffering into account in deciding whether the burdens exceed the expected benefits.

Now imagine that a patient with severe intellectual disability faced a similar set of difficult operations but lacked the mental capacity to understand her future and therefore she suffered differently. It is possible that intellectual disability could be a relevant factor in determining the level of benefit and burden that the patient would experience. In this case, it is conceivable that the person with intellectual disability could be said to suffer less. In that case, one might argue that two patients facing the same set of medical procedures experience different levels of benefit and burden and that, in this case, the one with intellectual impairment might suffer less from the surgeries. If so, the burdens and benefits might be such that the intellectually aware child should not receive the surgery, but the intellectually impaired child should receive them.

The morally relevant criterion is the comparison of benefit and burden. If the burden is less in a patient with intellectual disability, one might conclude that the same operation that a person without impairment could justifiably refuse would still be appropriate treatment for someone who would not suffer with the anticipation of knowing the long medical course ahead of him.

Needless to say, it is possible that in some cases, the intellectual disability could conceivably make the suffering worse because of a lack of understanding. In 1977, a man with severe intellectual impairment was deemed an inappropriate candidate for chemotherapy (which had only a modest chance of success) on the grounds that he could not understand why his trusted caregivers were "turning on him" and sticking him with needles repeatedly (Mass., 1977). In this case, it seems that the intellectual impairment was relevant in the judgment, and that the treatment presented a greater burden than it would have been to an intellectually able patient similarly situated.

What seems relevant here is that the same burden-benefit ratio that justifies forgoing treatments—including nutrition and hydration—in an intellectually normal person would justify the decision in a person with impairment (even if the intellectual status is relevant in determining the levels of burden experienced).

Conclusion

State laws and the Baby Doe Regulations are wrong if they require nutrition and hydration for all intellectually disabled persons, including babies. Almost all babies, including almost all babies with intellectual disabilities, require nutrition and hydration, but there are exceptions. If nutrition and hydration could be legitimately foregone in a baby or child without intellectual disabilities, it could also legitimately be foregone in one with such disabilities facing the same burden and benefit pattern.

References

Advance directives statutory links for states with Ascension Health ministries: State-by-state analysis of advance directive laws. (n.d.). Retrieved July 21, 2009, from http://www.ascensionhealth.org/ethics/public/issues/ADR_StatebyState_5305.pdf

California Chapter 1439, Code, Health and Safety, sec. 7185–7195 (Natural Death Act 1976).

Callahan, D. (1983). On feeding the dying. *The Hastings Center Report, 13*(5), 22.

Cruzan v. Harmon 760 S.W.2d 408 (Mo.banc 1988).

Duff, R. S., & Campbell, A. G. M. (1973). Moral and ethical dilemmas in the special-care nursery. *New England Journal of Medicine, 289*, 890–894.

Graber, G. C. (1979). Some questions about double effect. *Ethics in Science and Medicine, 6*(1), 65–84.

Gustafson, J. M. (1973, Spring). Mongolism, parental desires, and the right to life. *Perspectives in Biology and Medicine, 16*, 529–557.

Indiana Supreme Ct. (1982, May 27). In re Infant Doe, No. GU 8204-00 (Cir. Ct. Monroe County, Ind. April 12, 1982). *writ of mandamus dismissed sub nom.* State *ex rel.* Infant *Doe v. Baker*, No. 482 S 140 (Indiana Supreme Ct., May 27, 1982) (case mooted by child's death).

Kuehl, K. S., Shapiro, S., & Sivasubramanian, K. N. (1992). Should a school honor a student's DNR order? Case history of S. A. *Kennedy Institute of Ethics Journal, 2*, 1–3.

Larriviere, D., & Bonnie, R. J. (2006). Terminating artificial nutrition and hydration in persistent vegetative state patients: Current and proposed state laws. *American Academy of Neurology, 66*, 1624–1628.

Lynn, J., & Childress, J. F. (1983, October). Must patients always be given food and water? *The Hastings Center Report, 13*, 17–21.

Lyons, D. (1965). *Forms and limits of utilitarianism.* Oxford: Oxford University Press.

Marquis, D. B. (1991). Four versions of double effect. *Journal of Medicine and Philosophy, 16*, 515–544.

May, W. E., et al. (1987) Feeding and hydrating the permanently unconscious and other vulnerable persons. *Issues in Law and Medicine, 3*(3), 203–217.

Meilaender, G. (1984). On removing food and water: Against the stream. *The Hastings Center Report, 14*(6), 11–13.

New Jersey Superior Court. (1983). Chancery Division, In the Matter of Claire C. Conroy Essex County, Docket No. P-19083E, Decided February 2.

Pellegrino, E. D. (1995). Intending to kill and the principle of double effect. In T. L. Beauchamp & R. M. Veatch (Eds.), *Ethical issues in death and dying* (2nd ed., pp. 240–242). Englewood Cliffs, NJ: Prentice-Hall.

Pope Pius XII. (1984, Spring). The prolongation of life: An address of Pope Pius XII to an international congress of anesthesiologists. *The Pope Speaks, 4*, 393–398.

President's Commission for the Study of Ethical Problems in Medicine and Biomedical and Behavioral Research. (1983). *Deciding to forego life-sustaining treatment: Ethical, medical, and legal issues in treatment decisions.* Washington, DC: U.S. Government Printing Office.

Rawls, J. (1955). Two concepts of rules. *Philosophical Review, 44*, 3–32.

Sieger, C. E., Arnold, J. F., & Ahronheim, J. C. (2002). Refusing artificial nutrition and hydration: Does statutory law send the wrong message? *Journal of the American Geriatrics Society, 50*, 544–550.

Sulmasy, D. P. (2005, Summer). Terri Schiavo and the Roman Catholic tradition of forgoing extraordinary means of care. *Journal of Law, Medicine & Ethics, 33*, 359–362.

Superintendent of Belchertown State Sch. v. Saikewicz, 370 N.E.2d 417, 432 (Mass. 1977).

U.S. Department of Health and Human Services. (1985). Child abuse and neglect prevention and treatment program: Final rule: 45 CFR 1340. *Federal Register: Rules and Regulations, 50*(72), 14878–14892.

CHAPTER 12

The Persistent Vegetative State

DAVID L. COULTER

INTRODUCTION

Jennett and Plum (1972) coined the term "persistent vegetative state" (PVS) to describe the state of patients who were living a "merely physical life devoid of intellectual activity or social intercourse." Others had described similar patients and coined different terms prior to 1972 (Jennett, 2002, pp. 1–6), but Jennett and Plum's term became widely accepted and is generally used today. Broad usage, however, does not mean that all who use the term "PVS" are in agreement.

An attempt was made between 1992 and 1993 to bring some standardization to the diagnosis and prognosis of PVS. Five professional medical societies—the American Academy of Neurology, the American Academy of Pediatrics, the Child Neurology Society, the American Association of Neurological Surgeons, and the American Neurological Association—joined together to create the "Multi-Society Task Force on the Persistent Vegetative State." Each society sent two members to the Task Force,[1] which then reviewed the literature and developed a consensus report that was published in 1994 (Multi-Society Task Force on PVS, 1994). The report clarified the diagnosis, established diagnostic criteria, reviewed the causes, and described the types of pathological findings reported in the brain of patients with PVS. Prognosis was considered in terms of recovery of consciousness and recovery of overall functioning. Prognostic data were derived from analysis of 754 published cases of PVS (603 adults and 151 children). The Task Force explicitly confined its report to medical aspects of PVS, since it believed that it could find a broad consensus on these medical issues. It recognized that a similar consensus on the legal and ethical aspects of the problem did not exist and felt that these issues were best considered elsewhere. Similarly, this chapter will cover primarily the medical aspects of PVS.

The 1994 report of the Task Force still stands and has not been revised. Professional societies in the United States and elsewhere have adopted versions of the definition and criteria for diagnosis as described in the Task Force report (American Academy of

---

1. The author of this chapter was a member of the Task Force representing the Child Neurology Society.

Neurology, 1995; Royal College of Physicians, 1996). Two major concepts have been added in the past 15 years, however. First, the distinction between PVS and the "minimally conscious state" (MCS) has become more widely recognized. And second, functional neuroimaging has provided an opportunity to investigate subconscious activity in patients who seem to be in coma or PVS. These concepts will be discussed below.

DEFINITION OF PVS

According to the Multi-Society Task Force, "The vegetative state is a condition of complete unawareness of the self and the environment, accompanied by sleep-wake cycles, with either complete or partial preservation of hypothalamic and brainstem autonomic responses" (Multi-Society Task Force on PVS, 1994). PVS is not the same as coma, although coma may develop into PVS. In a coma, the patient is unaware and unresponsive but does not have sleep-wake cycles. Patients in a coma do not open their eyes spontaneously and do not appear to be awake, but patients in PVS do. Patients usually do not remain in coma for more than 2 to 4 weeks after an acute event. After that period of time, patients generally become conscious (eyes open spontaneously with awareness of the self and environment), or they enter a vegetative state (eyes open spontaneously with no awareness of the self or environment). Patients who are said to be in a "permanent coma" are usually in PVS.

The term "vegetative state" simply describes the condition of the patient at a given point in time and does not by itself indicate a prognosis. Jennett and Plum originally used the term "persistent" to describe patients who remain in a vegetative state for a long period of time (1972). Others have chosen to use the term "permanent" to describe the vegetative state in these patients. Thus, "PVS" has come to mean "persistent vegetative state" to some and "permanent vegetative state" to others. This confusion is unfortunate, because the two terms are not equivalent. *Persistent* means that the vegetative state has been present for a period of time and is still present. *Permanent* means that in the opinion of the user of the term, the patient is not likely to ever recover consciousness. Thus, "persistent vegetative state" is a diagnosis of the patient's present condition, while "permanent vegetative state" is a statement of the prognosis (Multi-Society Task Force on PVS, 1994). In general, a vegetative state that is still present 1 month after the onset of coma may be termed "persistent" but should not be considered "permanent" until sufficient time has passed to indicate that the likelihood of recovery is negligible.

DIAGNOSIS OF PVS AND RELATED CONDITIONS

The Multi-Society Task Force outlined criteria for diagnosis of a vegetative state, which are listed in Table 12.1. These consensus criteria convey the essence of the diagnosis, that the patient is "awake but unaware" and unable to respond to others. The criteria also note that patients in a vegetative state have preserved "vegetative" functions (such as breathing, circulation, digestion, and elimination), which may permit long-term survival with appropriate care. The criteria of the Royal College of Physicians (1996) are shown in Table 12.2 for comparison. The British criteria are in agreement on the basic concept but add some clarifying detail about the sort of findings that may be present. The "other

Table 12.1
Criteria for Diagnosis of the Vegetative State Multi-Society Task Force on PVS

1. No evidence of awareness of self or environment and an inability to interact with others

2. No evidence of sustained, reproducible, purposeful, or voluntary behavioral responses to visual, auditory, tactile, or noxious stimuli

3. No evidence of language comprehension or expression

4. Intermittent wakefulness manifested by the presence of sleep-wake cycles

5. Sufficiently preserved hypothalamic and brainstem autonomic functions to permit survival with medical and nursing care

6. Bowel and bladder incontinence

7. Variably preserved cranial nerve reflexes and spinal reflexes

Table 12.2
Criteria for Diagnosis of the Vegetative State: Royal College of Physicians
Three clinical criteria must be fulfilled:

1. No evidence of awareness of self or environment; no volitional response to visual, auditory, tactile, or noxious stimuli; no evidence of language comprehension or expression

2. Cycles of eye closure and opening simulating sleep and waking

3. Sufficiently preserved hypothalamic and brainstem function to maintain respiration and circulation

Other clinical features:

1. Incontinence of bladder and bowel; spontaneous blinking and usually retained pupillary and corneal responses

2. No visual fixation, visual tracking of moving objects, or visual response to threats

3. May have occasional movements of the head and eyes toward sound or movement and of trunk or limbs in a purposeless way

4. May have startle myoclonus or roving eye movements

5. May smile or may grimace to pain

clinical features" may be confusing to family members and inexperienced professionals, who may think that these occasional eye, face, or head movements are in fact indications of conscious awareness.

At what point do these occasional movements truly represent conscious awareness? This is the critical distinction between PVS and MCS. Consensus criteria for MCS are presented in Table 12.3 (Giacino, Ashwal, & Childs, 2002). The most important distinction is that in PVS there is absolutely *no* evidence of awareness or responsiveness

---

Table 12.3
Criteria for Diagnosis of MCS

1. Evidence of limited but clearly discernable awareness of the self and/or the environment, manifested by consistent, reproducible, or sustained performance of one or more interactive behaviors.

2. Interactive behaviors may include the following:

   A. Following of simple commands

   B. Verbal or gestural yes/no responses (regardless of accuracy)

   C. Intelligible verbalization

   D. Purposeful behavior (including movement or affective response) in a contingent relation to relevant stimuli, such as the following:

      1. Appropriate crying or smiling to relevant visual or linguistic stimuli

      2. Vocalization or gesture in response to questioning

      3. Reaching for objects in an appropriate direction and location

      4. Touching or holding objects by accommodating to the size and shape of the object

      5. Sustained visual fixation or tracking of a moving stimulus

---

whatsoever. If there is *any* credible evidence of awareness or responsiveness (as in Table 12.3), then MCS is a more likely diagnosis. The responsiveness of a person in MCS must be consistent and reproducible over time, and it must be interactive, that is, it occurs in response to an action by someone else. A person in PVS who is beginning to recover consciousness may initially show some very questionable responses that are not sufficient to establish the presence of conscious awareness. Over time, however, these responses may become more consistent and reproducible and thereby allow a diagnosis of MCS.

Diagnostic Problems

Two other conditions should be distinguished from PVS and MCS. One is the *locked-in state* in which the patient is completely conscious but paralyzed and unable to make any motor responses to indicate awareness of self and environment. It is well described in medical texts (Posner, Saper, Schiff, & Plum, 2007) but perhaps even better described in popular literature (Bauby, 1997). Generations of students and neurological trainees have failed their clinical exams because they did not look for evidence of a locked-in state in a patient who appeared to be completely unaware. Patients in a locked-in state can respond with great effort, and it is critical to recognize this fact when it is present.

The other condition that needs to be distinguished from PVS and MCS is *brain death*. Brain death is diagnosed when there is irreversible cessation of all functions of the brain, including the brainstem. The key distinction in patients with brain death is the absence of all brainstem function. If any brainstem functions are present (as in Tables 12.1 and 12.2), then PVS is a more appropriate diagnosis. Since brain death is sufficient to pronounce the patient dead, one should never diagnose brain death when there is even the slightest evidence of brainstem function. Although well-recognized criteria exist for diagnosing brain death, recent studies indicate that hospitals are inconsistent in the way that these diagnoses is made (Wijdicks, Rabinstein, Manno, & Atkinson, 2008).

Indeed, another cause for concern is the lack of precision with which the diagnosis of PVS is made. In several older studies, 15%–43% of patients initially diagnosed with PVS were eventually found not to be in a vegetative state (Andrews, Murphy, & Munday, 1996; Childs, Mercer, & Childs, 1993; Tresch, Sims, & Duthie, 1991). Sometimes a diagnosis of a vegetative state is made correctly, but insufficient time is provided to determine whether it will become permanent or not. In such cases, life support may be withdrawn from patients who might still have a prospect of recovering consciousness. Appropriate observation times are considered later.

The Task Force concluded that a diagnosis of a vegetative state could not be made in premature infants or in full-term infants less than 3 months of age due to the lack of validity of the diagnostic criteria before this age. The sole exception to this rule refers to infants who are born with a diagnosis of anencephaly, a severe congenital malformation in which the scalp, skull, and cerebral hemispheres are absent. Consciousness cannot develop because of the absence of these parts of the brain, but the presence of the brainstem in these infants means that they can survive in a permanent vegetative state.

CAUSES OF PVS

The Task Force recognized four categories of causes for PVS:

1. Severe developmental malformations other than anencephaly, such as hydranencephaly or lissencephaly. Infants with these conditions could be diagnosed with a vegetative state after 3 months of age.
2. Progressive neurological disorders, such as Tay-Sachs disease in children or Alzheimer's disease in adults. Individuals with these disorders may eventually reach a late stage of their disease in which consciousness is no longer present, and a vegetative state may be diagnosed.
3. Severe traumatic brain injury with initial coma that evolves into PVS.
4. Nontraumatic acute events, such as cardiac arrest, perinatal asphyxia, hypoxic-ischemic encephalopathy, near-drowning, suffocation, stroke, brain hemorrhage, cancer, meningoencephalitis, or poisoning

The pathology in cases of PVS relates to the etiology (Jennett, 2002). Evidence of thalamic damage is seen in 80%–95% of cases. In addition, diffuse subcortical axonal injury is present in 70% of traumatic cases, and diffuse laminar cortical necrosis is present in 65% of nontraumatic cases. The pathology in cases of severe developmental malformations and in cases of progressive neurological disorders reflects the specific underlying disease process.

PROGNOSIS

The Task Force reviewed the published evidence for recovery from PVS and identified 754 cases in which sufficient data were provided to be able to estimate the prognosis. These studies included 434 adults and 106 children with a traumatic etiology and 169 adults and 45 children with a nontraumatic etiology. The Task Force distinguished between recovery of consciousness and recovery of function. Recovery of consciousness occurred when the patient showed reliable evidence of awareness and the ability to interact with others. Recovery of function was assessed according to the Glasgow Outcome Scale (good function, moderate disability, severe disability, PVS, or death).

Recovery of consciousness occurred when the vegetative state had been present for less than 3 months following nontraumatic injuries and for less than 12 months following traumatic brain injuries (Multi-Society Task Force on PVS, 1994). After these periods of time had elapsed, recovery of consciousness was very unlikely to occur. Thus, the vegetative state could be considered to be *persistent* up until these periods of time had passed and to be *permanent* after these periods of time had passed.

This potential for recovery of consciousness is often unrecognized. Families may be told that the prognosis is hopeless when, in fact, the recommended observation periods (3 months after nontraumatic injury and 12 months after traumatic brain injury) have not yet passed (Payne, Taylor, & Stocking, 1996). Withdrawal of life support may then be recommended even though the patient still has a potential for recovery. Efforts to encourage organ donation from patients whose life support is being withdrawn may unintentionally cause families and caregivers to be unwilling to wait for the recommended observation periods.

Recovery of function is often incomplete. In the Task Force data, only 24% of adults and 27% of children who had been in a vegetative state for 1 month following traumatic brain injury were considered to be independent after 1 year (good function or moderate disability on the Glasgow Outcome Scale). Similarly, only 4% of adults and 6% of children who had been in a vegetative state for 1 month following nontraumatic brain injury were considered to be independent after 1 year. Late recoveries of consciousness have been reported (beyond the intervals noted earlier), but virtually always at a functional level of severe disability (Jennett, 2002; Multi-Society Task Force on PVS, 1994).

The Task Force concluded that the vegetative state could be considered to be permanent after 6 months of age in children with severe developmental malformations. The vegetative state could also be considered to be permanent after 3 months in patients with progressive neurological disorders. In these cases, recovery of consciousness or function is extremely unlikely.

Survival rates are difficult to measure. In the Task Force data, 34% of those in a vegetative state for 1 month were dead by 1 year after the causative event. Prolonged survival is not unusual, however, and depends on the quality of medical and nursing care. Clearly, survival rates are influenced by decisions to limit or withdraw care. When good care is provided, survival for 10 years or more is common.

Functional Neuroimaging

Positron emission tomography (PET) studies of patients in PVS have shown reductions in cerebral metabolic activity by 50% or more (Levy, Sidtis, & Rottenberg, 1987). In some patients with fragmentary behavior suggesting possible responsiveness, similar PET studies have demonstrated preservation of cerebral metabolic activity in brain regions possibly related to the observed behavior (Posner et al., 2007). PET studies in one patient who was in PVS 4 months following an attack of postinfectious demyelination demonstrated selective regional activation in the right occipital and posterior temporal areas, suggestively indicating minimal awareness without any behavioral evidence of responsiveness (Menon, Owen, & Williams, 1998). Functional magnetic resonance imaging studies in another patient who was in PVS 5 months after a traumatic brain injury showed imaging evidence of brain activity following the absence of any behavioral evidence of responsiveness, suggesting subclinical evidence for MCS (Owen, Coleman, & Boly, 2006). These studies have been controversial and their significance remains unclear. Much more research is needed to determine whether selective regional activation indicates nothing more than islands of relatively preserved circuitry in an otherwise devastated brain (and thus a permanent, rather than persistent, vegetative state) or alternatively represents early recovery from PVS to MCS: "It is critical, then, to identify residual capacity as opposed to isolated functional activity in the cortex. This will require prospective studies of large numbers of patients with early vegetative state, to determine if there are indices on functional imaging that can predict eventual improvement" (Posner et al., 2007, p. 372). Studies of this type have, however, not yet been organized.

TREATMENT

The basic elements of treatment for PVS involve comprehensive supportive care (Jennett, 2002). Nutrition and hydration typically require placement of a feeding tube. Although some nutrition may be swallowed orally by some individuals, it is not usually sufficient to maintain body weight and function. The choice of a nutritional product for chronic maintenance requires careful consideration of the individual's long-term metabolic needs. Periodic monitoring of body weight and laboratory tests to monitor metabolic levels, such as serum albumin levels, provides a measure of nutritional balance. Elimination usually requires assistance using stool softeners or other agents to promote regularity.

Coexisting medical problems must be addressed, such as diabetes or hypertension. If seizures are present, they should be treated appropriately. Individuals in a vegetative state are at risk for infections, especially respiratory and urinary tract infections. Measures to prevent infections are appropriate, and prompt treatment is essential to avoid septicemia and other complications. Skin care is critically important. Bedsores can develop quickly due to the immobility that is typically present and can become secondarily infected. Good nursing care requires frequent repositioning, monitoring for the emergence of pressure sores, and increasing interventions to prevent the sores from becoming open or infected.

Some form of physical therapy is generally required as part of comprehensive, supportive care. In order to avoid contractures, regular, frequent, daily movements of the extremities throughout the range of motion are essential. This is generally maintenance therapy and can be performed by nursing staff under the supervision of a physical therapist. It may be helpful to prevent complication from immobility by positioning the individual in supportive chairs and even possibly providing supportive weight bearing exercises. Once contractures develop, they can become extremely difficult if not impossible to reverse. Furthermore, contractures can cause significant problems in positioning the individual during waking and sleep. Medical treatment of spasticity with a variety of agents can hopefully prevent or minimize the development of contractures, but they are of limited usefulness once contractures have emerged.

Individuals in a persistent vegetative state may be transferred from an acute care unit to a rehabilitative unit as long as the caregivers believe there is a potential for the recovery of consciousness and function. When sufficient time has passed and recovery has not occurred, the individual may then be transferred to a chronic or long-term care facility. In some cases, the person may be able to return home if there are sufficient in-home nursing supports available to provide the needed care. The quality of care received in these long-term care facilities varies significantly from one program to another. One particularly exemplary facility is Santa Viola Hospital in Bologna, Italy. This is a small, relatively new, private hospital that cares for 30 to 40 patients in vegetative or minimally conscious states. All of the basic elements of supportive care described earlier are provided to the patients, and families are extensively involved on a regular basis. The atmosphere is light and stimulating, and the medical care is excellent. Unfortunately, programs of this quality are not widely available for many individuals in PVS.

A number of therapeutic interventions have been developed that seek to promote recovery of consciousness. Systematic sensory stimulation has been used for some time to try to prevent or reverse the chronic sensory deprivation that can develop over time. Whether or not this kind of external stimulation can promote recovery is harder to determine (Giacino, 1996). As with any such intervention, demonstration of effectiveness would require a randomized, controlled trial in which a large group of patients with fairly well-defined and comparable clinical situations are randomized to receive either the standard therapy that is usually provided or the standard therapy plus the intervention being studied. In the absence of such clear evidence of effectiveness, one can use common sense to apply those forms of sensory stimulation that make sense and are not excessively burdensome for the patient or the caregiver.

Direct electrical stimulation of the brain in patients in a vegetative state has been attempted in order to provide sensory stimulation more precisely to those parts of the brain that would seem to be important for arousal and awareness. Reports in the literature on this therapy are somewhat limited, however, and no randomized controlled trial is available for review. In one recent, long-term follow-up of deep brain stimulation for patients in a vegetative or minimally conscious state, 8 of 21 patients in a vegetative state became conscious and able to obey verbal commands but continued to exhibit severe disabilities. Four of five patients in a MCS recovered sufficiently to return to their own homes (Yamamoto, Kobayashi, & Kasai, 2004). Although these results appear somewhat encouraging, they have not been replicated sufficiently to justify a clinical recommendation for this type of therapy.

WITHDRAWAL OF CARE

At some point after the onset of the vegetative state, limitation or withdrawal of care may be considered. According to the American Academy of Neurology (1995),

> Physicians and the family must determine appropriate levels of treatment relative to the administration or withdrawal of medication and other commonly ordered treatments, supplemental oxygen and the use of antibiotics, complex

organ-sustaining treatments such as dialysis, administration of blood products, and artificial nutrition and hydration. Once PVS is considered to be permanent, a "do not attempt resuscitation" order is appropriate.

The ethical and legal aspects of limiting care in the United States, Great Britain and other countries are discussed extensively (Jennett, 2002). In general, the practice guideline quoted above is widely accepted in the United States but not necessarily in other countries.

The guideline notes that cardiopulmonary resuscitation (CPR) may not be appropriate when a patient is in a permanent vegetative state. "Permanent" is defined in the practice guideline according to the description provided earlier in this chapter: persistence of the vegetative state more than 3 months after a nontraumatic event and more than 12 months after a traumatic event. From an ethical perspective, individuals in a permanent vegetative state are not felt to have any long-term interests that would justify the imposition of any risk. Thus, the implication is that CPR cannot benefit the patient, since the patient will never recover consciousness anyway and can only impose a risk of injury or additional disability. From this perspective, an order to withhold CPR ("do not attempt resuscitation") makes sense. The family needs to agree with this approach, of course. The treatment team needs to be aware of the family's cultural, religious, social, and personal perspectives and must discuss the medical facts with the family in such a way that everyone understands the risks, benefits, and alternatives available. Once a decision is made to withhold resuscitation, the order needs to be written to clearly define for all involved exactly what is to be done or not done in the event of a life-threatening medical emergency.

In the same way, the treatment team needs to discuss with the family precisely what care should be provided in the event of a medical condition that may not be immediately life threatening. For example, if the patient develops a fever and respiratory distress, the family may elect to provide oxygen by mask and antipyretic treatment to ensure patient comfort but may also decide to defer antibiotics and "let nature take its course." The family would want to consider whether or not the patient should be moved to an acute care setting—such as a hospital emergency department—or should be allowed to remain in the chronic care setting. If the expectation is that the medical condition may be terminal, the treatment team and the family may decide together to allow the individual to die in the more comfortable chronic care setting, surrounded by familiar and loving people.

Considerable controversy surrounds the question of withdrawal of "artificial nutrition and hydration" as mentioned in the practice guideline. "Artificial" in this sense means that nutrition and hydration are provided by some means other than oral ingestion, usually by tube feeding. The practice guideline suggests that withdrawal of tube feeding may be appropriate in some situations, but it does not specify how this is to be determined. In fact, extensive literature has developed over the past 25 years concerning this topic. One of the key issues has been whether or not tube feeding constitutes medical treatment or not. Those who consider it a form of medical treatment argue that it can be withdrawn or withheld just like any other form of medical treatment. Those who consider it a form of basic care believe that it should be provided to all individuals out of respect for their human dignity and worth. Religious authorities have also differed on this point. For example, even though Pope John Paul II declared that he believed artificial nutrition to be a form of basic care, he did not invoke the full weight of papal authority and left the issue open for further discussion. These issues are discussed further in chapters 10 and 11.

One point upon which there should be general agreement is that once the decision has been made to withdraw artificial nutrition and hydration, both nutrition and hydration should be withdrawn. Continuing to provide hydration only prolongs the dying process and leads to starvation and wasting. When both are withdrawn, death usually occurs within a few days or weeks at the most.

Organ Donation

In the United States, all hospitals are strongly encouraged to do everything possible to encourage organ donation when patients are going to die. Continued accreditation depends on how well the hospital accomplishes this goal. Recently, hospitals have been asked to develop and implement protocols to increase organ donation by clarifying and streamlining the process of organ donation after life-sustaining treatment has been withdrawn. This is called "donation after cardiac death" (DCD) to distinguish it from organ donation after brain death. Once brain death has been declared, the patient is legally dead and organs can be removed for transplantation (assuming the patient or family gives consent). DCD does not involve brain death, however. DCD protocols involve withdrawing life-sustaining treatment, waiting for the heart to stop beating ("cardiac death") in order to declare the patient legally dead, and removing the patient's organs for transplantation (Steinbrook, 2007).

In order to be considered to be a candidate for DCD, the patient must be receiving life-sustaining treatment. This usually means that the patient is on ventilatory support; when the ventilator is "turned off," the patient's heart is likely to stop beating. Although some patients in a persistent vegetative state may be on ventilatory support, many are not, and so they would not be considered for DCD. (Withdrawal of artificial nutrition and hydration does not lead to death in a sufficiently predictable way to allow such patients to be considered for DCD.)

A further requirement before considering DCD is that the treatment team and family must have decided to withdraw life-sustaining treatment independent of the decision to pursue organ donation. Thus, the decision to withdraw life-sustaining treatment is not considered to be part of the DCD protocol. In practice, this means that the DCD process does not provide any consideration regarding the validity of the decision to withdraw life-sustaining treatment. For example, doctors might tell a family that their ventilator-dependent son, who is still in a vegetative state 3 months after a severe traumatic brain injury, will never recover and that the case is hopeless. Even though this prognosis is wrong, based on the data reviewed earlier in this chapter, the family may be convinced to withdraw ventilatory support and allow their son to die a cardiac death. Once that decision has been made, the patient would then be a candidate for DCD. Under existing DCD protocols, nothing would prevent the transplant surgeon from going forward and removing organs from the patient after his heart stops beating, even though he might have recovered consciousness eventually and lived a productive, meaningful life if treatment had been maintained.

This is not just a theoretical possibility, given the high rate of misdiagnosis of the vegetative state and the low rate of knowledge about prognosis by physicians and others described earlier. In theory, DCD could be a reasonable option for families when the diagnosis and prognosis are accurate and valid. In practice, however, existing DCD protocols provide no mechanism for preventing mistakes of this sort and thus represent a potential threat to the lives of patients with profound neurological disability. Certainly further refinement of DCD protocols could resolve this problem, and efforts will be needed to collect the data required to make this happen.

PERSPECTIVE

Individuals with intellectual or developmental disabilities (IDD) are rarely in a vegetative state. There are some severe congenital brain malformations or birth injuries that can cause a persistent vegetative state, and a vegetative state may develop after severe traumatic and nontraumatic events. Individuals with Down syndrome (as well as others with IDD) may develop a progressive dementia that may end in a vegetative state. In general, the diagnostic criteria described in Tables 12.1 and 12.2 are relevant for these individuals just as they are for the general population. In some situations involving people with profound disabilities at a low baseline level of functioning, loss of additional function may be difficult to determine, however, the diagnosis of the vegetative state is based on present functioning regardless of baseline. For example, a person with Down syndrome may never have had much speech, so "absence of language comprehension or expression" may not have much meaning as a criterion for the vegetative state. Nonetheless, this criterion must be met (together with all of the other criteria) before the person with Down syndrome can be diagnosed as being in a vegetative state.

The prognostic data reviewed earlier are based on published reports of individuals who did not have IDD before developing a vegetative state. Little or no data exist describing the outcomes when individuals with IDD experience a severe traumatic or nontraumatic event that causes coma and eventually leads to a vegetative state. Given the diagnostic difficulties noted earlier, collection of this data is not likely to occur in the near future. Thus, it is probably best to assume that the prognosis for recovery from the vegetative state is the same for individuals with IDD as it is for the general population. Although this is admittedly an assumption that is not based on published evidence, no evidence exists to support an alternative assumption, and the simpler proposition would seem more useful in general practice.

Making decisions about treatment may be complicated when individuals with IDD have not had an opportunity to express competent wishes regarding what they would like to be done in the event that they develop a vegetative state. Even though a fully competent "living will" or health care proxy may not be possible, the patient's long-term guardians, caretakers, friends, and others should be able to provide an indication of what the individual preferred and enjoyed when well. Issues related to the decision-making process are described in chapters 8 and 17. When this information about the patient's previous preferences is taken into account, the previous treatment considerations should be as relevant for individuals with IDD as they are for the general population.

Perhaps the greatest concern when individuals with IDD develop a vegetative state is the potential for premature withdrawal of life-sustaining treatment based on assumptions about when (or if) recovery will occur and what level of function is possible if the patient survives. Given the pressure on hospitals to increase organ donation and to implement protocols for DCD (Steinbrook, 2007), premature withdrawal of life-sustaining treatment is likely to occur for these individuals. The only way to prevent this from happening is through greater awareness regarding the criteria for diagnosis of the vegetative state, meticulous attention to ensure that these criteria are met, careful distinction from MCS, and strict adherence to published information regarding the prognosis for recovery of consciousness and function. Unfortunately, the literature suggests that many physicians do not have the information necessary to do this, and the DCD process provides no mechanism for preventing premature withdrawal of life-sustaining treatment, so continued vigilance is required.

Finally, the potential for functional neuroimaging to reveal preserved areas of presumably conscious awareness in patients who might appear otherwise to be in a vegetative state needs to be pursued through further research. The present state of this research is too preliminary to draw any conclusions regarding the possibility of recovery from a vegetative state. In the future, when a patient develops a vegetative state that persists long enough to question whether recovery will occur (and to question whether life-sustaining treatment should be continued), one hopes that well-validated techniques such as functional neuroimaging will be performed before life-sustaining treatment is withdrawn. One also hopes that new techniques will be developed to increase the possibility for recovery of consciousness and function, perhaps using new drugs, surgery, or other rehabilitative technologies. The search for better diagnosis and treatment of the vegetative state must go forward.

REFERENCES

American Academy of Neurology. (1995). Practice parameter: Assessment and management of patients in the persistent vegetative state. *Neurology, 45*, 1015–1018.

Andrews, K., Murphy, L., & Munday, R. (1996). Misdiagnosis of the vegetative state: Retrospective study in a rehabilitation unit. *British Medical Journal, 313*, 13–16.

Bauby, J.-D. (1997). *The diving bell and the butterfly.* New York: Vintage Books.

Childs, N. L., Mercer, W. N., Childs, H. W. (1993). Accuracy of diagnosis of persistent vegetative state. *Neurology, 43*, 1465–1467.

Giacino, J. T. (1996). Sensory stimulation: Theoretical perspectives and the evidence for effectiveness. *Neurorehabilitation, 6*, 69–78.

Giacino, J. T., Ashwal, S., & Childs, N. (2002). The minimally conscious state: Definition and diagnostic criteria. *Neurology, 58*, 349–353.

Jennett, B. (2002). *The vegetative state: Medical facts, ethical and legal dilemmas.* New York: Cambridge University Press.

Jennett, B., & Plum, F. (1972). Persistent vegetative state after brain damage: A syndrome in search of a name. *Lancet, 1*, 734–737.

Levy, D. E., Sidtis, J. J., & Rottenberg, D. A. (1987). Differences in cerebral blood flow and glucose utilization in vegetative versus locked-in patients. *Annals of Neurology, 22*, 673–682.

Menon, D. K., Owen, A. M., & Williams, F. J. (1998). Cortical processing in the persistent vegetative state. *Lancet, 352*, 1148–1149.

Multi-Society Task Force on PVS. (1994). Medical aspects of the persistent vegetative state. Part 1 and 2. *New England Journal of Medicine, 330*, 1499–1508, 1572–1579.

Owen, A. M., Coleman, M. R., & Boly, M. (2006). Detecting awareness in the vegetative state. *Science, 313*, 1402.

Payne, K., Taylor, R. M., & Stocking, C. (1996). Physicians' attitudes about the care of patients in the persistent vegetative state: A national survey. *Annals of Internal Medicine, 125*, 104–110.

Posner, J. B., Saper, C. B., Schiff, N. D., & Plum, F. (2007). *Plum and Posner's diagnosis of stupor and coma* (4th ed.). New York: Oxford University Press.

Royal College of Physicians Working Group. (1996). The permanent vegetative state. *Journal of the Royal College of Physicians London, 30*, 119–121.

Steinbrook, R. (2007). Organ donation after cardiac death. *New England Journal of Medicine, 357*, 209–213.

Tresch, D. D., Sims, F. H., & Duthie, E. H. (1991). Clinical characteristics of patients in the persistent vegetative state. *Archives of Internal Medicine, 151*, 930–932.

Wijdicks, E. F. M., Rabinstein, A. A., Manno, E. M., & Atkinson, J. D. (2008). Pronouncing brain death: Contemporary practice and safety of the apnea test. *Neurology, 71*, 1240–1244.

Yamamoto, T., Kobayashi, K., & Kasai, M. (2004). Deep brain stimulation for the vegetative state and minimally conscious state. *Acta Neurochirurgica Supplementum, 93*, 101–104.

PART IV

Social, Emotional, and Spiritual Considerations

CHAPTER 13

Applying the Dignity-Conserving Model

ZANA M. LUTFIYYA AND KAREN D. SCHWARTZ

I think there's a very good reason to extend the franchise, to widen the conversation, to democratize our debates, and to make disability central to our theories of egalitarian social justice. The reason is this: a capacious and supple sense of what it is to be human is better than a narrow and partial sense of what it is to be human, and the more partici-pants we as a society can incorporate into the deliberation of what it means to be human, the greater the chances that that deliberation will in fact be transformative in such a way as to enhance our collective capacities to recognize each other as humans entitled to human dignity.

—Bérubé (2003, p. 56)

This chapter will focus on a discussion of the implications of encouraging dignity at the end of life for people with intellectual and developmental disabilities (IDD). The dignity-conserving care model of palliative care (Chochinov, 2007; Chochinov, Hack, McClement, Kristjanson, & Harlos, 2002) will be used in this important analysis. This conceptual framework illustrates the potentially positive impact of a person's "dignity-conserving repertoire" on the potentially negative impact that illness-related and social concerns can have on an individual's dignity at end of life. The framework was devel-oped using interview data extracted from discussions with dying patients who did not have IDD. The intent of the research was to examine what the term "dignity" meant to patients and what experiences either supported or undermined their sense of the word (Chochinov et al., 2002).

The notion of treating patients with dignity is a fundamental responsibility of physi-cians under the Canadian Medical Association Code of Ethics (2004), a principle of medical ethics for the American Medical Association (2001), and a goal of the Canadian Hospice Palliative Care Association (2007). The American Association on Intellectual and Developmental Disabilities (2005) has also stressed the importance of dignity in its principles regarding caring at the end of life. In his discussion of dignity and end of life, Johnson (1998) refers to notions of worthiness, nobility, and honor—that is, treating people as if they are worthy and noble. Franklin, Ternestedt, and Nordenfelt (2006) have reviewed the literature on dignity from a nursing perspective. They have found that definitions of dignity acknowledge not only its subjective and multidimensional nature but also its internal (valuing of self) and external (valuing by others) aspects.

In considering end-of-life care and people with IDD, Chochinov et al.'s (2002) model is compelling in that it provides a new way of encouraging dignity in a group of people who have traditionally been highly devalued and stigmatized throughout their lives. This group of people is one for whom good health care has been problematic (Cooper et al., 2006; Melville et al., 2006) and who have been described as "disadvantaged dying" (Read, Jackson, & Cartlidge, 2007). For those who care provide end-of-life care for persons with IDD, the dignity-conserving care model will offer palliative care professionals and other caregivers the invaluable opportunity to move beyond devaluation and toward being treated with worthiness, elevation, honor, and nobility.

The chapter will begin with an examination of the concept of devaluation, because people with IDD are typically seen as devalued and are treated accordingly. This examination will include the socially devalued roles into which many people with IDD have been cast and the consequence of perception in this devaluation process. It will then explore the themes of dignity, social role valorization, and humanness in order to perceive and understand people with IDD differently and more positively. It will continue by briefly touching upon the barriers that stand in the way of people with IDD in the area of medical and end-of-life care. Finally, it will focus on the dignity-conserving care model and discuss its appropriateness as a strategy to minimize devaluation and to promote best practice in caring for people with IDD who are in fact at the end of their lives.

People With IDD and Devaluation

Social Devaluation

People with IDD have faced a long history of being devalued in Western societies. In his work on social role valorization, Wolfensberger (2000) has defined social devaluation as the process whereby certain individuals or groups are perceived as having less value than most others in that society. Not only is this process universal in its scope, but it also may be unconscious in its practice, making it all the more difficult to address. People who have been labeled as having an intellectual disability are perceived as lacking many of the characteristics that our society values so highly, and they are prime candidates for devaluation. The perception of a lack of value has very real consequences for those placed in that position, including few or no opportunities for decent housing, little chance at a proper education, poor—if any—employment possibilities, and inadequate health care (Wolfensberger, 1998).

Results of Devaluation

Wolfensberger (1998, 2000; see also Race, 1999) argues that "bad things" get done to people who are devalued. People who are devalued are often relegated to a low social status within society. Closely tied to this notion is the denial of rights that are afforded to other citizens or more valued members of a society and the failure to ensure that the rights of devalued people are adequately protected. This fosters the creation of a lower class of citizen or member—or a person whose citizenship is denied altogether.

Devalued people may be rejected by family, neighbors, and people in their communities, leading to feelings of abandonment and discontinuity. This rejection is demonstrated in the reluctance of valued members of society to associate with devalued members, resulting in a physical and social distancing between the two groups. Wolfensberger (1998) describes this phenomenon as a form of "exile" (p. 18).

Another way in which society reinforces the devaluing of people is the juxtaposition of devalued people against negative images in society (Wolfensberger, 1998). Of particular note here is the juxtaposition of people with IDD with people who are very ill or those who may be at, or near, death. This serves to conflate intellectual disability with death in our society.

Finally, devalued people may experience deindividualization—a loss of control over their lives, financial poverty, an impoverishment of world experiences, and risk for abuse and brutalization, all leading to wasted potential and wasted lives (Wolfensberger, 1998).

Devalued Social Roles

Significantly, Wolfensberger (1998) also contends that devalued people get cast into a number of devalued roles within society. These roles include (a) the alien or "other" (p. 14); (b) the subhuman or nonhuman, such as when they are referred to as in a "vegetative state"; (c) a menace or "object of dread"; (d) an object of ridicule; (e) an object of pity; (f) a burden of charity; (g) an eternal child; (h) a "sick, ill or diseased organism"; and (i) the "death-related and death-imagined roles" where "people who are not dying may be put into the dying role" (p. 15–16). Simply put, casting people into devalued roles provides a justification for treatment that is not tolerated among society's valuable and valued citizens.

Unconsciousness and Expectations

One of the most important reasons for considering devaluation and its effects on vulnerable people, including people with IDD, is its often unconscious and therefore undervaluated nature. This highlights the importance of bringing these unconscious reactions to light. If people become conscious of how they think and feel, they become free to examine why they hold these thoughts and beliefs. In the end-of-life care context, the usefulness of devaluation as a framework for understanding people with IDD can be reevaluated.

Closely related to the notion of unconscious beliefs are the expectations generally held about people with IDD. Because our society has tended to view these individuals as incompetent, there is little expectation that they will ever be able to accomplish enough to alter this status. Professionals may be under the mistaken impression that these people have no opinions or feelings about their end-of-life preferences and care. If these expectations are held deeply enough, palliative care professionals may not be able to acknowledge competence, even when it is clearly demonstrated.

Bérubé (2003), writing about his son, perhaps puts it best when he writes,

> It might be a good idea for all of us to treat other humans as if we do not know their potential, as if they just might in fact surprise us, as if they might defeat or exceed our expectations. (p. 53)

THE IMPACT OF DEVALUATION

Past

Whether consciously intended or not, social devaluation has had a tremendous impact upon the lives of people with IDD. Although a more detailed history of these issues has been explored in chapter 2, it is crucial to reiterate some of this history here. People with IDD have been discriminated against and excluded because they were considered to be "abnormal," which served to justify their unequal treatment in society (Reinders, 2000). Devaluation provided a rationale for the removal of people from family and community and their relocation to large- and small-scale institutions (Parmenter, 2001; Trent, 1994; Wolfensberger, 1975). This resulted in some shockingly inhumane treatment (Blatt & Kaplan, 1974; Ferguson, 1994; Rothman & Rothman, 1984; Wolfensberger, 1975). People were denied basic human rights, and they were presumed to be too incompetent to make even the most mundane decisions about their own lives, leading, ultimately, to a disqualification from fully participating in society (Angrosino, 1998).

Activist and championing advocate Gunnar Dybwad's (2000) haunting recollections are also worth quoting here:

> Thus I have a vivid memory of conditions that to most readers will only be historical facts which they have read. I saw first hand the dismal conditions in the overcrowded institutions which originated in good intentions, to give asylum and protection and quickly became warehouses to offer society protection from the so-called "mental defectives." I saw in the late 1930s, overcrowding with all its dire consequences was the major problem. . . . We are confronted with our own holocaust in the area of intellectual disability. The actual holocaust story is kept alive because of a strong belief that this is necessary to prevent a repetition in years to come. Likewise, the institutional horrors must be kept alive by eyewitnesses. . . . It must not be forgotten, it cannot be erased from our professional history. (pp. 432–433)

Present

Even today, as the end of the first decade of the 21st century approaches, the impact of continued devaluation, while not experienced by all people with IDD, is felt in numerous aspects of many people's lives. In medical contexts, Ali and Hassiotis (2008) note that the "suboptimal care" received by patients with IDD has been recognized in a report by the Joint Committee on Human Rights, which considers human rights issues in the United Kingdom (p. 570). The authors point to the problem of diagnostic overshadowing, where health care professionals attribute a health problem to the patient's intellectual disability. The British Disability Rights Commission discovered that patients with IDD were less likely to receive proper treatment and were more likely to die at a younger age than patients from outside that group (Ali & Hassiotis, 2008). Furthermore, MENCAP, a leading advocacy organization for people with IDD in Britain, looked into the deaths of six patients and found that they were the result of "poor medical practice" (Ali & Hassiotis, 2008, p. 570).

Genetics, bioethics, and end-of-life issues are also particularly sensitive for this group of people given that people without disabilities assume they would rather be dead than live their lives with a disability (Derksen & Chochinov, 2006).

When prevailing perceptions of people with IDD are expressed medically and pathologically as defect and deficit, the reaction is to fix, rehabilitate, cure, and eliminate. New advances in genetics make the ability to eliminate defects a reality. Yet these new technologies also contain echoes of a common refrain heard during the first half of the 20th century, when eugenics was in its heyday and the elimination of "mental defectives" became a driving and sustained social force.

Conversations about how to distribute limited resources and determinations of medical futility can affect people with IDD, particularly in light of perceptions that these people are less valued than other members of society. Thus, medical decisions about how aggressive medical management should be in pursuing life-sustaining approaches can have a serious impact on these individuals. Doctors and health care professionals, like all other members of our society, are not immune to the social influences that have been examined here. As Derksen and Chochinov (2006) explain,

> There is another contemporary experience, and that is when people with disabilities come into crisis and they may not be able to speak, or may otherwise be less able to defend or assert themselves. Doctors' perceptions and decisions still dominate, and this can be dangerous for persons with disabilities who are experiencing a health crisis. . . . As a result, we have the sense that doctors may not be our best friends when we most need them. (p. 178)

Contesting Devaluation

Not every person with IDD is highly devalued. There are many people who have loving relationships, welcoming homes, engaging work, and full lives. The question to answer is how do some individuals get past the societal devaluation to become valued citizens? It is argued that people with IDD can emerge from the depths of devaluation to the heights of dignity, both generally and in palliative care contexts. It is suggested that the key to altering perceptions can be found in the ideas of valued social roles (Wolfensberger, 1998, 2000) and the social construction of humanness (Bogdan & Taylor, 1998).

Valued Social Roles

Wolfensberger (1998) suggests that social roles are important because they help to define people and locate them within the larger world. Thus, the creation and establishment of valued social roles is vital because such roles lead to social acceptance and respect (Wolfensberger, 1998). One significant aspect to holding a highly valued role is that role's ability to overshadow less desirable characteristics.

There are many types of roles that people hold. Wolfensberger (1998) discusses eight common role domains—relationships; residence; occupation; education; recreation and leisure; civic identity; and participation, values, and culture. Holding valued social roles has been difficult for many people with IDD. Yet there is a great deal of simplicity to many valued roles, and, as will be illustrated in the next section, recognizing a person's valued roles at end of life helps promote and maintain their dignity. Social roles such as those of valued family member, neighbor, employee, union member, student, tutor, athlete, coach, organization member, board member, voter, taxpayer, volunteer, parishioner, arts patron, and music or book lover are all valued ways in which to identify people with IDD.

Notwithstanding the simplicity in recognizing these roles, such individuals are more likely to be perceived as holding negatively valued converse roles such as old maid, idler, special needs student, loser, welfare recipient, sponge, lost soul, and illiterate (Wolfensberger,

1998). Palliative care professionals can play a big part in recognizing some of the positive roles in their patients' lives, while at the same time promoting dignity while dying.

Elks's (1994) critique of the importance of valued social roles over valuing the person suggests that even people with highly valued roles may not have a personal identity that is highly valued within the culture or society. Although it is argued here that social roles play an important part in maintaining and encouraging dignity for people with IDD, it will also be suggested that relationships that recognize the humanness of these individuals is another key in preserving dignity at end of life.

Social Construction of Humanness

Bogdan and Taylor (1998) define humanness as the "taken-for-granted view" that people with IDD are "full-fledged human beings" (p. 246). This can be contrasted with other perspectives in which people with complex disabilities are looked upon as either not human or less than fully human. People with IDD become defined, not by their disability, but by their membership in the human community.

In their work analyzing the loving relationships between people who do not have a disability and people with significant and complex IDD, Bogdan and Taylor (1998) examine how people without disabilities in loving, caring, and accepting relationships with people identified as "severely disabled" define these people (p. 242). These long-term relationships are defined as close and affectionate.

Bogdan and Taylor's (1998) work suggests several "mental constructions" held by the people without disabilities in these relationships. In the first construct, the partner with a disability is seen as a thinking human being by their loved ones—contrary to popular social assumptions that reasoning and thinking actually define a human being. Even for loved ones who could not communicate with oral speech, their partners without disabilities felt they were more intelligent than they might appear, and they relied on the sounds and movements made by the person with a disability as evidence of intelligence. The deep bond between the people in these relationships allows the partner without a disability to "just know" what the other is thinking and feeling (p. 249, referencing Goode, 1994).

Contrary to popular social assumptions that consider people with IDD to be unable to reason, the partner with a disability is seen as a thinking human being. It is interesting to note the belief in the innate intelligence of the partner with a disability—notwithstanding social, medical, and professional opinions to the contrary: "Clinical perspectives are based on different ways of knowing and seeing than the perspectives of people involved in intimate relationships with people with disabilities" (Bogdan & Taylor, 1998, p. 250).

The second mental construct identified by Bogdan and Taylor (1998) is the ability of the partners without a disability to see individuality in their partners with disabilities. Thus, the partners without disabilities were able to identify and discuss those characteristics of their partners with disabilities that set them apart from other people and make them distinctly who they are.

More specifically, partners without disabilities spoke of the personality of their loved ones with a disability. Words such as "profoundly retarded" and "developmentally disabled" were not part of their vocabulary. However, descriptors such as "silly, fun, shy, live wire, bright, appreciative, nice, likable, calm, active, kind, gentle, wonderful, amusing, pleasant and good company" (Bogdan & Taylor, 1998, p. 251) were abundantly evident. Partners without disabilities also mentioned the likes and dislikes of their partners with disabilities, which both confirms individuality and reinforces the bonds in the relationship. Humanness also comes through when people without disabilities discuss the life histories of their partners with disabilities. Bogdan and Taylor (1998) note that the telling of life histories may involve two distinct chapters in the life of the person with a disability: the first being life before the relationship with the partners without disabilities and the second being the formation of the relationship, involving significant improvement in the life of the person with a disability. Paying close attention to personal appearances is yet another way of seeing the loved one with a disability as an individual. Thus things like hairstyle, clothing, makeup, and the like present a more "normal" version of the person with a disability to outsiders and construct an identity in keeping with the definition set by the partner without a disability.

Thirdly, the people without disabilities saw their partner as a reciprocating and contributing member of the relationship (Bogdan & Taylor, 1998). Some of the benefits of the relationships that people without disabilities discussed were the enjoyment of spending time with their partner with a disability, the belief that these relationships made them better people, and a feeling of worth in making a contribution to the lives of the partners with disabilities.

Finally, people without disabilities were able to successfully create a place for their partner with a disability in their family and/or social circle, as well as in their daily routines and rituals (Bogdan & Taylor, 1998). Such inclusion facilitated greater community presence and acceptance. In addition, absences of the partner with a disability from these routines and circles were noted and lamented. Rather than being devalued, people with significant and complex needs become, in the bosom of family and friends, "someone like me" (p. 257).

THE DIGNITY-CONSERVING MODEL OF CARE

The Model

The notion of looking beyond the condition to see the human being is a central theme in Chochinov et al.'s (2002) dignity-conserving care model of palliative care. As a result of this qualitative work, the researchers uncovered what they describe as three major dignity categories, each with its own set of themes and subthemes. Some explanation about these dignity categories and how they operate together on the concept of a person's dignity at end of life will now be examined.

In collecting data for this research, Chochinov et al. (2002) asked patients with advanced cancer questions to promote a discussion of dignity. These questions included (a) how patients defined the term dignity in terms of their experience, (b) what things both supported and undermined the patient's sense of dignity, (c) what specific experiences compromised or supported dignity, (d) what life occurrences would lead to feelings of a loss of a sense of dignity, (e) how patients felt about the notion that life without dignity is not worth living, and (f) whether patients felt dignity was something within themselves or something given and/or taken away by others.

The three categories that emerged from the data analysis were (a) illness-related concerns, (b) the social dignity inventory, and (c) the dignity-conserving repertoire. Illness-related concerns "are those that derive from or are related to the illness itself, and threaten to or actually do impinge on the patient's sense of dignity" (Chochinov et al., 2002, p. 435). The social dignity inventory refers to the "social concerns or relationship dynamics that enhance or detract from a patient's sense of dignity" (p. 439). The dignity conserving repertoire includes both "a way of looking at one's situation that helps promote dignity" and "personal actions that can bolster or reinforce one's sense of dignity" (p. 437).

Illness-Related Concerns

Illness-related concerns involve two themes: the level of independence and symptom distress. Within the theme of independence, two subthemes emerge: cognitive acuity and functional capacity. Within the theme of symptom distress, there are also two subthemes: physical distress and psychological distress. Psychological distress includes medical uncertainty and death anxiety. Figure 13.1 illustrates these themes and subthemes.

The notion of level of independence centers around a person's reliance on others. In our society, independence, health, and the appearance of physical strength are greatly valued, whereas dependence and reliance on others to perform certain tasks are viewed as a failure or weakness (Toombs, 2004). Chochinov et al. (2002) note that "diminished cognitive capacity" and the need to ask for help play a large role in the "fracturing" of the personal dignity of patients (pp. 435–436).

The physical distress experienced by some people causes them to wish for death over pain. As one gentleman is quoted as saying, "Sometimes I hurt so much, I'd like to take all my pills and get it over with so I wouldn't hurt" (Chochinov et al., 2002, p. 436). Psychological distress also impacts and threatens dignity. Medical uncertainty is "the anguish associated with not knowing, or being unaware of aspects of one's health status or treatment" (p. 436). Death anxiety is "the worry or fear specifically associated with the process or anticipation of death and dying" (p. 436).

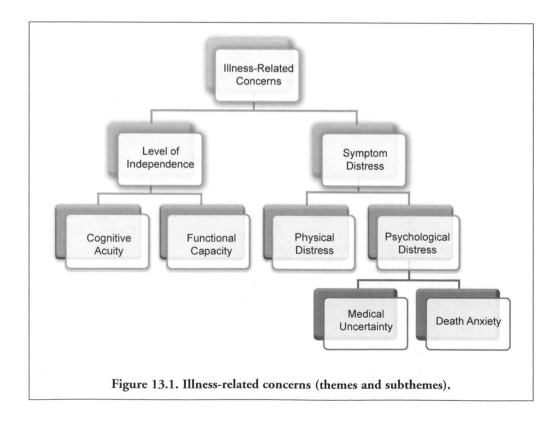

Figure 13.1. Illness-related concerns (themes and subthemes).

Social Dignity Inventory

Depending upon the person's perspective and circumstances, this category may serve to impinge on dignity or, in the case of certain themes, help to conserve it. There are five themes contained in the social dignity inventory: privacy boundaries, social support, care tenor, burden, and aftermath concerns. These are illustrated in Figure 13.2.

When personal privacy becomes a matter of a more "public" domain, a patient's dignity can become significantly compromised. For example, a participant confirmed, "I still feel like I like my privacy" (Chochinov et al., 2002, p. 439). Another participant echoed this feeling by saying, "Things like not being able to go to the bathroom myself. Oh to me, that would take everything away from me because I am so modest" (p. 439).

The social support a person has can serve to maintain or enhance dignity at end of life. For some people, knowing they have family or friends that they can rely on helps them and may act as a buffer against other indignities. An older gentleman participant expressed this sentiment when he emphasized, "Well it doesn't matter how bad things get. I know that my family is there and I'm very lucky. Not everybody's family is supportive" (Chochinov et al., 2002, pp. 439–440). Similarly, the attitudes of others can affect that person's dignity when care is being provided.

Care tenor is defined by Chochinov et al. (2002) as the attitude of others when they interact with patients. How this attitude is manifested either promotes or negatively impacts upon patient dignity.

The notion of being or becoming a burden is also significant to this discussion and is tied to ideas of being reliant on others for things like personal care. An older woman who participated in the study was worried about having "to depend on people just to look after me, to wash me, to take me to the bathroom . . . clean me up. . . . I know this happens but I wish it didn't happen to me" (Chochinov et al., 2002, p. 440).

Aftermath concerns are those worries that a person might have about what will happen to loved ones after their death and the effect their death will have on these people. For example, a patient with lung cancer expressed his concern about his children after he dies. He said, "Well I've got four young children. They're all at home still . . . and I'm really concerned about . . . their future" (Chochinov et al., 2002, p. 440).

Issues in the social dignity inventory can act in conjunction with illness-related concerns to significantly reduce dignity in patients at the end of their lives. Yet for some

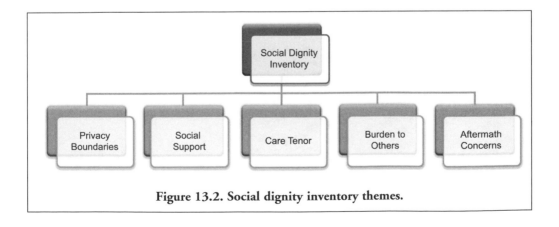

Figure 13.2. Social dignity inventory themes.

people, some or all aspects of the social dignity inventory can help to counterbalance loss of dignity and even maintain it. Social support and an awareness of privacy issues and care tenor can have a positive effect. Similarly, care providers who are conscious of helping to ease feelings of being a burden and stress about aftermath concerns can help patients balance the negative effects of illness-related problems.

Dignity-Conserving Repertoire

Chochinov et al.'s (2002) final category is called the dignity-conserving repertoire. The two themes within this category are (a) dignity-conserving perspectives, which involve how people *look* at their situation, and (b) dignity-conserving practices, which are things people can actually *do* that may reinforce their dignity. Figure 13.3a illustrates the sub-themes in the dignity-conserving perspectives while Figure 13.3b illustrates the subthemes in the dignity-conserving practices.

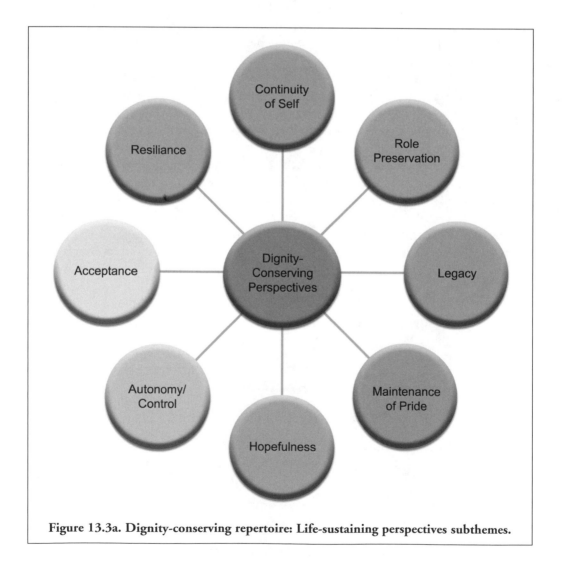

Figure 13.3a. Dignity-conserving repertoire: Life-sustaining perspectives subthemes.

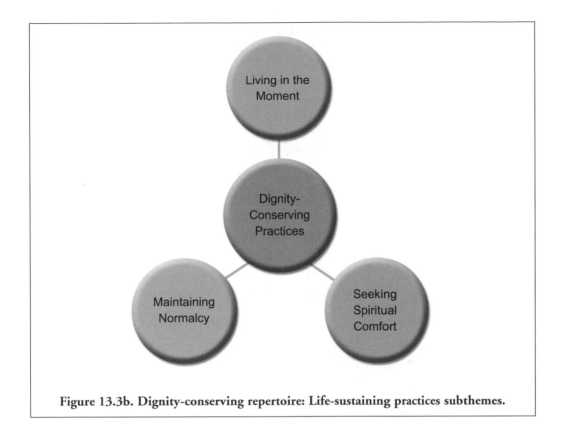

Figure 13.3b. Dignity-conserving repertoire: Life-sustaining practices subthemes.

The authors note that the dignity-conserving perspectives are individual to each patient and reside within the person. They are not hierarchical in terms of importance, and different perspectives may, alone or in conjunction with other perspectives, have more or less effect on different patients. Even more importantly, the themes and subthemes represented here "likely mediate, or in some instances even buffer the extent to which their sense of dignity is maintained rather than fractured in the face of their advancing illness" (p. 438).

Dignity is a crucial concept in the field of end-of-life care: "Prior studies have documented loss of dignity as the most common response given by physicians when asked why their patients had selected euthanasia or some form of self-assisted suicide" (Chochinov et al., 2002, p. 442). These prior studies include a national survey on physician-assisted suicide in the United States (Meier et al., 1998). The ability to maintain and even bolster people's dignity may lead to better mental health and a better death, while ensuring that they live their final days maintaining a sense of their self-worth as fellow human beings.

End-of-Life Care and People With Intellectual Disabilities

There are some significant issues facing the success with which dying patients with IDD have been able to access and receive palliative care. Botsford (2000) has written that—like the people themselves—the dying, death, and grief experienced by people with IDD have been devalued. Read et al. (2007) suggest that people with IDD are not necessarily able to access the palliative care they might need. Tuffrey-Wijne, Bernal, Butler, Hollins, and Curfs (2007) emphasize that the provision and appropriateness of the end-of-life care for people with IDD is not well known and these individuals have, in fact, been "totally excluded" from palliative care (p. 81).

Current research has demonstrated that there are a number of issues involving the provision of palliative care for people with IDD that are unique to this group. Palliative care issues for and about people with IDD include (a) problems in identifying symptoms in a timely fashion, resulting in late diagnosis, (b) difficulty communicating with patients, (c) issues of disclosing diagnoses and prognoses, (d) presentation of symptoms and assessment of pain and other symptoms, (e) ethical issues involving competence to give consent and make other end-of-life decisions, (f) making the decision to move from home to hospice facilities, (g) knowing what patients want and need, (h) piecing together fragmented medical histories, (i) patient knowledge of health matters, (j) poor health screening, (k) understanding spiritual needs, and (l) overcoming disempowerment in life (Read, 2005; Read et al., 2007; Tuffrey-Wijne, 2003; Tuffrey-Wijne, Hogg, & Curfs, 2007).

Read (2005), Read et al. (2007), and Tuffrey-Wijne, Hogg, and Curfs (2007) have discussed some examples of best practice when caring for patients with IDD at end of life. These include (a) ensuring that services and staff are well supported and have knowledge of palliative care issues; (b) being attentive to the patient's needs; (c) being committed to person-centered care; (d) promoting strong collaboration between health care staff, service staff, and families; (e) being open and providing full disclosure to patients; and (f) having palliative care professionals who understand people with IDD.

Dignity-conserving care involves an understanding of how care professionals see the patient (Chochinov, 2002). Thus, "when dying patients are seen, and know that they are seen, as being worthy of honor and esteem by those who care for them, dignity is more likely to be maintained" (p. 2259). Caring for people with IDD at end of life is no exception. Yet there is very poor understanding of what people with IDD need and what their end-of-life experiences have been. Tuffrey-Wijne, Hogg, and Curfs (2007) argue that relevant and appropriate care means gaining more insight into what these patients value, want, and need as they near the end of their lives.

Tuffrey-Wijne, Bernal, et al.'s (2007) work has demonstrated that people with IDD are capable of thinking about and discussing the topics of death and dying. Participants with IDD were recruited to discuss end-of-life issues. The researchers used the Nominal Group Technique (a single-question technique) to elicit responses to a picture of a woman resting in a chair and the following question: "This is Veronica. Veronica is very ill. She is not going to get better. The doctor knows that she is going to die. What do you think people should do to help Veronica?" (p. 82). The participants were able to discuss the question and consider issues of illness and dying. As the authors remind us, "They were not only able to give their opinions and show an ability to think about a wide variety of issues that may be of importance in end-of-life care, but *relished the opportunity to do so*" (p. 85, emphasis added).

APPLYING THE DIGNITY-CONSERVING CARE MODEL TO PATIENTS WITH IDD

Given what is known about people with IDD, their devaluation and forced positioning into devalued roles, our tendency to confirm these roles and make negative assumptions about them, the importance of dignity at end of life, and the issues facing palliative care providers who care for people with IDD, does Chochinov et al.'s (2002) dignity-conserving model of care have relevance to them? Although it may be comfortable for practitioners to argue that palliative care for people with IDD should be separate from or different than palliative care for the general population, Read (2005) argues against this idea, suggesting that these patients actually have much in common with the rest of the population.

One pressing concern in the literature on people with IDD and palliative care is the need to educate and familiarize end-of-life care providers with issues that might relate to these people. Botsford (2004), in a study surveying directors of American organizations providing services to older adults with IDD, concludes that there is a need for education and resources on end-of-life care for individuals, family, caregivers, and health care providers. The authors further note the need for more staffing, policies to provide better end-of-life care, and more research on improving end-of-life care for these individuals. Furthermore, Tuffrey-Wijne, Hogg, and Curfs (2007) discuss in their recent literature review that a number of studies have found that health care professionals do not have much experience caring for patients with IDD. A study by Slevin and Sines (1996) showed negative and stereotypical attitudes toward people IDD among nurses in a hospital setting, using both quantitative attitude measurements and qualitative interviews. Research by Lindop and Read (2000) pointed to the need for professionals to better understand the concept of IDD (Tuffrey-Wijne, Hogg, & Curfs, 2007).

How can the dignity-conserving care model be applied to people with IDD? To answer this question, the model must be reviewed again to determine how palliative care professionals can use it to promote dignity for these people. In recalling the model, there are three dignity categories: the illness-related concerns of level of independence (cognitive acuity and functional capacity) and symptom distress (physical and psychological); the social dignity inventory comprising of privacy boundaries, social support, care tenor, burden to others and aftermath concerns; and dignity-conserving repertoire, which includes dignity-conserving perspectives (continuity of self, role preservation, legacy, maintenance of pride, hopefulness, autonomy/control, acceptance, and resilience) and dignity-conserving practices (living in the moment, seeking spiritual comfort, and maintaining normalcy). Each category will now be explored to see how it can be used to promote dignity for these individuals at the end of life.

Illness-Related Concerns

The very first theme in this category involves the notion of independence and the threat of end-of-life realities to that notion. Yet independence is also the very concept that challenges our perceptions of people with IDD. Do people for whom dependence is a daily reality mourn a loss of independence at end of life? It is suggested that it is dangerous to believe that people with IDD do not have independence simply because they may be dependent on some people to help them with some things. Independence, like competence, may be better understood not as a global construct but as something more specific to particular events or situations. It may be very devastating for a person with IDD to realize that, after having spent considerable time and effort learning a particular skill, they can no longer accomplish the task due to their illness. Thus, it is important for palliative care professionals to recognize the demoralizing effects of this type of loss, as they would for any other person.

Discussing symptoms and prognoses directly with patients with IDD is necessary in order to provide and receive better end-of-life care. Professionals must acknowledge that there are patients who would and will benefit from conversations about what to expect in terms of illness trajectory and potential treatments. Furthermore, some patients may be facing death anxiety yet may not be able to discuss their feelings when no one expects their desire to have such a conversation. Communication becomes even more vital when pain alleviation is the goal. Cases where patients with IDD have been misdiagnosed or not treated when their pain is misinterpreted as a behavioral issue have been reported (Tuffrey-Wijne, 2002, p. 223). These patients are certainly not immune from the effects of physical distress. Telling people what is happening, even when they may not understand, encourages them to be treated as adults rather than as children. Recognizing and assisting with illness-related concerns can help individuals maintain valued social roles and dignity.

Social Dignity Inventory

Given the importance of reconciling the social dignity inventory themes with dignity conservation and affirmation, end-of-life care professionals can play a significant role in helping to maintain the dignity of people with IDD. Again, negatively held preconceived notions must be actively challenged, and positive ones must be maintained. For example, a carer might dismiss concerns of encroaching on the privacy of people with IDD because such encroachment may have been part of that person's life before illness struck. However, not all people require assistance with personal care, and those who do require it may still feel that their dignity is compromised because of such a need. This feeling may result in a response that is simply assumed by professionals to be another example of bad behavior.

Chochinov et al. (2002) found that social support is also critical to maintaining a sense of dignity. Families can play an enormous role in actively advocating for treatment of their family member. Unfortunately, in medical settings, families may also feel vulnerable and thus find it difficult to find their voice in a process dominated by professional opinions and decision making. For some people with IDD, family may be absent or nonexistent. These situations demand that palliative care providers make extra efforts to determine who is involved in the support networks for these people and calling upon that support. They may be required to search beyond traditional family roles. Yet such an endeavor is likely to encourage dignity and make the end of life more meaningful to those people. It is also an opportunity for carers, family, and friends to assure the person that he or she is not a burden and that engaging with him or her is beneficial for everyone.

Care tenor is another theme that involves attitudes of care professionals. This concept refers to "the attitude others demonstrate when interacting with the patient" (Chochinov et al., 2002, p. 440). It is within this context that assumptions about competence and ability to see the humanness of the patient become a priority. Recognizing the humanity of the patient and actively drawing upon and enhancing all possible valued social roles not only helps to support dignity but also provides a model of behavior for other carers to emulate.

Finally, people with IDD may also be thinking about aftermath concerns, or "the worry or fears associated with anticipating the burden or challenges that one's death will impose on others" (Chochinov et al., 2002, p. 440). Carers must anticipate that some people will need to talk about their death and what that will mean for the family and friends left to mourn them.

Dignity-Conserving Repertoire

Chochinov et al. (2002) have demonstrated the positive effects on dignity that a dignity-conserving repertoire can have on people at end of life. It is argued that this repertoire can also have affirming effects on people with IDD. The key to the repertoire for these individuals is the ability of professional carers, family, and friends to assist the individual in gaining these perspectives and practicing them. This requires a real knowledge of the person in order to best promote the dignity-conserving strategies. This process can also be aided by encouraging people with IDD, in a way and at a pace tailored to their needs and capacities, to consider end-of-life issues within a normative context during their lives and by recording these preferences for possible use in the future.

As Chochinov et al. (2002) pointed out, not all of the repertoire categories will be relevant or necessary for all people. Yet some perspectives are particularly appropriate to vulnerable people. It is easy to see how role preservation can play an essential part in dignity conservation. By concentrating on the valued roles the person has accumulated over his or her lifetime, end-of-life professionals can encourage these individuals to function in such roles rather than focusing solely on the paucity of roles or the role of the sick and/or dying person. Even if the individual has not had the opportunity to acquire many valued roles, the end of life can still be a time to encourage positive roles. This will allow for a continuity of self or a renewed interest in self during illness and can also serve as a starting point for considering the lasting legacy of the person. All human beings have the potential to leave a legacy, including those who have IDD. Knowing the person and developing relationships with that person's support network can also help to maintain pride and hopefulness. There can be a continued purpose to life as well as an anticipation of good things when end-of-life professionals can appreciate that the vulnerable person has worth and value as a human being.

Conclusion

One effective way to familiarize carers with people with IDD is to use the dignity-conserving model to emphasize the humanness and basic human needs of all people at end of life. Employing this model will discourage devaluation and encourage end-of-life professionals to preserve dignity and facilitate "the ideal, proper death" for people with IDD, which, as Johnson (1998) argues, "will be different for everyone, yet often dependent on others" (p. 343). If, as Johnson (1998) suggests, communication between patient and professional is a key element of end-of-life care, the dignity model is an ideal way to facilitate this process, fostering "a respect for the worth of all persons" and acknowledging the "humanizing responsibility" in "dealing with the wants and needs of dying patients" (p. 350).

Acknowledgments

The preparation of this chapter was supported by the Canadian Institutes of Health Research New Emerging Team Grant on End of Life Care and Vulnerable Populations held by Harvey M. Chochinov, Deborah Stienstra, Joseph M. Kaufert, and Zana M. Lutfiyya.

REFERENCES

Ali, A., & Hassiotis, A. (2008). Illness in people with intellectual disabilities. *British Medical Journal, 336*(7644), 570–571.

American Association on Intellectual and Developmental Disabilities. (2005). *Position statement on caring at end of life*. Retrieved March 3, 2008, from http://www.aaidd.org/Policies/pos_end_of_life.shtml

American Medical Association. (2001). *Principles of medical ethics*. Retrieved March 3, 2008, from http://ama-assn.org/ama/pub/category/2512.html

Angrosino, M. V. (1998). Mental disability in the United States: An interactionist perspective. In R. Jenkins (Ed.), *Questions of competence* (pp. 25–53). Cambridge: Cambridge University Press.

Bérubé, M. (2003, Spring). Citizenship and disability. *Dissent, 50*(2), 52–57.

Blatt, B., & Kaplan, F. (1974). *Christmas in purgatory: A photographic essay on mental retardation*. Syracuse, NY: Human Policy Press.

Bogdan, R., & Taylor, S. J. (1998). The social construction of humanness: Relationships with people with severe retardation. In S. J. Taylor & R. Bogdan (Eds.), *Introduction to qualitative research methods: A guidebook and resource* (3rd ed., pp. 242–258). New York: John Wiley & Sons.

Botsford, A. L. (2000). Integrated end if life care into services for people with an intellectual disability. *Social Work in Health Care, 31*(1), 35–48.

Botsford, A. L. (2004). Status of end of life care in organizations providing services for older people with a developmental disability. *American Journal on Mental Retardation, 109*(5), 421–428.

Canadian Hospice Palliative Care Association. (2007). *Annual report, 2006–2007*. Ottawa: Canadian Hospice Palliative Care Association.

Canadian Medical Association. (2004). *Code of ethics*. Retrieved March 3, 2008, from http://www.cma.ca/index.cfm/ci_id/44274/la_id/1/htm

Chochinov, H. M. (2002). Dignity-conserving care—a new model for palliative care. *Journal of the American Medical Association, 287*(17), 2253–2260.

Chochinov, H. M. (2007). Dignity and the essence of medicine: The A, B, C, and D of dignity conserving care. *British Medical Journal, 335*, 184–187.

Chochinov, H. M., Hack, T., McClement, S., Kristjanson, L., & Harlos, M. (2002). Dignity in the terminally ill: A developing empirical model. *Social Science & Medicine, 54*, 433–443.

Cooper, S.-A., Morrison, J., Melville, C., Finlayson, J., Allan, L., Martin, G., & Robinson, N. (2006). Improving the health of people with intellectual disabilities: Outcomes of a health screening programme after 1 year. *Journal of Intellectual Disability Research, 50*(9), 667–677.

Derksen, J., & Chochinov, M. H. (2006). Disability and end-of-life care: Let the conversation begin. *Journal of Palliative Care, 22*(3), 175–182.

Dybwad, G. (2000). Mental retardation in the 21st century. In M. L. Wehmeyer & J. R. Patton (Eds.), *Mental retardation in the 21st century* (pp. 431–433). Austin, TX: Pro-Ed.

Elks, M. (1994). Valuing the person or valuing the role? Critique of social role valorization. *Mental Retardation, 32*(4), 265–271.

Ferguson, P. M. (1994). *Abandoned to their fate: Social policy and practices toward severely retarded people in America 1820–1920*. Philadelphia: Temple University Press.

Franklin, L.-L., Ternestedt, B.-M., & Nordenfelt, L. (2006). Views on dignity of elderly nursing home residents. *Nursing Ethics, 13*(2), 130–146.

Goode, D. A. (1994). *A world without words: The social construction of children born deaf and blind*. Philadelphia: Temple University Press.

Johnson, P. R. S. (1998). An analysis of dignity. *Theoretical Medicine and Bioethics, 19*, 337–352.

Lindop, E., & Read, S. (2000). District nurses' needs: Palliative care for people with learning disabilities. *International Journal of Palliative Nursing, 6*, 117–122.

Meier, D. E., Emmons, C.-A., Wallenstein, S., Quill, T., Morrison, R. S., & Cassel, C. K. (1998). A national survey of physician-assisted suicide and euthanasia in the United States. *New England Journal of Medicine, 338*, 1193–1201.

Melville, C., Cooper, S.-A., Morrison, J., Finlayson, J., Allan, L., Robinson, N., Burns, E., & Martin, G. (2006). The outcomes of an intervention study to reduce the barriers experienced by people with intellectual disabilities accessing primary health care services. *Journal of Intellectual Disability Research, 50*(1), 11–17.

Parmenter, T. R. (2001). Intellectual disabilities—*Quo vadis?* In G. L. Albrecht, K. D. Seelman, & M. Bury (Eds.), *Handbook of disability studies* (pp. 267–296). Thousand Oaks, CA: Sage.

Race, D. G. (1999). *Social Role Valorization and the English experience*. London: Whiting & Birch.

Read, S. (2005). Learning disabilities and palliative care: Recognizing pitfalls and exploring potential. *International Journal of Palliative Nursing, 11*(1), 15–20.

Read, S., Jackson, S., & Cartlidge, D. (2007). Palliative care and intellectual disabilities: Individual roles, collective responsibilities. *International Journal of Palliative Nursing, 13*(9), 430–435.

Reinders, H. S. (2000). *The future of the disabled in liberal society: An ethical analysis*. Notre Dame, IN: University of Notre Dame Press.

Rothman, D. J., & Rothman, S. M. (1984). *The Willowbrook wars: A decade of struggle for social justice*. New York: Harper & Row.

Slevin, E., & Sines, D. (1996). Attitudes of nurses in a general hospital towards people with learning disabilities: Influences of contact, and graduate-non-graduate status, a comparative study. *Journal of Advanced Nursing, 24*, 1116–1126.

Toombs, K. (2004). Living and dying with dignity: Reflections on lived experience. *Journal of Palliative Care, 20*, 193–200.

Trent, J. W., Jr. (1994). *Inventing the feeble mind: A history of mental retardation in the United States*. Berkeley, CA: University of California Press.

Tuffrey-Wijne, I. (2002). The palliative care needs of people with intellectual disabilities: A case study. *International Journal of Palliative Nursing, 8*(5), 222–232.

Tuffrey-Wijne, I. (2003). The palliative care needs of people with intellectual disabilities: A literature review. *Palliative Medicine, 17*, 55–62.

Tuffrey-Wijne, I., Bernal, J., Butler, G., Hollins, S., & Curfs, L. (2007). Using nominal group technique to investigate the views of people with intellectual disabilities on end-of-life care provision. *Journal of Advanced Nursing, 58*(1), 80–89.

Tuffrey-Wijne, I., Hogg, J., & Curfs, L. (2007). End-of-life and palliative care for people with intellectual disabilities who have cancer or other life-limiting illnesses: A review of the literature and available resources. *Journal of Applied Research in Intellectual Disabilities, 20*, 331–344.

Wolfensberger, W. (1975). *The origin and nature of our institutional models*. Syracuse, NY: Human Policy Press.

Wolfensberger, W. (1998). *A brief introduction to Social Role Valorization: A high-order concept for addressing the plight of societally devalued people, and for structuring human services* (3rd ed.). Syracuse, NY: Training Institute for Human Service Planning, Leadership & Change Agentry, Syracuse University.

Wolfensberger, W. (2000). A brief overview of social role valorization. *Mental Retardation, 38*(2), 105–123.

CHAPTER 14

End of Life Through a Cultural Lens

Tawara Goode and Patricia Maloof

What could be more universal than death? Yet what an incredible variety of responses it evokes.

—Metcalf and Huntington (1991, p. 24)

Introduction

The 21st century is sometimes described as the century of "people on the move." It is estimated that 1 out of every 35 people in the world is an international migrant, meaning more than 200 million people are living outside their home countries (Koser, 2008). In 2000, about 35 million, or almost 20% of these people, lived in the United States (Koser, 2008).

The United States is one of the most diverse societies in the world. This diversity spans such variables as age, race, ethnicity, language, religion, socioeconomic status, and geographic region. In a press release from the U.S. Census Bureau in May 2007 (U.S. Census Bureau, 2007a), it was noted that the minority population in the United States has reached 100.7 million, which means that one out of every three people in the United States self-identified as a member of a minority group. Census data show the composition of the U.S. population in 2006 to be: White, 66.38%; Hispanic, 14.8%; Black, 13.4%; Asian, 4.98%; American Indian and Alaskan Native, 1.5%; and Native Hawaiian and other Pacific Islander, 0.34%. (Total population adds to 101.4% because the Census Bureau reported populations as "alone" or "in combination." See U.S. Census Bureau, 2007b, table 1.)

Given the scope of this nation's diversity, it is understandable that the provision of holistic, quality health care requires the capacity to respond to numerous cultural differences at both the individual and system levels. In the United States, culture is usually only associated with ethnicity or race. The authors believe it is essential that this narrow perception of culture be expanded, with culture viewed and understood as multidimensional, and that ethnicity represents only one of these dimensions. Wenger (1991) describes culture as a system of collectively held values, beliefs, and practices of a group that guides decisions and actions in patterned and recurrent ways. From this viewpoint, the conceptualization of culture extends beyond the boundaries to include

219

groups that are not defined solely by ethnicity, such as professional associations, organizations, and systems. For the purposes of this chapter, it is important to think of culture in its broadest sense. For example, consider the culture of the U.S. legal system, institutions of higher education, or systems of services and supports such as the health care system. The cultural characteristics of each of these systems are complex, multifaceted, and hierarchical. While seemingly constant, each system is also dynamic—responding to social, economic, political, and technological changes that are taking place in both the internal and external environments.

This chapter explores cultural beliefs and influences that often converge when an individual is faced with end-of-life decisions within the contexts of the legal system, the health care system, community and social networks, spirituality or the faith community, and the family. This chapter addresses each of these systems beginning with that which is most public and visible (the legal system) and concluding with the ones that are more private vis-à-vis an individual, that is, family (Iltis, 2004). Examples are provided that describe how the cultural variables of each system may impact an individual with an intellectual or developmental disability (IDD). Suggestions on how to address myriad cultural differences in end-of-life decisions are offered for administrators, educators, health policy makers, service providers, and advocates.

While not all inclusive, Figure 14.1 illustrates how an individual with IDD may interact with multiple systems regarding end-of-life decisions.

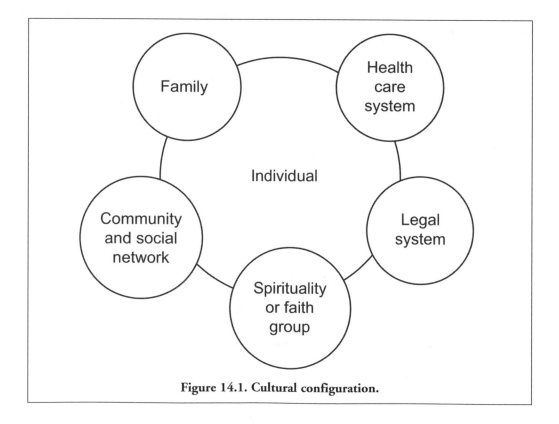

Figure 14.1. Cultural configuration.

FRAMING THE ISSUE: THE DYNAMICS OF CULTURE

Defining and Exploring Culture

Hundreds of definitions of culture seek to explain a known but at times elusive concept that encompasses and forms everyone's life. Culture provides the lens through which we view, interpret, and find meaning in the world in which we live. Culture structures perceptions, shapes behaviors, and defines our sense of reality. Culture defines health and well-being. It also defines and determines the manner in which we recognize and cope with illness and disability. Culture frames attitudes and beliefs about death and determines mourning rituals. It is not uncommon that under stress, a person relies on aspects of culture that have long been neglected or thought of as unimportant. The cultural beliefs and practices of families, and the communities in which they live, are assets and a great source of strength to a person with IDD throughout life and at the time of death.

The guiding definition of culture for this chapter is that of the National Center for Cultural Competence (2001), Georgetown University Medical Center:

> Culture is an integrated pattern of human behavior that includes thoughts, communications, languages, practices, beliefs, values, customs, courtesies, rituals, manners of interacting, roles, relationships and expected behaviors of a racial, ethnic, religious, social or political group; the ability to transmit the above to succeeding generations; it is dynamic in nature.

A Focus on Cultural Variables

This chapter does not use specific examples from cultural groups because of the risk of stereotyping the particular group mentioned and of possibly losing the significance of the concept for groups not mentioned. It is the opinion of the authors that it is better to start with a more generic approach to note broad categories and then explore how the specific group and the individual relate to these larger concepts. For example, Hall (1981) classifies cultures as low context and high context. Low context cultures emphasize independence, the importance of an individual in his own right, and a future time orientation. These cultures highly value individual rights and choice. Direct communication is acceptable, with the spoken and written word as the major means of communication. High context cultures value interdependence and relationships with others with a present-time orientation. There is less emphasis on the spoken word. A message can be conveyed indirectly, such as demonstrating feelings by actions rather than voicing them.

Locus of control is another variable in understanding cultures. An internal locus of control is preferred by most Western cultures and is at the heart of medicine in the United States. Self-determination is paramount, with the individual controlling his life based upon the choices he makes. In contrast, many other cultures embrace an external locus of control whereby it is thought the individual has little control over the events in his life, and much of it is determined by fate.

Bowman (2004) addresses other cultural variables related to the perception of moral order. Typically, Western cultures value autonomy rather than paternalism. Competition is highly valued and encouraged. This contrasts with many non-Western cultures where the focus is on harmony, equilibrium, and a world view that opposites are complementary and not competitive (such as the roles of males and females in a society).

Thus, drawing upon these descriptions, it is easy to see how cultural differences may arise related to autonomy and decision making regarding who should be informed of diagnoses and to what degree of disclosure and who should make end-of-life decisions. Multiple systems that operate from differing cultural orientations can converge when this decision making involves an individual with IDD, at times resulting in ethical dilemmas and conflict.

The Language-Culture Link

Language is one of the most symbolic aspects of any culture and carries messages far beyond the literal meaning of individual words. Within it, culture is encoded. Values, beliefs, attitudes, and shared subtleties are interwoven in such a way that individuals can express and share their deepest and most profound feelings. Symbols of communication go beyond words and include nonverbal communication such as gestures, silence, space, and touch. This complex structure becomes a mental map (Fisher, 1988) shared by all within the same culture. Meaning is understood within context, and in most instances, much goes unspoken—but it is understood by members who share a culture. Within this mental map are shared beliefs regarding concepts of health and illness, prevention and etiology of disability or disease, and treatment options (Fisher, 1988).

Within the health care system, it is not unusual that mental maps are not congruent or equally shared among all parties. This is particularly evident in the language used to describe death and end of life by people who are ill and their families, health and mental health care clinicians, clinical and administrative personnel in hospitals and other health care settings, or clergy and spiritual advisers. Miller (2002) provides a poignant explanation of the dynamics and power of language:

> Language is in every way an antidote to our fears and anxieties and general paralysis on the subject of death and dying. . . . Once we find the common ground of language, we can develop treatment plans, erect facilities for the comfort of the dying, ratify laws that assist the dying, argue ethical standard regarding the treatment of the dying, take comfort from others, and begin to heal. Without language we can do none of these. (p. 24)

Communicating with and on behalf of a person who has IDD can span a broad range of needs and preferences in the delivery of health care and mental health services. Understanding diagnoses, decision making regarding consent for treatment, following through on treatment, and completing advance care directives are all influenced by the capacity to communicate with and on behalf of an individual who experiences dementia, an intellectual disability, a language or speech disorder, a sensory disorder (such as hearing loss, low vision, or blindness), traumatic brain injury, or a serious mental illness. In the opinion of the authors, in order to create an environment that values and respects every person and that is more inclusive of people with disabilities, concerted attention must be directed toward establishing and implementing policies, practices, and procedures that effectively address the complexity of communication in this nation's health and mental health care systems.

THE LEGAL SYSTEM

Legislation and Social Activism

While legislation and media coverage are only two examples of the public, or external, elements of culture, they reflect and are based upon values that are mostly identified as part of the internal culture. Federal and state legislation address numerous concerns related to access to health care, language access in health care provisions, patient rights and responsibilities, and end-of-life decision making. Title VI of the Civil Rights Act of 1964 asserts that national origin (i.e., language and lack of fluency in English) should not be a barrier to receiving quality health care and provides specific ways to address this. The American Hospital Association adopted the Patient's Bill of Rights in 1973. The consumer-rights movement of the 1970s may have helped to influence a shift that gave more control over decision making to the person who is ill, while lessening that of the health care provider (Giger, Davidhizar, & Fordham, 2006). The Joint Commission on Accreditation of Health Organizations (JCAHO), the largest and oldest accrediting entity in the United States for health care, has made numerous references to the need to consider diversity when providing quality health care.

Social activism also contributed to the passage of the Americans With Disabilities Act (ADA) in 1990. While earlier disability legislation largely focused on support and benefits for those who could not work, this new legislation enabled people with disabilities to work and participate more fully in society (Seligman & Darling, 2007, p. 7).

Legislation as an Expression of Cultural Values

The great amount of media attention given to such court cases such as *Cruzan* (*Cruzan v. Director*, 1990) and Quinlan (Rowell, 2000) brought to the public awareness the need to better address end-of-life care and related decisions. Following these and other decisions, the Patient Self-Determination Act (PSDA) was passed in 1991. Giger, Davidhizar, and Fordham (2006) discuss the basic values on which this act is based and include (a) patient autonomy, (b) informed consent, (c) truth telling regarding information provided openly to people who are ill by health professionals, and (d) an individual's control over the dying process. While the basic premise of the PSDA is that decision making is a personal decision—a notion clearly acceptable to many—nevertheless, implementation has been difficult because of challenges presented by different cultural perspectives. This chapter will briefly consider each of these as they relate to cultural values and potential areas of incongruence.

Autonomy

The concept of autonomy includes the role of the individual within his larger cultural setting. For high context cultures that foster social interdependence rather than individual independence, the concept of autonomy may feel incongruent, incompatible, inconsistent with their world view, and conflict with traditional beliefs and practices. Decisions for individuals are made by taking into consideration the interests of the larger group (extended family or community) as well as the individual. Simultaneously, each—both the larger group and the individual—has mutual responsibilities and provides support to one another. A death is a loss for the family and the community. If a culture values a family-centered rather than an individual-centered model of decision making, then expecting a person to make such decisions on his own will not feel empowering but instead, will run the risk of making the person feel isolated and burdened. A strategy to work within this framework is to ask a person his preference (i.e., does he want to be informed of his condition or not and if he does not want to know, then who should be informed? Blackhall, Murphy, Frank, Michel, & Azen, 1995; Candib, 2002).

In family-centered models, decisions may be based on group consensus. Harmony of the group is more highly valued than the personal desires of an individual. While elders are often responsible for decisions, as they age, family members assume the responsibility for their health care decisions. This is based on respect for elders and the desire to relieve them of the burden of decision making.

Autonomy and decision making are also influenced by gender roles. This may be encountered when the individual is a female under the guardianship of a male. In many cultures, males routinely make decisions for and on behalf of their wives, daughters, sisters, and other female relatives. A female's decision may be overruled by that of her husband or father if she is not in agreement with the male decision maker (Klessig, 1992, p. 318).

Respect for authority, particularly in terms of the role and expertise of the health care provider, can also enter into the question of autonomy and decision making. If a person or family member seems indecisive, it may be due to the expectation that the physician should tell them what to do because of the trust and respect bestowed on the role of the physician. In some cultures, a strong concept of courtesy exists. It is considered impolite or disrespectful to disagree openly with a physician; even if family members do not agree with the recommendation of the physician, they may not say anything to the contrary. In addition, in high context cultures where social relationships are paramount, the physician may be seen as an extended family member and be expected to make the decisions. In the larger U.S. society, characterized as low context—in which some members may think autonomy signifies personhood (Bowman, 2004) and where "I" is capitalized in the written language—it is easy to see that the concept of autonomy presents cultural challenges.

Informed Consent

Informed consent can be complicated by the use and understanding of language, particularly the legal terms used in such documents. There are 311 languages spoken in the United States. Of these, 162 are indigenous and 149 represent languages of immigrants (National Virtual Translation Center, 2007). Responding to such language diversity presents challenges in any health care setting.

The importance of a trained, competent, and/or certified interpreter cannot be underestimated because discussion of a person's health or mental health care involves much more than a simple lexicon of translated terminology. Words that are thought to be easily understood because they are so commonly used in English may not carry the same meaning in another language. For example, "hospice" is well known within palliative care, and it may be expected that the word and concept are readily understood by most people. In 2006, there were 4,500 hospice programs in the United States. Yet, in an article from the Kansas City Star, a hospice chaplain explains that, in Spanish, the word for "hospice" means a place much like an asylum or an orphanage and does not connote the services that are provided by health care workers or social workers to a person at home. Instead, the word implies that the family member will be removed from family and familiar surroundings (Franey, 2008). This example emphasizes that translations cannot be literal; they must take into consideration cultural contexts of the message that is being conveyed. Research conducted by Hablamos Juntos, a ground breaking national project funded by the Robert Wood Johnson Foundation, documents that the overall quality of most translated Spanish language documents is poor (Hablamos Juntos, 2006). These issues have obvious implications for granting informed consent for individuals who speak a language other than English.

While some individuals feel more comfortable with family members serving as interpreters, it is not a safe practice in health and mental health care settings, and it is illegal in jurisdictions such as California to have a minor serve in the role of an interpreter. There are numerous reasons why family, friends, and minors should not serve in this role including lack of knowledge of medical terminology, no control of the quality of interpretation, risk of liability, issues associated with confidentiality, and the inappropriateness of burdening children/youth with a professional responsibility.

When a person has low literacy in English as well as in his or her language of origin, the challenge of communication is even more daunting. However, miscommunication is not only relegated to those who speak languages other than English. An Institute of Medicine (IOM) report (IOM, 2004) on health literacy in 2004 estimates that nearly 90 million people (i.e., nearly half of all adults) have difficulty in understanding basic health information. In a fact sheet issued by the National Academy on an Aging Society (1998), it was estimated that low health literacy skills accounted for about $73 billion in additional health care expenditures in 1998, $30 billion for those who were functionally illiterate and $43 billion for those who were marginally illiterate.

The Agency for Healthcare Research and Quality (AHRQ) commissioned an evidence report regarding the relationship between literacy and health (Berkman et al., 2004). Based on this study, individuals with limited health literacy appear to have a higher rate of hospitalization and are less likely to understand emergency department discharge instructions. This same report also indicated that people with low literacy skills are less likely to seek or receive preventive care, understand informed consent forms, comprehend their children's diagnoses, understand medication instructions for themselves and their children, and be less knowledgeable about the health effects of smoking, diabetes, asthma, human immunodeficiency virus (HIV), and postoperative care. These same authors conclude that "low reading skills and poor health are clearly related" (Berkman et al., 2004, p. 6).

For a person with IDD, it may be even more difficult to understand fully all that is required in signing an informed consent document. It may also present uncertainties and dilemmas on the part of individuals with low health literacy who are legally entrusted with the responsibility to make decisions on behalf of a person with IDD. In many instances, parents of children with special needs have expressed to service providers their difficulty in understanding the complexities presented in the Individual Educational Plans (IEP) that have been developed for their children in the school system.

When it comes to decision making, government agencies that serve as legal guardians for individuals with disabilities usually have a policy in place that must be followed. For family members, caretakers, and legal guardians making a life and death decision on behalf of someone when they may not know the individual's wishes presents a complexity of burdens with medical, personal, and familial dimensions (Braun, Beyth, Ford, & McCullough, 2008). Research by Braun et al. (2008, p. 273) indicates that surrogates face burdens that are "common across race and ethnicity," but the authors also note that few studies have been conducted on differences among racial and ethnic groups when it comes to surrogate decision making in relation to end of life. They suggest that coping strategies may vary by race or ethnicity, and awareness of these may be important to a better understanding of the uncertainty and burdens faced by surrogates.

Truth Telling

Truth telling allows for a person to participate actively in end-of-life decisions. The general acceptance of such disclosure has only become commonly accepted in North American culture within the last 40 years (Giger et al., 2006). Ideally, an advance directive will ensure that the individual's wishes about end of life are followed. However, such a document is viewed with skepticism by many. For those who distrust the medical system because of historic abuses or who are fearful because of perceived negative public sentiment toward certain minorities, there is concern that such a document may legalize neglect (Giger et al., 2006) or may be used as a way to deny care (Mitty, 2001).

Newcomers to the United States may be unaccustomed to the importance of putting end-of-life decisions in writing, and they may be reluctant to execute these documents since such discussions and understanding in a home country did not require a written formality—or such discussions did not customarily take place at all. But it is not only newcomers to the United States who may be reluctant to sign an advance directive. There are many other cultural groups with long-standing roots in the United States that are resistant to this practice. It is estimated that 80% of patients who are admitted to U.S. hospitals do not have an advance directive (Searight & Gafford, 2005). To approach an ill person with the expectation of signing forms about treatment when death is imminent would be considered insensitive. In addition, people in many cultures believe that language and thought can shape reality. It is important to think positively for good results, and talking about bad things can bring on unwanted results (Carrese & Rhodes, 1995). Therefore, to speak openly of a terminal disease or an impending death may cause a person to lose hope and may even bring about or hasten death.

For those people who think it is inappropriate to raise the future prospect of an illness, one strategy that has been suggested is to use a third-person hypothetical format (Carrese & Rhodes, 2000). Some health care providers have developed the strategy of "partial disclosure," that is, words such as tumor, cyst, and inflammation are used, which the individual can accept at face value or come to understand its truer meaning without the word "cancer" ever being used (Candib, 2002). While this approach may be culturally responsive, it may have legal implications in some health care settings.

These points of view can present a major dilemma for a health care provider who believes it is a professional and ethical responsibility to fully disclose all information to the ill person. Fan (1997) refers to family determination and Candib (2002) calls for the need to rework the notion of autonomy to one of "autonomy-in-relation," or recognition of the family context of autonomy. Decision making thus comes from one's connectedness as a family member and not from separateness as an individual (Candib, 1995). Candib (2002, p. 226) calls for the recognition that health care providers are also "culture-bound" by their approach and that "assumptions about truth telling and the end of life are not universally applicable or appropriate."

Individual Control Over the Process of Dying

The emphasis on the individual right to make choices seemingly presents the option that death can be defied or at a minimum prolonged. However, for many, death is more readily accepted as a natural part of life. Rather than viewing death as the opposite of life, many view death as the opposite of birth, a journey between two worldly events in time (Desai, 2000). From this point of view, "end of life" as a concept does not exist. Attitudes toward death and suffering differ remarkably and are greatly influenced by cultural and spiritual beliefs. For example, some cultures believe all life is sacred and only the Divine can intervene, and other cultures question whether longevity or prolonging of life is desired over quality of life.

Legislation, including those laws related to health care, is based upon the underlying assumptions and values of any cultural system. While for many, these decisions may seem obvious and pose no inherent difficulties in acceptance, for those who view the system from other cultural perspectives, incongruities and challenges may arise.

THE HEALTH CARE SYSTEM

A "culture of medicine" exists within any health care system and its influence permeates throughout, including the selection of students, curricula content, value placed on technology, communication style, quality of life, roles of providers and patients, and many more variables (McGaghie, 2002). This section will explore the nature of the culture of biomedicine in the United States, its emphasis on technology, institutional policies and structures, brain death as a cultural construct, and the use of alternative medicine.

The Culture of Biomedicine

As the world economies industrialized, as people moved farther away from their families and places of birth, as jobs became more specialized, and as preparation of the dead grew into a large mortuary industry, death and dying became increasingly "medicalized" and removed from the home. In the United States, only about 23% of people actually die at home, however, many more state this as a preference (Mitty, 2001). Kapp (2000) supports this figure, estimating that 80% of the two million people who die in the United States every year die in health care institutions.

"Biomedicine," the prevailing medical viewpoint in the United States, is commonly characterized as a cultural system (Spector, 1985, pp. 70–71). Keeping in mind the definition of culture provided earlier in the chapter, it is possible to see that biomedicine also has its own set of values, beliefs, language, communication styles, practices, manners of interacting, roles, relationships, and expected behaviors. Let us consider examples of a few of these. Communication style and language were addressed in the sections on truth telling and informed consent. As a belief system, there are standardized definitions of health and illness based largely on a mind-body dichotomy and with an emphasis on the disease and the individual. A high value is placed on technology, and there is a strong reliance on surgical and therapeutic interventions. Values also include cleanliness, promptness, adherence or compliance, and organization. Goals often relate to prolonging life versus a high quality of life, and trying to save lives while minimizing any permanent disability (Iltis, 2004). Standard practices include prevention measures, such as immunizations, and diagnostic procedures, such as an annual physical exam, mammography, and biopsy, are common.

There are specific procedures ("practices") around birth and death. Within biomedicine, there are definitive "cultural" practices around death and dying, and "physicians act in accord with deeply held values" (Koenig & Gates-Williams, 1995). A person with IDD will require support to navigate through such a system. It can be equally difficult for the surrogate decision maker who is burdened with the worry, guilt, or pressure from other family members to make the right decisions.

While it is often assumed that biomedicine, or "Western" medicine, is homogenous across North America and Western Europe, it, too, does not exist in a social vacuum and reflects the values of the countries in which it is found. Helman (1990, pp. 63–68) compared studies of doctors in the United States and Europe and noted how they reflect the underlying cultural values of their respective societies. Differences were found in the leading diagnostic categories and in the types of medications prescribed, but disparities in the health of the populations were not sufficient to explain the marked variations among these countries. Feldman (1992, p. 348) explains differences in structure, values, and practices between the French and U.S. systems of health care, noting that Western medicine is "not a single uniform medical system but a multiplicity of related systems, each arising out of its own cultural and historical context." Hahn and Gaines (1985) and Payer (1988) provide additional explanations regarding biomedicine as a cultural entity and Ohnuki-Tierney (1994) discusses "biomedicine as Western culture," noting differences in the types and rates of organ transplants.

People who are ill and their family members are not the only ones who experience conflicts surrounding cultural values. Providers are socialized into biomedicine, but they, too, "carry value systems that relate to their past experiences, upbringing, and ethnic identity" (Klessig, 1992, p. 319). Through medical training, many providers come to regard their traditional cultural beliefs with skepticism, while others are at least able to understand how a person may hold traditional beliefs but still seek care within the biomedical field. And, according to Chattopadhyay and Simon (2008, p. 171), "the same physician with the same moral sensibility may practice ethical medicine differently in two different sociocultural contexts."

Health care providers receive the same cultural messages as the rest of society toward individuals with disabilities—negative stereotyping, misinformation, and valuation of a poorer quality of life (DeLisa & Thomas, 2005; Seligman & Darling, 2007). Estimates indicate that one in five, or 20% of the U.S. population, has a disability of some kind (DeLisa & Thomas, 2005, p. 6, 10). Nevertheless, few professionals have had direct experience, whether in their personal lives or in their training with individuals with disabilities (Seligman & Darling, 2007, p. 287), and medical curricula devote little time to issues related to disabilities (DeLisa & Thomas, 2005). This presents significant challenges not only to treatment and care but also to how the lives of people with IDD are valued in the health care system. Whose life is more valuable as choices are made? DeLisa and Thomas (2005, p. 10) recommend strongly that a disability curriculum should be integrated into the training of health care providers, saying that "it is imperative to raise the level of awareness and, consequently, the level of understanding about disability issues within the medical professions."

Technology

Technology, a hallmark of biomedicine, has contributed to difficulties in decision making around life support—whether to start it or not, and if started, whether to discontinue it. Klessig (1992) documents major differences among various groups when it comes to starting or stopping life support. For a person who believes that God alone determines the time of birth and death, then a moral responsibility exists to care for one's body. Based on this belief, the seeking of medical help can be justified, as medical technology can be viewed as a "gift" from God. From this cultural viewpoint or belief system, there is no right to die since the time of death is determined by God. Even if a family agrees to discontinue life support, a strong belief in astrology may lead to a request to postpone this action until an auspicious date so that the children of the dying person will have a positive future rather than suffer a negative fate (Galanti, 1997). In some cases, demanding the maximum care available for a loved one is felt to be a sign of the family's love and caring, even in the face of what appears to be insurmountable odds. In cultures where filial piety, or loyalty to one's parents, is strong, children believe they owe their lives to their parents, are responsible for them, and must preserve their lives no matter the cost. At the same time—keeping in mind religious and traditional views regarding compassion, justice, and concern for the family as a unit—a person may decide against life supporting technology because of the economic or emotional hardship it may present for the family (Klessig, 1992, pp. 318–319). So even within the same culture and the same family, cultural imperatives can present difficult decisions. When values compete, even within the same culture, there are no easy answers. The complexity, dynamics, and emotional burdens of such decisions are no different in families whose loved ones have IDD.

Institutional Policies and Structures

Nearing the time of death, institutional policies and structures designed with efficiency and the individual as the focus may pose difficulties related to cultural and religious beliefs. For example, visiting hours are limited in many health care institutions. Particularly for surrogate decision makers, this may challenge opportunities for communicating with health care providers and adds the extra burden of scheduling around work and other family responsibilities while trying to understand the diagnosis, treatment options, and changing responses of the person who is ill.

Along with limited visiting hours, the design of hospital rooms does not accommodate visits from large groups of family members. This is especially true in the intensive care units when a person may be near death. For cultures that have "loud" expressions of grief with wailing upon the death of a loved one or those that have traditions of playing musical instruments such as a flute or drum, such practices may conflict with the cultural practice and norms of the quiet, hushed tones in most hospitals. In such a case, with a bit of advanced preparation, arrangements can be made to move the person who has died and the family members into a chapel or other designated space where the family can mourn in a manner to which they are accustomed without disturbing others around them (Galanti, 1997, p. 111).

Family members may insist on lighting a candle or burning incense at the time of death to guide the spirit to heaven, a potentially challenging request due to fire code regulations and the use of oxygen in the room. Some families may wish to turn the body toward a certain direction as death approaches. Many buildings, including hospitals, have windows that do not open and may present a structural barrier for some families. For those who believe a soul cannot be free until it can escape to the outside, family members may request that the body be carried outside for a short period of time so that the soul can be released. Some families may want to burn the mattress and anything worn by the person who died, while others may request that burial include amputated body parts, if they are available.

Although beliefs and practices surrounding end-of-life and death rituals present ethical and legal dilemmas for health care systems, providing accommodations and reaching compromise are desirable alternatives for families. For example, parents or caregivers may place an amulet or blessed string on a child for protection and to aid in recovery, most often around the neck or wrist. Depending upon placement and the severity of the child's condition, it may interfere with treatment. If at all possible, such items should not be removed without consulting the parents. A compromise may be reached such as hanging the amulet on the wall over the bed, placing it under the mattress, or attaching it to a visible part of the bed without it being in the way of treatment.

Brain Death as a Cultural Construct

All health care systems, including biomedicine and the technology associated with it, do not exist outside of culture but are rooted within it. The definition and discussion of brain death as a cultural construct—or, in the words of Ohnuki-Tierney (1994), a "new cultural institution"—are based upon the premise that in Western culture, the brain is the seat of "reason." Emerging from the prominence that 17th century philosophers placed on rationality, the brain was the seat of rational thought. The well-known phrase "Cogito ergo sum" (I think therefore I am) brings into question the personhood of an individual with IDD; the brain became the defining criteria for the value of a person. Not all cultures place paramount emphasis on the brain. It is the dichotomy of "being" versus "doing." For some, a person may have multiple souls located in various major organs. Or, a person may have one soul, which is not centered in the brain but may leave the body after death through the head. Even while a person is still alive, surgery or blood tests may release a spirit, and fright may cause a soul to be lost, resulting in an illness or disability in Western terminology. Relatives often have difficulty in accepting the diagnosis of brain death, preferring to wait for the physical signs of the cessation of breathing or of the lack of a pulse or heartbeat. Ohnuki-Tierney (1994) speaks of the time before the development of the diagnosis of brain death when an "inactive brain" was viewed as the "prolongation of life" rather than the "prolongation of the process of dying," as it has come to be known. For many cultures, the former remains the more commonly accepted view.

During the 1960s and 1970s, more than 30 sets of criteria defining brain death were in existence, but none of them were exactly the same. In 1981, the Uniform Declaration of Death Act (UDDA) attempted to standardize the criteria. Still, when it comes to end-of-life decisions, the diagnosis is not straightforward since it ultimately involves discussion and negotiation among the major participants (health care providers, recipient patient and/or family, donor and/or family, third party payers, etc.). As Angrosino refers to "context-specific interactions," he states that "the decision to declare brain death is a social act that occurs in various ways depending on shifting circumstances; it is not purely an exercise of neutral biomedical technology" (Ohnuki-Tierney 1994, p. 243). This is an extremely complex issue, and the equivalence of brain death with death is generally, but not universally, accepted (Bernat, 2004). There remains no global agreement on diagnostic criteria, as a review of the brain death guidelines for adults in 80 countries demonstrated (Wijdicks,

2002). There are some religious beliefs that do not accept brain death to be the equivalent of death. New Jersey and New York have passed legislation to deal with this issue (Inwald, Jakobovits, & Petros, 2000).

Alternative Medicine

According to the World Health Organization (WHO), traditional medicine is defined as the

> health practices, approaches, knowledge and beliefs incorporating plant, animal and mineral based medicines, spiritual therapies, manual techniques and exercises, applied singularly or in combination to treat, diagnose and prevent illnesses or maintain well-being. (Bagozzi, 2003)

In the United States, adaptations of traditional medicine are called "complementary" or "alternative" medicine (CAM), and there is a National Center for Complementary and Alternative Medicine (NCCAM) housed within the National Institutes of Health. Popularity for alternative medicine is increasing throughout the world and in the United States, 42% of the population has used CAM at least once, and the annual CAM expenditure is estimated at $2,700 million (WHO, 2002).

Alternative medicine options abound in the United States, and many practices and practitioners come from cultural or religious communities. Beliefs and behaviors around death do not change easily, and in times of crisis, many find comfort in cultural and religious traditions. Traditional healers may be consulted for treatment of a person with disabilities or for a person who is terminally ill at any stage of an illness. Consultation with a traditional healer may occur simultaneously with health care received within the biomedical system. Often times, consultation at the end of life is not so much to heal but to provide comfort within a culturally and socially meaningful context. For some, it is thought that a specialist will help the soul find its way after death.

COMMUNITY, SOCIAL NETWORK, AND FAMILY

Definitions of health, illness, and recognition of disability are defined by a community, with the sociocultural context adding meaning to a clinical diagnosis. This section will address how communities lend cultural interpretations to disability and their implications for end-of-life decisions.

Definition of Community

There are many definitions for community, but a key factor in culturally and ethnically diverse communities is that not all members are always clustered or living closely together geographically. For purposes of this chapter, community is defined as "a body of persons of common interests scattered through a larger society" (Goode, 2001).

Definitions of Disability

Definitions of disability vary—they may be clinical or social. For the National Institute on Disability and Rehabilitation Research (NIDRR), disability "is the result of an interaction between characteristics of the individual and those of the natural, built, communications (IT), cultural, and social environments" (NIDRR, 2008). However, disability is often socially defined within one's community. In some cultures, there may be no specific words to identify a particular disability, or the acceptance of it may be such that a new role for the person is defined and accepted. For example, a diagnosis of epilepsy may be understood within an ethnic community that the person is the host of a healing spirit, the seizures are proof of special powers, and this person is expected to become a shaman (Fadiman, 1997).

Cultural Perceptions and the Causes of Illness and Disability

Cultural beliefs regarding disability vary greatly. Table 14.1 lists some cultural beliefs for the causes of illness and disability worldwide. It is not intended as an all-inclusive list but rather as an example of the complexity around this topic within many cultural communities.

Even if parents understand the clinical etiology, they may still explain its occurrence within a meaningful sociocultural context. For example, Seligman and Darling (2007) recount the case of a family whose child was diagnosed with Schwartz-Jampel syndrome— "an autosomal recessive disorder characterized by short stature, skeletal abnormalities, generalized myotonia [muscles that cannot relax], ocular anomalies, and a unique facies [a distinct facial bone structure]" (Viljoen & Beighton, 1992, p. 59). Although the parents were educated and understood autosomal recessive transmission, the mother still expressed the belief that a severe fright had caused the gene mutation in the fetus.

Folk or traditional explanations hold much symbolism for the believer and provide a sense of comfort in that understanding the cause gives a person some control over the situation and suggests ways to prevent recurrence in another child.

Table 14.1
Cultural Beliefs of Causes for Illness and Disability

- Air, wind
- Accident of nature
- Angry deity or deities
- Ancestors and other ghosts
- Chastisement or punishment of God or other deity for bad acts of parents
- Disruption of equilibrium in the body—cold, heat, other humors
- Evil eye or other malevolent forces
- Fright
- Gift or blessing from God or other deity
- Intrusion by an object
- Karma
- Loss of soul(s)
- Mischievous spirits
- Possession by an evil spirit
- Sorcerers or witches who have cursed the child or parents
- Taboo broken by the mother during pregnancy

Disability within a community may be accepted as a fact of life; there may be a belief that the person can be cured by rituals or through the use of certain medicines, and acceptance may or may not exist that a person with disabilities can contribute to his community and lead a productive life in a role as defined by the community (Blankenship & Madson, 2007). Family responses to a loved one's disability may also vary widely. For some, a stigma is attached to the disability and the person is hidden away. It may be thought that marriage or other opportunities (e.g., business) may be adversely affected by how others view a particular disability. For others, a cultural tradition that includes a strong sense of family may make it easier to accept and care for a person with special needs. Families who have immigrated to the United States explain how lonely and isolated it can be to care for a family member with a disability compared to the situation in the home country. In the United States they often feel isolated, with no one coming to visit the family caretakers or the person who needs care. They contrast this with the home situation where there are more relatives, where family members live closer to each other, and where every day someone is visiting, even if for a short time. This provides support for the caregiver as well as the person with a disability.

Grief

Grief, the emotional response to a loss, differs from the concept of bereavement or mourning, the "culturally patterned behavioral response to a death" (Andrews & Boyle, 1995, 366).

Social experiences of individuals from minority cultural groups, including those who experience disability, can greatly influence end-of-life decisions and responses to grief. Centuries of discrimination, unlawful experimentation, and access to care issues can all contribute to the level of trust placed with the provider and the health care system and can influence the end-of-life choices that are made (Dufy, Jackson, Schim, Ronis, & Fowler, 2006).

Refugees and certain other immigrants fit into the designation as noted by Irish, Lundquist, and Nelson (1993, p. 188) of having experienced "chronic" losses—"homeland, personal belongings, family members, economic status, professional identity, cultural traditions, language, and sense of self." There may be unrealistic expectations of the capabilities of medicine in the United States, particularly, of the medical technology available, so that certain types of losses may not be expected to happen. The sense of loss can be spread across multiple dimensions within these migrant communities. The loss of any person may raise the issue of unresolved grief, personally and community-wide. If an elder—the bearer of traditions and the community historian—dies, then much is being lost and forgotten in this new country. The loss of a child may be seen as the loss for the future of the community and not just an individual family's loss. Traditional burial practices and mourning rituals may not be possible so far away from the country of origin, making it harder to process the grief.

Just as the expression of grief varies widely around the world, so do explanatory models of death and the nature of the afterlife. Questions and differing ideas regarding what happens after death abound. Table 14.2 lists only a sample of some of these thoughts that can be found worldwide.

Table 14.2

Cultural Thoughts and Questions Regarding Death and an Afterlife

- Did witchcraft cause this death, and if so, how can I compensate for that? Witchcraft accounted for the death, and someone must compensate for it.

- The soul of the dying person will be reincarnated in the body of the next baby who is born into the family or the community.

- The soul of the dying person will join with the person standing closest at death.

- How can I appease the ghost of the dead person when it is difficult to carry out the appropriate rituals so far from my home country? The ghost of the dead person needs to be appeased, which may be difficult so far away from one's home country.

- The dead will come back to visit on certain days each year and I will be certain to offer them the appropriate food and respect.

- An autopsy may prevent reincarnation.

- How can I agree to an organ donation when my loved one will need it when she enters the next life? The dead person's soul requires the presence of their organs, and so families cannot consent to organ donation.

Note. Adapted from "Cross-cultural variation in the experience, expression, and understanding of grief," by P. Rosenblatt, 1993, in D. Irish, K. Lundquist, and V. Nelson (Eds.), Ethnic variations in dying, death, and grief: Diversity in universality. *New York: Taylor & Francis, with additions by the authors.*

In some high context cultures, parents take on the name of a child after his birth, such as "Mother of . . ." or "Father of . . ." (followed by the name of the child). In low context cultures, such as the United States, parenthood is not characterized with this informal name recognition. The expression of loss in the English language is clearly defined as widow or widower when a spouse dies, but such recognition does not exist in the English language for a parent who suffers the loss of a child. How, then, is one's loss publicly acknowledged and recognized? Referring to the importance of language, Miller (2002, p. 19) explains how the lack of a formal name in the English language for a person who has lost a child is immensely important. Language and culture are integrally linked. The absence of such a term in the English language may express a belief that a child should not precede her parents in death. There is no single word in English to share the experience of the loss of a child as there is in other cultures. For many families, the lack of clear, concise language adds to their grief, as they are forced to use many words or to tell their story of their child's death. Karla F. C. Holloway (2009), a noted researcher who has examined African American mourning and death rituals, acknowledges the absence of this term in the English language. In a recently published article, Holloway suggests the use of a Sanskrit word, *vilomah*, which means "against a natural order," to describe a parent who buries a child rather than a child who buries a parent.

It is not uncommon for parents of children (including adult offspring) with IDD to frequently encounter those who may not share the same mental map about the worth and value of their loved ones. Parents encounter well intentioned people who say, "It was for the best . . . he had such a difficult life," or "Fortunately she was not aware of what was happening to her—that must be such a relief for you." These kinds of interactions shed light on how cultural perceptions of disability and the process of grief may collide in the everyday encounters that parents and caretakers experience in the loss of a loved one with IDD.

SPIRITUALITY OR FAITH GROUP

Discussion about the relationship between spirituality or religion and health has grown enormously over the last several decades in the field of health care. As this debate continues, health care providers are increasingly aware of the support and challenges that religion and spirituality may provide the individual and family members. While there are many definitions of both terms—"religion" and "spirituality"—the general consensus in the literature is that spirituality is the more general term, encompassing religion for some but able to stand alone for others without attachment to a particular faith group.

Culture and religion are intertwined. Many members of cultural groups do not consciously differentiate between the two. For these individuals, it is more than the box they mark on a paper—instead, it is like the "air I breathe," guiding actions throughout the day. Their well-being is composed not only of physical and mental health but also of the unity of mind, body, and spirit. Religion permeates daily life with no real separation of the sacred from daily living. Others compartmentalize religion and spirituality, seeing them as very private and something that one does not talk about. Some profess no real sense of spirituality or religion in their lives at all. Variation exists within the same faith group across cultures, and individual interpretation lends still further diversity.

In Western medicine, over the last several decades, spirituality and religion lost prominence in healing and healers are no longer regarded as religious specialists. However, there is now renewed interest in further exploring this potential relationship. Providers and scholars are starting to develop the paradigm of the "biopsychosocial-spiritual" model of health with application to multiple health issues, specifically to end-of-life concerns as discussed by Sulmasy (2002) and Maloof (2008).

For parents and caregivers, the response to having a child with a disability or special needs can vary greatly from one culture and religious group to another, and even within any given culture or group. Seligman and Darling (2007, p. 29) present several ways that families may view having a child with special needs: (a) the child's disability is seen as a blessing and an indication of the family's strong emotional strength, (b) the child's disability is seen as good luck or as a blessing from "God" (or a higher being) because he was deemed particularly special, and (c) a child's disability may be viewed as a punishment from God for past sins that may be those of a family member or that of the child in a past life.

Caregivers may seek solace in religion (Seligman & Darling, 2007, p. 29) because (a) religion helps them to accept their child's disability more easily, (b) the child's disability may encourage them to look for more of a connection with God and for support within a faith community, and (c) God is giving them an opportunity to become better people.

A challenge may arise in these examples if the parent or caregiver is angry with God for his or her family member's situation, and this anger can generate a great deal of guilt that may be difficult to reconcile.

A great deal of variation relates to end-of-life decisions. Not all religions view pain and suffering as having a redeeming value for the next life, but some do. In such a case, if a spiritual cause is attributed to the illness or disability, there may be the preference to try and prolong life. For a person of deep faith, suffering and pain may provide the opportunity to demonstrate ones faith and put trust in "God." For the believer in "karma," it is not acceptable to end one's life early, because one's work in this life must be completed and the consequences of past deeds must be worked out or the suffering is carried over into the next life. To a believer, miracles are always possible and one must not lose hope. This latter belief is often mentioned as a reason to request life-prolonging technology in the face of what is clinically seen as an insurmountable illness.

The United States is often characterized as a "death defying culture" (Giger et al., 2006, p. 7). Compared to references such as fighting an illness, battling against cancer, or even viewing death as the enemy, in other cultures, death is a transition with the family and community being supportive during the dying process. Life may be viewed as a "journey between two temporal events, birth and death" (Desai, 2000). The body may be viewed as a house or a jacket for ones spirit that is discarded as one completes this temporal journey.

Religion: A Source of Comfort and Conflict

The American Academy of Pediatrics (AAP, 2000) acknowledges that spirituality is encompassed within good pediatric palliative care and recommends that a spiritual advisor be included as a member of the provider team. However, there is also concern about the potential negative impact of spiritual and religious beliefs. An example may be that parents will choose to withhold treatment based upon such beliefs, such as their refusal to allow immunizations, antibiotics, or blood transfusions, or the substitution of prayer for medical treatment, to name a few. The AAP (1997) Committee on Bioethics has issued a statement that recommends that health care providers "show sensitivity to and flexibility toward the religious beliefs and practices of families" and seek to make collaborative decisions. Nevertheless, the AAP "opposes religious doctrines that advocate opposition to medical attention for sick children" (p. 280).

Religious rights and freedom of parents versus the state's responsibility to ensure a person's health and well-being is an ongoing debate, especially for children. Four states (Hawaii, Nebraska, North Carolina, and Massachusetts) have no religious immunity in criminal and civil codes (Larabee & Sleeth, 1998). Five states have a religious defense for homicide (Arkansas, Ohio, Iowa, Delaware, and West Virginia), and most states allow for a religious defense related to charges of child death, neglect, or abuse (Gordon, 2000). However, even with these religious exemptions, in most states, the state or the courts still hold the power to order medical treatment for a child who needs it (Gordon, 2000).

Conflicts between religious traditions and laws in the United States may also arise as members of communities try to perform certain rituals from their home countries. For example, in the United States, a healer who uses the sacrifice of animals such as a chicken or a cow in a religious healing or funeral ritual will be in violation of public health laws and can be charged with cruelty to animals. If the remains of the animals are left in public areas such as on the beach, laws regarding littering, dumping, or waste disposal will have been violated.

Religion can pose a challenge on an individual, family, or faith-group basis if it is thought that the disability is a punishment from God. A parent who feels angry with God because her child has IDD may experience guilt about such feelings, making it all the more difficult to cope, and perhaps leading to a feeling of alienation from the very community on which she would have relied for help. Even within a family, not all members may profess the same religion, posing challenges for religious leaders who wish to develop memorial services without alienating any family members.

CONCLUSION

Perhaps this chapter raises more questions than it answers—and that is acceptable. It is the intent of the authors to provoke reflection, to stimulate thought, and to encourage dialogue on viewing end of life through a cultural lens. No human behavior is 100% predictable, and even within a single social or ethnic group there is variation. Particularly during a crisis around illness and end-of-life decisions, a person's thoughts may seem incongruent and confused, and relying on traditional beliefs and practices may provide solace—but then even these are open to individual interpretation. As health, mental health, and disability professionals, the important thing is to know not only one's discipline but also oneself. From there, being well grounded, knowing what questions to ask, and taking the time to listen and reflect on the answers is critical. Even if one does not agree with the individual's or family's perspective, self-knowledge and dialogue provide a foundation of understanding on which to build support of and respect for the end-of-life decisions that are made. The authors leave you with the following quote as a pathway to thinking about and responding to diversity throughout the circle of life, which for many cultures includes death:

> Diversity generally understood and embraced is not casual liberal tolerance of anything and everything not yourself; it is not polite accommodation. Instead, diversity is in action—the sometimes painful awareness that other people, other races, other voices, other habits of mind, have as much claim on the world, as you do. . . . And I urge you, amid all the differences present to the eye and mind, to reach out to create the bond that . . . will protect us all. We are meant to be here together. (Chase, 1989, p. 36)

RECOMMENDATIONS

The National Center for Cultural Competence embraces a conceptual framework and model of achieving cultural competence adapted from Cross, Bazron, Dennis, and Isaacs (1989). Cultural competence requires that organizations

- have a defined set of values and principles and demonstrate behaviors, attitudes, policies, and structures that enable them to work effectively cross-culturally;
- have the capacity to (a) value diversity, (b) conduct self-assessment, (c) manage the dynamics of difference, (d) acquire and institutionalize cultural knowledge, and (e) adapt to diversity and the cultural contexts of the communities they serve;

- incorporate the previous in all aspects of policy making, administration, practice, and service delivery and involve systematically consumers, key stakeholders, and communities.

Cultural competence is a developmental process that evolves over an extended period. Both individuals and organizations are at various levels of awareness, knowledge, and skills along the cultural competence continuum.

Using this framework, the following strategies are offered to policy makers, administrators, practitioners/service providers, educators, and advocates across the multiple disciplines that are concerned with or involved in end-of-life decisions for individuals with IDD and their families.

Value Diversity

- Ensure that your organizational philosophy recognizes the diversity of cultural expressions, traditions, and norms associated with the end of life.
- Actively seek and include individuals from diverse cultural and linguistic groups as members of your organization's advisory committees and governing boards.

Conduct Self-Assessment

- Assess the extent to which your organization's existing policies, structures, procedures, and practices take into consideration the beliefs and practices related to death and end of life for cultural groups served.
- Assess awareness and knowledge of cultural expressions, traditions, and norms associated with death and end of life of your organization's staff, faculty, students, and volunteers.
- Introduce instruments and tools for self-assessment of values and attitudes of staff, faculty, students, and volunteers about cultural practices related to the end of life.
- Assess the extent to which your organization's curricula, in-service training/professional development, and continuing education activities

  - include content on (a) cultural perceptions of illness and disability, (b) cross-cultural communication skills, and (c) cultural beliefs and practices related to death and end of life;
  - provide opportunities for research in these areas; and
  - include individuals from culturally diverse groups as guest lecturers to share their knowledge and experiences.

- Assess the degree to which your academic institution and faculty contribute to the body of knowledge on cultural practices related to death, end of life, and individuals and families impacted by IDD.

Manage the Dynamics of Difference

- Use existing structures, or establish new ones, to explore and resolve ethical dilemmas associated with end-of-life decision making and differing cultural viewpoints.

- Offer conflict resolution and mediation to address cultural differences related to end-of-life decision making, policy, and practices.
- Ensure that designated staff are knowledgeable and skilled in conflict resolution and mediation processes that take culture, language, and power dynamics into consideration.
- Enlist the assistance of religious and spiritual advisors and cultural brokers in problem solving and dispute resolution.
- Ensure that language differences are addressed through the provision of language interpretation services, translation services, sign language interpretation, and information in alternative formats for individuals and families who need or prefer this level of assistance.
- Attend to issues associated with literacy, health literacy, and mental health literacy of individuals, families, and communities served.

Acquire and Institutionalize Cultural Knowledge

- Offer forums for staff, faculty, students, and volunteers to
  - share knowledge and experiences related to cultural practices, traditions, and norms associated with death and end of life; and
  - receive training, mentoring, and consultation to enhance knowledge and skills necessary to interact with and support culturally and linguistically diverse individuals and their families.
- Establish relationships with community-based organizations, faith-based and spiritual organizations, and advocacy organizations to provide information about cultural beliefs and practices associated with death, end of life, and grieving.
- Establish policies that specifically address cultural preferences in end-of-life decisions. Ensure that all staff are knowledgeable and have received training in the procedures and practices to implement such policies.
- Develop and implement policies and allocate resources to advance and sustain organizational, cultural, and linguistic competence.

Adapt to Diversity and the Cultural Contexts of Communities

- Revisit existing policies and practices related to end of life to determine if they present barriers for the cultural communities served. The review process should include diverse perspectives, such as those representing the views of individuals with disabilities and their family members, community members, and advocates.
- Identify and modify those policies and practices that promote cultural congruence in end-of-life care and support, with the exception of those that would violate legal and regulatory requirements.
- Identify space or rooms within your health care organization's buildings/facilities that can be used for end-of-life and death rituals (e.g., chanting, burning incense, playing music, large families, wailing, or dance).

CHECKLIST TO FACILITATE THE DEVELOPMENT OF CULTURALLY AND LINGUISTICALLY COMPETENT POLICIES, STRUCTURES, AND PRACTICES

The following checklist is designed to guide the integration of cultural and linguistic competence in the complex set of issues surrounding end of life for individuals who have IDD, their families, and the systems that provide them with services and supports.

Does your program, organization, institution, or system have the following?

- A vision or mission that articulates values, principles, and rationale for cultural and linguistic competence
- A mission or vision that values communities as essential allies in achieving overall goals and objectives
- Policies that support the integration of culture in the provision of care, services and supports, education and research, or advocacy
- Supporting policy and structures to ensure the meaningful participation of a diverse cadre of individuals with disabilities, their family members, or caretakers in planning, implementation, and evaluation activities
- Supporting policy and structures that delineate community participation in planning, implementation, and evaluation activities
- Policies and allocated resources (both fiscal and personnel) to ensure compliance with all relevant federal, state, or local mandates governing language access (e.g., interpretation services, translation services, and signage)
- Policies and practices that are responsive to the health and mental health literacy needs of individuals, families, and communities
- A policy and allocated resources to ensure compliance with disability related federal, state, and local mandates
- A policy and allocated resources to support professional development and in-service training (at all levels) to enhance knowledge and skills related to cultural and linguistic competence
- A policy and a process to keep abreast of and examine emergent demographic population trends and their relevance for the provision of care, services and supports, education and research, or advocacy

REFERENCES

American Academy of Pediatrics (AAP), Committee on Bioethics. (1997, February). Religious objections to medical care. *Pediatrics, 99*(2), 279–281.

American Academy of Pediatrics (AAP), Committee on Bioethics and Committee on Hospital Care. (2000). Palliative care for children. *Pediatrics, 106,* 351–357.

American Hospital Association. (1973). *A patient's bill of rights.* Revised October 21, 1992. Retrieved July 15, 2009, from http://www.patienttalk.info/AHA-Patient_Bill_of_Rights.htm

Andrews, M., & Boyle, J. (1995). *Transcultural concepts in nursing care.* Philadelphia: J. B. Lippincott.

Bagozzi, D. (2003). *Traditional medicine. World Health Organization. Fact Sheet No. 134.* Retrieved July 20, 2009, from http://www.who.int/mediacentre/factsheets/fs134/en/

Berkman, N. D., DeWalt, D. A., Pignone, M. P., Sheridan, S. L., Lohr, K. N., Lux, L., et al. (2004). *Literacy and health outcomes. Evidence Report/Technology Assessment No. 87* (Prepared by RTI International–University of North Carolina Evidence-based Practice Center under Contract No. 290-02-0016). AHRQ. Publication No. 04-E007-2. Rockville, MD: Agency for Healthcare Research and Quality. Retrieved July 2, 2009, from http://www.ahrq.gov/downloads/pub/evidence/pdf/literacy/literacy.pdf

Bernat, J. (2004). Ethical issues in the perioperative management of neurologic patients. *Neurologic Clinics 22*(2), viii–ix, 457–471.

Blackhall, L. J., Murphy, S. T., Frank, G., Michel, V., & Azen, S. (1995). Ethnicity and attitudes toward patient autonomy. *Journal of the American Medical Association, 274*(10), 820–825.

Blankenship, D., & Madson, N. (2007). *Resource guide for serving refugees with disabilities.* Washington, DC: U.S. Committee for Refugees and Immigrants.

Bowman, K. (2004). What are the limits of bioethics in a culturally pluralistic society? *Journal of Law, Medicine, and Ethics, 32*(4), 664–669.

Braun, U., Beyth, R., Ford, M., & McCullough, L. (2008). Voices of African American, Caucasian, and Hispanic surrogates on the burdens of end-of-life decision making. *Journal of General Internal Medicine, 23*(3), 267–274.

Candib, L. (1995). *Medicine and the family: A feminist perspective.* New York: Basic Books.

Candib, L. (2002). Truth telling and advance planning at the end of life: Problems with autonomy in a multicultural world. *Families, Systems & Health, 20*(3), 213–228.

Carrese, J., & Rhodes, L. (1995). Western bioethics on the Navaho reservation: Benefit or harm? *Journal of the American Medical Association, 274,* 826–829.

Carrese, J., & Rhodes, L. (2000). Bridging cultural differences in medical practice: The case of discussing negative information with Navajo patients. *Journal of General Internal Medicine, 15,* 92–96.

Chase, W. (1989, Fall). The language of action. *Wesleyan LXII, 2,* 36.

Chattopadhyay, S., & Simon, A. (2008). East meets west: Cross-cultural perspective in end-of-life decision making from Indian and German viewpoints. *Medicine, Healthcare & Philosophy, 11*(2), 165–174.

Cross, T., Bazron, B., Dennis, K., & Isaacs, M. (1989). Towards a culturally competent system of care. Volume 1. Washington, DC: Georgetown University Child Development Center, CASSP Technical Assistance Center.

Cruzan v. Director, Missouri Department of Health, 110 S. Ct. 2841 (1990).

DeLisa, J., & Thomas, P. (2005). Physicians with disabilities and the physician workforce: A need to reassess our policies. *American Journal of Physical Medicine and Rehabilitation, 84,* 5–11.

Desai, P. (2000). Medical ethics in India. In R. Veatch (Ed.), *Cross-cultural perspectives in medical ethics.* Sudbury, MA: Jones and Bartlett.

Dufy, S., Jackson, F., Schim, S., Ronis, D., & Fowler, K. (2006). Racial/ethnic preferences, sex preferences, and perceived discrimination related to end-of-life care. *Journal of the American Geriatrics Society, 54,* 150–157.

Fadiman, A. (1997). *The spirit catches you and you fall down: A Hmong child, her American doctors, and the collision of two cultures.* New York: Noonday Press.

Fan, R. (1997). Self-determination vs. family determination: Two incommensurable principles of autonomy. *Bioethics, 11,* 309–322.

Feldman, J. (1992). The French are different—French and American medicine in the context of AIDS: Cross-cultural medicine—a decade later [Special issue]. *Western Journal of Medicine, 157,* 345–349.

Fisher, G. (1988). *Mindsets: The role of culture and perception in international relations.* Yarmouth, ME: Intercultural Press.

Franey, L. (2008, January 2). Crossroads hospice reaches out to Hispanic community. *Kansas City Star,* p. B1.

Galanti, G. (1997). *Caring for patients from different cultures.* Philadelphia: University of Pennsylvania Press.

Giger, J., Davidhizar, R., & Fordham, P. (2006). Multi-cultural and multi-ethnic considerations and advanced directives: Developing cultural competency. *Journal of Cultural Competency, 13*(1), 3–9.

Goode, T. (2001). *Policy brief 4: Engaging communities to realize the vision of one hundred percent access and zero health disparities: A culturally competent approach.* Washington, DC: National Center for Cultural Competence, Georgetown University Child Development Center.

Gordon, Dianna. (2000, March). When faith healing fails. *State Legislatures Magazine, 26*(3), 26.

Hablamos Juntos. (2006). *Developing better non-English materials: Understanding the limits of translation.* Retrieved July 21, 2009, from http://www.hablamosjuntos.org/resource_guide_portal/pdf/Brief-NonEngl-Final.pdf

Hahn, R., & Gaines, A. (Eds.). (1985). *Physicians of Western medicine: Anthropological approaches to theory and practice.* Dordrecht, The Netherlands: D. Reidel.

Hall, E. (1981). *Beyond culture.* New York: Doubleday.

Helman, C. (1990). *Culture, health, and illness.* London: Wright.

Holloway, K. (2009, May 25). Parents deserve word to convey loss of a child: Name needed for mourning that goes against natural order. *Atlanta Journal-Constitution.* Retrieved June 26, 2009, from http://www.ajc.com

Iltis, A. S. (2004). Bioethics: The intersection of private and public decisions. *Journal of Medicine and Philosophy, 29*(29), 381–388.

Institute of Medicine. (2004). *Health literacy: A prescription to end confusion.* Washington, DC: National Academy Press.

Inwald, D., Jakobovits, I., & Petros, A. (2000). Brain stem death: Managing care when accepted medical guidelines and religious beliefs are in conflict. Consideration and compromise are possible. *British Medical Journal, 320*(7244), 1266–1267.

Irish, D., Lundquist, K., & Nelson, V. (1993). Conclusions. In D. Irish, K. Lundquist, & V. Nelson (Eds.), *Ethnic variations in dying, death, and grief: Diversity in universality.* New York: Taylor & Francis.

Kapp, M. (2000). Ethical considerations and court involvement in end-of-life decision making. In K. Braun, J. Pietsch, & P. Blanchette (Eds.), *Cultural issues in end-of-life decision making.* Thousand Oaks, CA: Sage.

Klessig, J. (1992). The effects of values and culture on life-support decisions: Cross-cultural medicine—a decade later [Special issue]. *Western Journal of Medicine, 157,* 316–322.

Koenig, B., & Gates-Williams, J. (1995). Understanding cultural difference in caring for dying patients: Caring for patients at the end of life [Special issue]. *Western Journal of Medicine, 163,* 244–249.

Koser, K. (2008, March 18). *Dimensions and dynamics of contemporary international migration.* Paper prepared for the conference on Workers Without Borders: Rethinking Economic Migration, Maastricht Graduate School of Governance, Maastricht, The Netherlands.

Larabee, M., & Sleeth, P. (1998). *Faith healing raises questions of law's duty—belief or life?* Retrieved July 2, 2009, from http://www.positiveatheism.org/writ/deadbabies.htm

Maloof, P. (2008). *Body/mind/spirit: Toward a biopsychosocial-spiritual model of health.* Retrieved July 15, 2009, from http://www11.georgetown.edu/research/gucchd/nccc/body_mind_spirit

McGaghie, W. (2002) Assessing readiness for medical education: Evolution of the medical college admission test. *Journal of American Medical Association, 288*(9), 1085–1090.

Metcalf, P., & Huntington, R. (1991). *Celebrations of death: The anthropology of mortuary ritual.* New York: Cambridge University Press.

Miller, S. (2002). *Finding hope when a child dies: What other cultures can teach us.* New York: Simon & Schuster.

Mitty, E. (2001). Ethnicity and end of life. *Reflections on Nursing Leadership, 27*(1), 28–31, 46.

National Academy on an Aging Society. (1998). *Fact sheet: Low health literacy skills increase annual health care expenditures by $73 billion*. Retrieved July 2, 2009, from http://www.agingsociety .org/agingsociety/publications/fact/fact_low.html

National Center for Cultural Competency (NVCC). (2001). *Process of inquiry—communicating in a multicultural environment*. Retrieved July 24, 2009, from http://www.nccccurricula.info/ communication/C2.html

National Institute on Disability and Rehabilitation Research (NIDRR). (2008). *Office of Special Education and Rehabilitative Services—Frequently asked questions (FAQs) about NIDRR*. Retrieved July 2, 2009, from http://www.ed.gov/about/offices/list/osers/nidrr/faq.html

National Virtual Translation Center. (2007). *Languages spoken in the U.S.* Retrieved May 4, 2008, from http://www.nvtc.gov/lotw/months/november/USlanguages.html

Ohnuki-Tierney, E. (1994). Brain death and organ transplantation: Cultural bases of medical technology. *Current Anthropology, 35*(3), 233–254.

Payer, L. (1988). *Medicine and culture: Varieties of treatment in the United States, England, West Germany, and France*. New York: Henry Holt.

Rosenblatt, P. (1993). Cross-cultural variation in the experience, expression, and understanding of grief. In D. Irish, K. Lundquist, & V. Nelson (Eds.), *Ethnic variations in dying, death, and grief: Diversity in universality*. New York: Taylor & Francis

Rowell, M. (2000). Christian perspectives on end-of-life decision making: Faith in a community. In K. Braun, J. Pietsch, & P. Blanchette (Eds.), *Cultural issues in end-of-life decision making*. Thousand Oaks, CA: Sage.

Searight, H., & Gafford, J. (2005). Cultural diversity at the end of life: Issues and guidelines for family physicians. *American Family Physician, 71*, 515–522.

Seligman, M., & Darling, R. (2007). *Ordinary families, special children: A systems approach to childhood disability*. New York: Guilford Press.

Spector, R. (1985). *Cultural diversity in health and illness*. Norwalk, CT: Appleton-Century-Crofts.

Sulmasy, D. (2002). A biopsychosocial-spiritual model for the care of patients at the end of life. *The Gerontologist, 42*, 24–33.

Title VI of the Civil Rights Act of 1964. 42 U.S.C. § (2000d et seq).

U.S. Census Bureau. (2007a). *Minority population tops 100 million*. Retrieved May 5, 2008, from http://www.census.gov/Press-Release/www/releases/archives/population/010048.html

U.S. Census Bureau. (2007b). *Table 1: National characteristics*. Retrieved July 24, 2009, from http://www.census.gov/Press-Release/www/releases/archives/cb07-70tbl1.pdf

Viljoen, D., & Beighton, P. (1992). Schwartz-Jampel syndrome (chondrodystrophic myotonia). *Journal of Medical Genetics, 29*, 58–62.

Wenger, A. F. (1991). The role of context in culture-specific care. In P. Chinn (Ed.), *Anthology on caring*. New York: National League for Nursing Press.

Wijdicks, E. (2002). Brain death worldwide: Accepted fact but no global consensus in diagnostic criteria. *Neurology, 58*(1), 20–25.

World Health Organization (WHO). (2002). *Traditional medicine strategy 2002–2005*. Retrieved July 24, 2009, from http://whqlibdoc.who.int/hq/2002/WHO_EDM_TRM_2002.1.pdf

Chapter 15

Spirituality Issues and Strategies

Crisis and Opportunity

William Gaventa

Introduction: Challenge and Opportunity

One of the familiar spiritual symbols from Eastern traditions is the Chinese character for "crisis," consisting of characters for both "challenge" and "opportunity." Professionals, families, friends, and caregivers who work with people with intellectual and developmental disabilities (IDD) simply cannot deal with end-of-life issues and experiences without encountering profound spiritual feelings, questions, and opportunities. The challenges come from the ways that IDD relates to our own understandings of spirituality; our own conceptions of how people with IDD deal with grief and loss; and the ways that issues of grief, loss, and death pervade our systems of care even without being named and addressed. This chapter will thus first provide a framework for understanding spirituality and IDD and the ways that end-of-life issues raise both universal and unique spiritual questions in the world of IDD.

Those questions and challenges also provide multiple opportunities for deepening and broadening our understandings of spirituality and care and for addressing the spiritual needs and gifts of the people we support as well as our own. It also allows us to develop strategies that help balance times of loss and crisis with opportunities for honoring relationships, celebrating gifts, and strengthening both community and commitment. In so doing, we are able to begin to address spiritual needs and gifts in the final stages of life, before the end, while simultaneously developing skills and ways to honor the spiritual needs of everyone concerned and involved when death does come. Those areas will be the focus of the last half of the chapter.

Dealing with death and end-of-life issues and the spiritual issues involved is at once profoundly individual and communal, personal and professional. It is an area that cannot be explored without raising our own experiences, thoughts, feelings, and beliefs regarding death and end-of-life issues. Thus, it calls for both human and professional skills at their best. We must be able to support others with skill and sensitivity when there are so many questions, feelings, and different traditions, while recognizing how our own journeys shape our ability and skill to support others at this critical time.

Spirituality and Intellectual Disabilities

Spirituality can be succinctly defined in a twofold definition: first, the experience that one has with whom or what one calls sacred and holy, and second, the ways that we make meaning and purpose in human life (Gaventa, 2006). It is related to—but not the same as—religion, with "religion" usually differentiated by being a particular tradition and organized collection of rites, rituals, and beliefs that shape and guide a spiritual journey. Spirituality can also be described as connection: connection with oneself; connection with others in relationships and community; connection with what one believes to be Holy or God; connection with time, such as one's ancestors or hopes for the future; and connection with those personal and communal places that hold a sense of sacredness and meaning for us.

The relationship between spirituality and religion leads directly into some of the challenges related to recognizing and addressing spirituality in systems of support and services for people with IDD. Barriers exist in both understandings of policy and in professional practice. In areas of policy, spirituality is

- often understood as a private matter, not public;
- separated from other areas of care because of understandings of church and state issues; and
- understood as "religion" and thus not part of "scientific" understandings of care, research, or practice.

One of the most important barriers for people with IDD, though, has been the equation of spirituality with reason and intellect; if people cannot "understand" in "typical" ways, how can they be spiritual or understand religion? The irony with this barrier is that caregivers and friends of every kind can cite examples of spiritual qualities, such as hope and love, in the lives of people with IDD. New researchers are exploring spirituality as understood by people with IDD (Swinton, 2001, 2002) and are thus helping to dispel myths that spirituality, religion, faith, and the non applicability to people with IDD because of assumptions about their ability to understand or reason.

Those policy barriers are also reflected in professional practice, when becoming and being "professional" is understood as separating one's professional self from one's spiritual or religious identity (Gaventa, 2005). That model of professional identity came about for a good reason: a reaction to the dangers of proselytizing and spiritual abuse by professionals. However, the walling off of spirituality from professional identity and practice has also led to reluctance and uncertainty over how to address spiritual and religious issues that come up in practice, a lack of capacity to address the huge diversity of spiritual and religious practices and traditions among patients, and, indeed, a paradoxical fear of the power of spirituality with a resulting inability to utilize it effectively in planning and delivering systems of care and support.

That paradox is deepened when we recognize the ways that core spiritual questions and issues are reflected in the primary values espoused and embedded in both policy and practice: independence, productivity, integration, and self-determination. The relationship between values, spiritual questions and themes, and practice is illustrated in Table 15.1.

Table 15.1
Values, Spirituality, and Practice

Policy value	Core spiritual theme	Addressing fundamental human/ spiritual question	Western answers and practices
Independence	Identity	Who am I?	Self made, own person, growth, development
Productivity	Purpose, calling, vocation	Why am I?	Employment, volunteering, making a difference
Integration	Community connection	Whose am I? Who do I belong to?	Community inclusion, participation, citizenship
Self-determination	Choice, control, power	How do I shape my own destiny? Why do bad things happen?	Advocacy, rights, empowerment

There are ways in policy and practice of addressing those core questions and themes, just as there are multiple ways the core questions are addressed in religious, spiritual, and cultural traditions. One of the direct implications of these multiple avenues is that one can approach the importance of addressing spiritual dimensions of care from a number of perspectives throughout the life span, not just at the end of life. At a minimum, they include the following:

1. Tapping into the power of what people consider to be sacred in their own lives, whatever one might think or believe about their own spirituality or faith
2. Assessing and utilizing the ways that people find meaning, what is important to them, how they cope, and how they connect with others
3. Being culturally sensitive and competent in dealing with the spirituality at the heart of many cultural traditions
4. Encouraging self-determination by enhancing and supporting choice, the right to participate in spiritual and religious practices, and the opportunity to receive from, and give to, a spiritual community
5. Paying attention to the spirituality and sense of calling of staff and caregivers and the ways this spirituality impacts, and is impacted by, their work
6. Enhancing the "souls" of organizations, the factors that make for good morale, vision, and commitment (Gaventa, 2006)

Within that definition and framework of spirituality one can quickly move beyond some of the traditional barriers to integration of spirituality to see how spirituality might be addressed and utilized in end-of-life issues. Before doing so, however, the diverse ways that end-of-life issues and experiences in IDD challenge our understandings of spirituality, values, and practice will be explored.

DEATH AS DENIER, GRIEF ON GRIEF

If independence, productivity, inclusion, and self-determination are indeed the values we hold dear, and those that shape policy and practice, then it is not hard to see death and end of life as the antithesis, the denier of the values we follow as well as the people that we cherish. Aging and end of life is a destroyer of independence, often taking people who have been striving all their lives for more independence back on a "downward" path toward dependence and loss of identity. Everyone struggles with productivity and purpose as they retire and move into old age and the final stages of life. Professionals and others in the health service system know these difficulties. We should allow people with IDD to have the equivalent of "retirement." Aging, infirmity, and certainly death take one away from participation and community. It raises the questions around "why"—the "why" of illness and loss, the "why" of death itself—questions that challenge any assumptions we make about personal and professional power and control.

In older systems of care that focused more on institutional settings rather than community, end of life and death had their own real and symbolic impact. One of the author's first jobs was as Protestant Chaplain at Newark State School in upstate New York, a facility whose history has partially been immortalized in some of the pictures in Blatt and Caplan's (1974) *Christmas in Purgatory*. As a young chaplain, death in the facility was often a reminder of loneliness and the loss of connection with the community. How many chaplains and social workers got calls saying, "Would you please inform the patient that his (or her) mother or father died?" (often followed by "several months ago"). I never forgot one of my first funerals, in one of the facility chapels, with four male residents present who were paid to be pallbearers (the best paying job on the campus) and one staff member sent from the living unit. Performing a funeral made no sense, since they are really for the living, unless one took a justice perspective (i.e., this person deserves what we would do for anyone else). They certainly were experiences of abandonment—an end-of-life congruity with a life of being abandoned—even when that was cloaked as the best of professional, social, and family care.

When families did become involved at the time of death, their grief was shaped by the history of ambivalence, uncertainly, love, woundedness, loss, and, perhaps, guilt about institutionalizing their child even when it was in an era of doing so based on professional advice. I remember two experiences in particular. In the first, I remember the shock and pain of one family when I took them to see the grave, which was in a lovely rural countryside but had a number marker rather than a gravestone. The second was a family who tore into a young physician who was trying to explain to them the death of their daughter from ingesting a rubber glove because of her pica behavior. I did not understand the depth of their anger, especially since they had been very infrequent visitors, until it occurred to me they were yelling at the doctor who presumably caused the IDD by misuse of forceps during delivery. It was as though 26 years had been stripped away.

Too often in institutional settings, however, deaths were evidence of the lack of good care when one hears the stories of ex-residents for whom friends suddenly disappeared, or deaths being the real result of direct abuse or neglect. Similar judgments may be made in newer systems of care focusing on community settings, especially when "incidence of death" or "mortality rate" is used in the arguments over the question "Which is better, institution or community?"

In current community-based systems, the loneliness at the end of life is still too often a reflection of loneliness during life and is evidence of disconnection that can happen even while living "in the community." One of the troubling calls the author receives is when an agency makes contact because there has been a relatively sudden death of someone living in a group home, and they are seeking any kind of help from someone experienced in dealing with grief and IDD. The problem is that I am usually a stranger, not a local clergyperson, congregational member, or hospice chaplain who already knows the person, their friends, and the staff. The disconnection between staff and family may also still be there, with each making assumptions about the other's lack of care and concern. All of that is compounded when routine medical care becomes an end-of-life issue when community-based health care systems, hospitals, and doctors don't know the patients either, or when assumptions about the patient's quality of life end up impacting decisions about treatment that might be routine for someone else.

The emotional and spiritual impact on caregivers, whether direct care staff, families, or professionals, may even be more intense in a modern system focused on growth, development of potential, and progress. Expressed feelings may cluster around a sense that death is a double injustice (i.e., "Why did they have to die? They already had the bad luck of having a disability. That was enough to deal with—why this?"). That intensified anger in response to the "why?" of grief gets heightened further when death shatters our illusions of control and our usual denial of the fragility of life. Death becomes the ultimate "unusual incident," and the system responds with questions and investigations about cause and responsibility. Too often the underlying assumption seems to be that it was someone's fault, which is reinforced when abuse or neglect is involved. Whatever the case, the "grief" of suspicion, investigation, and paperwork gets piled on top of and mixed in with the need to grieve in more typical ways, making effective spiritual response even harder.

Addressing the grief and loss with other "consumers," family members, staff, and friends often presents additional challenges. Far too many staff and agencies report the experience of having a family member call about a death outside of the institution, but expressing the desire that the person within the institution not attend the funeral. Staff and family alike make assumptions about someone's capacity to understand or to handle what is happening, ironically at a time when everyone might be struggling with those questions. "They can't understand" overlaps with "We don't want to cause them more pain," with the result that no one makes a real effort to address the grief involved. Systemic pressures to move on, to fill the empty bed or program slot, and to not give anyone the time to recognize and feel the empty places in homes, programs, and hearts compounds the problem. Unrecognized or unaddressed grief, in Granger Westberg's (1997) classic phrase, is "grief denied, but only delayed, and grief delayed is grief denied." Grief denied or delayed may manifest in inappropriate behavior, either on the part of individuals with IDD or on the part of staff whose unresolved grief may lead to disillusionment and departure. In the face of all the problems of staff turnover and change, it is easy to forget sometimes the profound and deep connections that exist between many staff and people with IDD. Dealing with death is often a very new experience for younger staff or an extra challenge when staff come from many different cultural backgrounds with a variety of ways of understanding death and the corresponding variety of rituals for grief and mourning.

There are, of course, stories and experiences that are far different and just as powerful on the positive side as these are on the negative. But it is not hard to see how aging, the end of life, and death—in a system based on values of growth, developing potential, and enhancing of life—may be interpreted as the ultimate denier of possibilities for someone. This can be evidence of failure on the part of caregivers or programs, and it may be the antithesis of presence, participation, and membership in community. Thankfully, person-centered planning as specified by Kingsbury (2005, 2008) provides a much more effective and humane response to aging and end-of-life issues, just as our society as a whole is learning that planning for end-of-life issues is a way to address both anticipated and unanticipated issues as one approaches death. These issues are even more important for people with IDD and those who care with and for them. They face a bigger health system focused on healing, fixing, and curing—one in which death is also seen as the enemy to be held off and one in which disability is seen as evidence of medical failure or a "fate worse than death." It is, to use a metaphor from literature and film, the makings for a perfect programmatic and spiritual storm, one in which people with IDD and their caregivers may be tossed about and overboard quite easily. It is then, also, an opportunity to predict its coming, and thus plan ahead, and in so doing, learn how to live and love in even more effective professional, programmatic and personal ways.

Re-Visioning Spirituality at the End of Life

Spirituality, spiritual issues, and spiritual practices at the end of life for people with IDD is more than assisting an individual with issues related to his or her own death, dealing with grief and loss, and providing appropriate ways to mourn. Spirituality should be infused into all major life events, in addition to times that may focus on end-of-life issues.

One of the first opportunities for spiritual influence is to revise the values that guide our system of supports. Moving toward and through the end of life with people with IDD does not mean giving up on independence, productivity, inclusion, and self-determination. Rather, it may provide an opportunity to be very faithful to those values, with new understandings of what success or progress might mean. The core question of independence or of "Who am I?" changes to the question of "Who have I been?" Productivity moves from "Why am I?" to "What difference can I now make, and what difference have I made?" Inclusion, the "Whose am I?" question, becomes "Who remembers me?" and "Whose have I been?" As someone loses capacity and control, the self-determination question changes to "How can those who support and love a person ensure that all possible choices are heard and honored in those end times?"

One of the core functions of spiritual traditions and rituals at the end of life is that of remembering. As people age and move toward the end of life, remembering and rehearsing—rather than doing—may take center stage. It may take many forms as people remember connections to the past, to the present, and, indeed, the dreams or hopes one might still have for the future. It may be a recalling of important relationships, a desire to reconnect with them, or a wish to visit important places in one's life one last time. If someone is losing memory toward the end of life, it becomes a time when caretakers may help them remember who they are by maintaining activities, foods, belongings, and relationships that are part of someone's identity. Stated another way, if people are dealing with dementia, the job of the community of care becomes that of "re-menting" (Swinton, 2007).

Specific planning activities around end-of-life issues—like advance care directives, DNRs, and even preplanning of funerals—become not only ways to think about medical treatment and funeral plans but also ways to remember what has given a person's life meaning. It is important to determine how others may be able to honor those values and that person at, during, and after someone dies. Moving toward the end of life thus potentially means connecting with older relationships while also having new people come into someone's life, such as hospice teams. These changes are opportunities to build new relationships, new partnerships, and new collaborations between professional services; faith communities; and current and previous staff, families, and friends.

Those acts of re-visioning and remembering mean a shift for professionals and other caregivers in order to embrace, professionally and personally, a number of paradoxes. Aging and the end of life always have their own set of conflicting or paradoxical experiences, as they are seen culturally and spiritually as a time for both

- honor and indignity;
- blessing and curse;
- growth and decay;
- wisdom and senility; and
- engagement and renunciation. (Park Ridge Center, 1999)

But there are other paradoxes faced by caregivers, especially professionals, as aging and end of life invites us to hold together what sometimes seems like opposites:

- We are professionals, but we are also friends and sometimes surrogate family, especially if we have known someone for years.
- The challenge moves from "doing for" others to simply "being with" others.
- There are new needs to care for, but it is also a time to celebrate the gifts of a person's life.
- Professionals who work in the field of IDD provide specialized supports and services, but toward the end of life, they may be challenged to give what they know to others, especially if others are being invited or called into a relationship with the person needing support.

Perhaps the largest challenge for professionals who have focused on helping people learn, grow, and develop is to recognize their own limits and be professional enough to invite others to help maintain the kind of care and support that is needed. This may include calling in and utilizing hospice teams; working with hospital and medical staff in new ways; or building new relationships with clergy, family, or others. It does not necessarily mean "handing over the care" but perhaps seeking new ways to support the direct care staff, families, friends and professionals who are the immediate community around a person moving toward the end of his or her life.

PREPARING FOR THE END

There has been, and continues to be, an explosion of research and resources related to spirituality, aging, and the end of life, although not much of that has focused particularly in the arena of IDD. There has been much focus on issues in aging in IDD, with only recent increased attention to end-of-life concerns and the emotional and spiritual needs in dealing with death and dying (Blackman & Todd, 2006; Gaventa & Coulter, 2005; Kauffman, 2005; Luchterhand & Murphy, 1998). Thus, in order to look at the spiritual tasks of preparation, we need to look at research and resources from the wider population.

In a resource manual titled *The Challenges of Aging: Retrieving Spiritual Traditions*, the Park Ridge Center (1999) looked across spiritual traditions at the core spiritual tasks of aging, as envisioned or lived out in different religious and cultural traditions. They identify five "unique" tasks of aging:

1. Reaffirming covenant obligations to community
2. Blessing (How have our lives been a blessing? Where do we now give our blessing?)
3. Believing and practicing honor toward those who are aging and treating them with dignity, respect, and appreciation
4. Maintaining faith in the face of loss and grief
5. Reconciling discordant experiences (e.g., letting go, reconnecting, and forgiving)

Those tasks of aging provide a very useful framework for thinking about how we might support people with IDD and their significant others as they move toward the end of life.

Covenant Obligations to Community

Our systems of support and services have professed and focused on community inclusion. The questions to ask now are the following: Who is part of someone's community? Is it family, direct care workers, professionals, individuals with whom they live, friends, and/or others in the community? What communities of interest (sports, clubs, etc.), faith, work, and place have been important to them? What might the person we are supporting want to do with those current and past connections? What might they want to do in relation to the person who is in the final stages of life? Are there ways that those relationships involve a sense of covenant, of wanting to maintain a connection even toward the end, or of wanting to do things one feels obliged to do—or wants to do—before it is too late?

Exploring those questions could lead to any number of responses. It might involve looking through picture albums or getting pictures of old friends and important places. It may mean revisiting places where one grew up or lived. If it is early enough, it may mean thinking about ways one can still make a contribution to people or groups that have been important to them. It may mean doing something one has always wanted to do.

For example, if people have not had the opportunity to be involved in a religious community that respects their choice and tradition, it is never too late to start. In Ira Wahl's film, *Best Man*, the sequel to *Best Boy*, the protagonist's cousin Philly, in his 70s, has his Bar Mitzvah, an event that creates a whole new set of relationships for him in a synagogue. Helping someone get involved in a religious community also introduces him or her to a clergyperson and practices that may turn out to be incredibly valuable as someone gets older and more infirm. Clergy and congregation members often visit people when they are hospitalized, provide spiritual supports such as prayer and bringing the Eucharist, or more. There are two important points here: help get people involved at whatever stage in their life and support their participation, so when the decline due to aging or failing health comes, that community can respond in addition to the supports in the service system. Doing so prevents point two: It is much harder to arrange for effective spiritual supports at the moment of crisis or a sudden death if connections have not already been made.

One of the communal acts of remembering that is often not available to people with IDD is that of reunion. Others have class reunions, military reunions, and school reunions. Many of the adults whom our system currently supports lived together in institutions before moving to community settings. What about providing them the opportunity for reunion? In less dramatic ways, there are now wonderful stories of agencies that honor the wishes of someone's friends in a group home to visit a sick or dying friend in a nursing home or hospital on a regular basis if they have had to move.

Giving and Receiving Blessing

The act of asking for a blessing from one's elders, or the opportunity to give one's blessing as an elder, is an ancient spiritual tradition. In disability services, that can happen in a number of ways:

- In helping people get included in faith communities, look for ways that they can do something to contribute to that community so they have the opportunity to feel that they are helping others. There are multiple kinds of volunteer jobs in congregations and other settings. Having the opportunity to give enhances self-esteem, and it often feels like a blessing to others who receive, or observe, people with developmental disabilities enjoying the opportunity to give, not just receive.
- One of the tasks of aging and the final stages, if not earlier, is for us to let people know the gifts and strengths we see in them, and how their lives have blessed us. We are already getting better at identifying key strengths and gifts in the people we support. Many of us, in whatever kind of caregiving role, have had our lives profoundly impacted and blessed by people with intellectual disabilities. But we rarely tell them so. One example of this was begun by Aaron Jager, the chaplain at Eastern Christian Children's Retreat in northern New Jersey, when he started ritualizing the act of recognizing gifts by giving a certificate of appreciation to the adults with multiple disabilities who are served by his agency. Using his own observation, his conversations with staff, and simple certificates from an office supply store, he produced certificates like the one in Figure 15.1 and then initiated a period of the annual Individual Habilitation Plan when it was presented. The impact on family, staff, and "consumer" has frequently been profound.

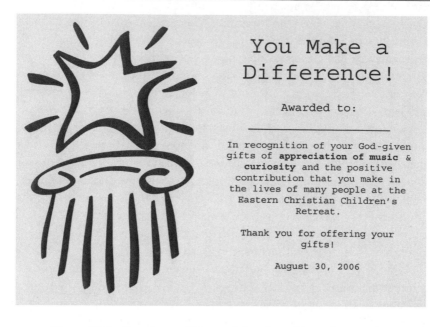

Figure 15.1. Sample certificate celebrating gifts and strengths.

- Beyond our affirmation of "their" blessing to us, how might we help them give a blessing to others in the final stages of their life? What might someone want to do for someone else? Or—if we indeed have moved to being able to help an individual and his or her family think about advance care directives or funeral planning—what might they want to "will" someone or some organization? Does someone want others to have a possession that might help them remember the relationship? For example, a sensitive parent of a person who died in New Jersey remembered to ask the staff and fellow residents in the group home, before they did the usual boxing up of possessions to give to the family, whether or not anyone wanted a memento. Indeed, one of his best friends wanted his Yankees cap.

Restoring Honor in Aging

"Honor your father and mother, that your days may be long on the earth" is, of course, one of the Ten Commandments. Up until the "youth culture" took over, honor toward elders was much more visible, but it is still there, in many ways. There are many ways in which honoring still takes place for community elders, grandparents, senior members of congregations, and others

How then might service systems for those with IDD embody that attitude and value? It is, first of all, an attitude of respect, honoring people's choices, and perhaps figuring out ways to let people do things they want to do even if it is programmatically inconvenient. Many support agencies are working on ways for people to "retire" if they so choose. Maintaining vocation or employment goals, if someone does not want to do so or because it is seen as the only option, is both unimaginative and antithetical to the values of choice and self-determination.

Other strategies could involve helping people write and develop their life story, a process that has received much more attention in Europe than in the United States. Most of the people supported by agencies have long medical or treatment records. How might staff, families, or volunteers help turn those into life stories, with pictures of people, places, and events that one can see, review, and show to others? How might systems revision "aging consumers" as "survivors" and "veterans"? Many have survived decades of programmatic changes, moves, staff turnover, and more. Could we tap them, and their stories, to be part of training teams to help new and younger staff learn more about the history of services and supports? Finally, as in the task of giving blessing, can professionals and caregivers figure out ways to tell people who are aging and moving through the end stages of life what "they" have meant to "us?"

Maintaining Faith in the Face of Loss

End of life is a time to pay special attention to spiritual beliefs and practices. That is as simple as ensuring that people have the opportunity to practice their own faith and develop relationships with spiritual leaders and communities. These relationships can assist in areas where professional staff may feel uncomfortable, such as helping people prepare through prayer and scriptures, daily and/or weekly rituals, engaging in rituals of loss and mourning, and ensuring that individuals have the opportunity to participate in funerals and events of their friends and colleagues. As appropriate, we also honor individuals by giving them the opportunity to deal with their own anticipatory grief. Resources like the *Books Beyond Words* (Hollins & Blackman, 2003) are ones that friends and counselors can utilize to look and talk through what happens when people are sick and die. If people have not had the opportunity or support to develop a relationship with a faith community, and it is their desire to do so, this would be the time, both for support of the individuals themselves and then for friends and staff during and after death.

The importance of connection to faith communities also means that agency staff and caregivers are not alone in their caregiving responsibilities. Clergy visits, congregational outreach, hospital visits, and a huge variety of spiritual practices are often expected and valued parts of illness and end-of-life time periods for members of faith communities. Staff, fellow residents, and friends of the person who is ill or dying may also appreciate that support. For that to happen, though, it means clergy and members of faith communities need to get to know someone because he or she has been a part of their community.

Reconciliation

The final spiritual challenge of aging is reconciliation and dealing with discordant experiences—things that people may want to say or do with others before it is too late. Some of the strategies previously mentioned also address this. By helping people to tell their own stories, in pictures and words; by helping people reconnect with distant family members, former staff, or old friends; by visiting or reuniting with special places and experiences; and by helping people be "at home," wherever that is, our service systems can provide opportunities for people to address, and sometimes resolve, old questions and feelings. As a former chaplain in a residential facility, I often had the opportunity to participate in someone's funeral. When asked to do a eulogy, it was often my attempts to weave together the unique qualities and strengths of someone's life that provided a way for staff and families to see the person and each other in new ways and to let go of old resentments or feelings of guilt when they realized how much their family member, or "their" consumer, had touched others. The question for me is how we might help those kinds of things happen before someone dies, so the person feels and experiences the emotional and spiritual resolution.

The hospice movement has produced a simple yet profound version of the five things one might need to say or feel before one's death, as part of the process of saying "good-bye." These help us to think about what a community of care can and should do in honoring the spiritual dimensions of care:

- "I forgive you."
- "Please forgive me."
- "Thank you."
- "I love you."
- "Good-bye."

So one of the questions might very well be, Who needs to see someone before they die? It might not be easy, but how can we support people, such as former staff, relatives, coworkers, friends from within and outside an agency, and others, to be part of opportunities for leave-taking, saying, "Thank you and good-bye," and simply being present, as appropriate, on someone's last journey? I know of group home staff and friends who have made commitments to visit someone at least weekly if they have been transferred to a nursing home or hospital. Making or writing card and participation in common rituals like prayer and other activities can be ways of bringing closure and supporting everyone in their feelings of loss and grief.

Anticipatory Grieving: Making Space

If we pay attention to the spiritual tasks of aging, then we have already made major strides toward assisting individuals and their friends with preparations and anticipatory grieving. There are other things we can do, which may mirror what happens for "typical" people, but also may teach a wider world about how one can deal with the spiritual dimensions of end-of-life care.

- *Training and educating wherever possible.* There are now curricula and resources (Hollins & Blackman, 2003; Steinman, 2006; Stern, Kennedy, Sed, & Heller, 2000) to support training and educational opportunities about death and loss. Those are valuable and important, but we also need to recognize that there are multiple teachable moments when questions and issues can be addressed. Television shows, news about deaths of famous people, or deaths of family members of both staff and consumers all provide opportunities for people to discuss questions and feelings and to discover what individuals may or may not need or want as they think about their own end of life.

- *Building relationships with local resources.* It is crucial to build relationships with local resources so that those called in to comfort and support in times of death and loss are not strangers but hopefully trusted advisors, clergy, and friends. When that is not the case and someone dies, if the clergyperson who is called upon to perform a funeral does not know the person or much about IDD, there is a very real chance that the services will not be conducted in ways that honor the person or meet the needs of the individuals involved. In the Syracuse, New York, region, for example, the Developmental Disabilities Service Office has an active Grief Response Team that includes clergy and professionals from other disciplines who can respond to individual situations as well as provide training and consultation.

- *Assessing, addressing, and honoring spiritual practices.* Being intentional about assessing spiritual interests and traditions for the people we support through person-centered planning or other forms of program planning is a first step toward building interests and connections that can be supportive in times of loss and grief. Those assessments need to be followed with supports that address the identified interests and goals (e.g., helping someone get to a congregation for its worship and community activities) and doing what it takes to honor the spiritual practices that someone has identified as important for them.

- *Holding in-services on dealing with death, grief, and loss.* For many, simply talking about the end of life, grief, and loss is not easy. These in-services may provide a beginning, as well as a way to outline policy and planning by an agency and to build relationships with local resources (e.g., the in-service could be done by a clergyperson or hospice chaplain who has begun to know the people served by an agency). They may also provide a way for staff to talk about how they might support each other when one of the people they support is dying. Figuring that out and sharing the care and support helps avoid the kind of resentments that can also happen in families when one or two family members feel like the rest of the family has been neither present nor supportive.

- *Planning ahead, explicitly, with individuals and their families.* That can involve end-of-life planning processes, but much earlier, doing what Jeff Kauffman (2005) calls "loss assessments." When someone comes into the services of a particular agency, the professional staff could talk with the person and family about the losses that have already occurred in someone's life and how the person and family have dealt with them in order to learn about the cultural and religious traditions that they practice. That would also be an opportunity for an agency to lay out its policies and practices (e.g., telling families that when someone close to the individual dies, this is what the agency tries to do, this is how staff will help, and this is why they believe it is important for people to participate in the rites and rituals that allow for grieving and support).

WELCOMING AND SHARING THE GRIEF

Both before death and when it happens, the first spiritual challenge to caregivers is to recognize and welcome grief. It can be expressed in all kinds of feelings and all kinds of behaviors. The biggest danger is ignoring or suppressing grief, for it is one of the most normal of human feelings and experiences. I used to have staff who asked about individuals who frequently talked about the death of a relative or pet, even though it happened years before. They wondered if that was evidence of their inability to understand or deal with death. I sometimes wondered that as well, but I came to recognize that those questions and feelings were one way of asking and saying, "Who have you lost?" At one level, beyond all the labels and disabilities, we are the same.

Thus, our challenge is to create safe places and opportunities for people to share, live out, and address their own grief and loss. In his book, *Helping Adults with Mental Retardation Mourn*, Jeff Kauffman (2005) outlines four key strategies for provider agencies and professionals:

1. *Provide accurate and honest information to friends and staff, with the time and support needed by others to help process it.* People deal with feelings and questions in very different ways and at different speeds. There is no one way that this should happen. Deal with the questions and feelings that people have, not what we might think they should have.

2. *Enable maximum involvement in the social and spiritual activities surrounding death.* That means doing what we need to do to enable people to participate in wakes, in funerals, to visit cemeteries, write cards, and participate in memorial activities. If family members have concerns, help them to know that staff will provide supports. If people cannot participate in those activities, or even when they can, agencies may also plan and carry through on memorial services and activities within a group home, day program, workshop, or agency as a whole. One of the services I remember best is the one where everyone helped make the funeral flowers out of colored paper.

3. *Keep individuals connected with the staff or others who are their key supporters.* When we grieve, we don't turn to everyone. We turn to the people we trust most. Do what is needed to support that supporter, as they provide the anchor for a person during the hardest times of grief.

4. *Maximize the opportunities for the expression of grief and condolences.* As already stated, cards, gifts, planting trees, cemetery visits, and anniversary rituals are all typical channels for expressing grief and condolences. One great irony, in my experience, is that we who worry about the capacity of people with IDD to handle grief and death often discover that "they" are better at handling it than we are, or that they do or say things that are profoundly helpful to others. It is also important to remember that grief is not often resolved quickly, and that those opportunities for expressing grief may need to go on, as they do for many, for years.

Luchterhand and Murphy (1998) outline ways for support individuals with IDD and their families. Steinman (2006) writes a fictional story of the death of someone in a group home, with guidelines for how that story may be used by staff and friends. There are a growing number of resources that caregivers, support providers, and friends have at their command to use.

Endings and Beginnings

At the International Association for the Scientific Study of Intellectual Disability Conference in Montpelier in 2004, there were at least 10 sessions with several presentations in each session dealing with end-of-life issues, death, and grief involving people with IDD, their caregivers, and friends. It simply pointed to the attention paid in other countries that preceded some of the attention that was just starting in the United States and has since grown in quantity and quality. That growth could be seen as a reflection of spiritual maturity by the system of care as a whole, recognizing not only that people grow older but that death, too, is a part of the "normal" life cycle rather than a byproduct of inadequate or unjust care.

As outlined in this chapter and evidenced in the very production of this book, the crises and challenges presented by end-of-life experiences for people with IDD are also opportunities for developing and celebrating a wider network of caregiving relationships, finding creative ways to share and support each other in times of loss and death, and honoring both the unique and common qualities that individuals with IDD share with many others. They can provide opportunities for the best of what it means to be professional (i.e., chances not to fix and cure, but to journey with others, to deal with the tough questions and feelings that disability and death raise for us, to recognize and celebrate those holy moments and miracles of accomplishment and growth, to recognize and give thanks for the meaning and gifts that others have brought to us, and, at times, to sacrifice and give up for the sake of others). For both health care systems and individuals, good endings can become good beginnings. Mourning can lead to remembering and renewal. In all of the major spiritual traditions of the world, new life and meaning comes in and through the journey of facing death. Perhaps, if "we" let "them," people with IDD can be our guides on that journey as well.

References

Blackman, N., & Todd, S. (2005). *Caring for people with learning disabilities who are dying.* London: Worth Publishing.

Blatt, B., & Kaplan, F. (1974). *Christmas in purgatory. A photographic essay on mental retardation.* Syracuse: Human Policy Press.

Gaventa, W. (2005). A place for all of me and all of us: Rekindling the spirit in services and supports. *Mental Retardation, 43*(1), 48–54.

Gaventa, W. (2006). Defining and assessing spirituality and spiritual supports: Moving from benediction to invocation. In H. Switzky & S. Greenspan (Eds.), *What is mental retardation: Ideas for an evolving disability in the 21st century* (pp. 151–166). Washington, DC: American Association on Intellectual and Developmental Disabilities.

Gaventa, W., & Coulter, D. (Eds.). (2005). *End of life care: Bridging disability and aging with person centered care.* Binghamton, NY: Haworth Press.

Hollins, S., & Blackman, N. (2003). *When somebody dies.* London: Gaskell/St. George's Hospital Medical School. Retrieved September 25, 2009, from http://www.rcpsych.ac.uk/publications/booksbeyondwords.aspx

Kauffman, J. (2005). *Guidebook on helping persons with mental retardation mourn.* Amityville, NY: Baywood.

Kingsbury, L. A. (2005). Person centered planning and communication of end-of-life wishes with people who have developmental disabilities. *Journal of Religion, Disability, and Health, 9*(2), 81–90.

Kingsbury, L. A. (2008). *People planning ahead: Communicating healthcare and end of life wishes.* Washington, DC: American Association on Intellectual and Developmental Disabilities.

Luchterhand, C., & Murphy, N. (1998). *Helping adults with mental retardation grieve a death loss.* Philadelphia: Taylor & Francis.

Park Ridge Center. (1999). *The challenge of aging: Retrieving spiritual traditions.* Chicago: The Park Ridge Center for the Study of Health, Faith, and Ethics.

Steinman, M. (2006). *The geese and the peanut butter chocolate ice cream: The grieving gifts to the Lexington street community—a resource to help individuals with developmental disabilities and people who support them grieve the death of loved ones.* New Brunswick, NJ: The Elizabeth M. Boggs Center on Developmental Disabilities. Retrieved September 25, 2009, from http://rwjms.umdnj.edu/boggscenter/products/prod_info.htm#grief

Stern, H. L., Kennedy, E. A., Sed, C. M., & Heller, T. (2000). *Person-centered planning for late life: A curriculum for adults with mental retardation.* Chicago: RRTC Clearinghouse on Aging and Developmental Disabilities, Institute on Disability Human Development, University of Illinois.

Swinton, J. (2001). *A space to listen: Meeting the spiritual needs of people with learning disabilities.* London: The Mental Health Foundation.

Swinton, J. (2002). A space to listen: Spirituality and people with learning disabilities. *Learning Disability Practice, 5*(2), 6–7.

Swinton, J. (2007). Forgetting whose we are: Theological reflections on personhood, faith and dementia. *Journal of Religion, Disability, and Health, 11*(1), 37–63.

Westberg, G. (1997). *Good grief: A constructive approach to the problem of loss, 35th anniversary edition.* Minneapolis: Fortress Press.

CHAPTER 16

Struggling With Grief and Loss

KENNETH J. DOKA

INTRODUCTION

One of the most significant trends for the past 40 years has been the increasing longevity of individuals with intellectual and developmental disabilities (IDD). Medical advances in both the understanding and the treatment of IDD and deinstitutionalization from the larger facilities where individuals with IDD were generally warehoused have increased their life expectancy. Most individuals with IDD—with exception of those with Down syndrome—now have a near-normal lifespan, and even persons with Down syndrome may expect to live well into midlife.

Along with the trend toward increased longevity, there have been significant strides in normalizing the lives of individuals with IDD. Many of them now live within the community in group homes, with family members, in special assisted-living facilities, or even on their own. They have, as other people do, created and sustained attachments to a variety of persons—family members, fellow residents and consumers, staff members, coworkers, members of their faith communities, and other friends.

One of the prices of such attachments is that individuals with IDD experience loss just like everyone else. They are now likely to outlive their parents. Loss inherently is a part of communal living as staff members and other residents relocate or die. In fact, individuals with IDD may experience significant secondary losses that may complicate grief. The death of a parent or caregiver, for example, may necessitate a change in residence leading to a range of losses that might include friends, neighbors, and employment.

In short, individuals with IDD experience grief.

People with mild IDD may even experience a sense of grief and loss over their disabilities—a lingering sense of loss over the fact that they are perceived as different from others. Grief is a reality of life for all persons whether or not they experience IDD.

Families of individuals with IDD experience grief as well. Certainly they may experience a deep sense of grief and loss when a family member with IDD dies. They may even experience an ongoing sense of loss over the disability itself. Roos (2002) identified *chronic sorrow*, or a continuing sense of loss that may surge at different moments. For example, parents may experience a profound sense of loss when they learn their child has an intellectual disability—sometimes even prior to their child's birth. This sense of loss continues throughout the child's life, possibly spiking when peers without disabilities experience transitional events such as graduations or weddings. It is, as Bruce and Schultz (2001) note, a continuing or *nonfinite* loss.

A basic and welcome assumption of this book is that an effective end of life needs to address the ongoing reality of loss. The chapter begins by exploring grief reactions in individuals with IDD, their families, and caregivers. A second focus of the chapter reviews the ways to assist individuals with IDD and significant others in dealing with loss. The chapter then concludes by addressing the possibilities and need for grief education.

Grief Reactions in Persons With IDD

There is a Buddhist proverb that states, "We are like all others, some others, no others." That is an excellent way to think of the grieving reactions of individuals with IDD. Individuals with IDD generally grieve in the same ways as others who experience a loss. That is part of our common humanity. Yet, the nature of IDD may potentially create unique issues in the experience of grief—hence, there may be characteristics of the grieving process that are shared by others with similar cognitive characteristics. Finally, every experience of grief is unique, based upon the characteristics of the person and the relationship to the person who died.

Like all others, individuals with IDD experience physical, cognitive, emotional, behavioral, and spiritual manifestations of grief. Grief reactions can be experienced on a physical level. Grieving individuals may convert grief into a range of physical reactions such as nausea, headaches, or other bodily aches or pains. This is especially true with individuals with IDD. Here, emotional manifestations may easily be converted and interpreted as physical symptoms. Anxiety, for example, might be expressed as stomach pains. Moreover, physical symptoms elicit care, concern, and support from others at a distressing time. In working with individuals with IDD during a time of loss, it is essential to continually assess their physical state.

In addition to physical responses, there is a range of affective responses to loss. These can include such emotions as anger, guilt, jealousy, anxiety, sadness, or regret, among many others. Some deserve special mention. It is not unusual for other residents, consumers, or staff members to become the focus of displaced anger. Guilt, too, is a common reaction. Again, this is especially true for some individuals with IDD, as they may have limited understanding of causality.

There also may be cognitive reactions. In the initial phases of grief, people may be in shock—disbelieving or denying—and unable to process information. Throughout the grieving process, individuals may find their concentration or span of attention is impaired. They may process information less effectively. It is not unusual for health professionals or others to be asked the same question or to provide certain information repeatedly. Individuals may experience impaired judgment. In persons with impaired cognition, these changes can be profound. In some cases, such as after the loss of a guardian, it is critical to temper any assessment of an individual with IDD with recognition that such an assessment will likely be affected by the loss.

Behaviors may be influenced as well. Grieving individuals may seem lethargic or hyperactive. Daily patterns such as sleeping or eating may change. For example, it is not unusual for individuals with IDD to experience sleep disorders. They may engage in risky behaviors such as substance abuse. They may exhibit acting-out behaviors—appearing angry, lashing out to others, or withdrawing. In short, grieving individuals may behave in quite uncharacteristic ways. Individuals with IDD may become quite resistant to any changes in routine; they may protest if someone, for example, sits in their regular seat. When significant changes occur, individuals often become resistant to the minor changes in things that they can control. This may result in compulsive behaviors in which they become rigid in the attempt to keep whatever they can from becoming unstable. Such changes in regular behavior should be included in assessments of grief.

Finally, individuals can have a range of spiritual reactions. They can struggle with profound spiritual questions. Guilt or anger can have a cosmic focus as persons vent their anger at their idea of a deity or feel the disease or death is a punishment for some supposed sin.

There is no timetable for grief. Over a period of years, most individuals find a lessening of painful thoughts and emotions and a return to their previous levels of functioning. In fact, some individuals may even do better in time as their loss creates a developmental push by creating within the individual the need to learn new skills or insights. However, this does not preclude that fact that, even over time, individuals may experience surges of grief at special times such as holidays, anniversaries, or at events in which the presence of the deceased is profoundly missed. Nor is there any particular sequence or stages within the grieving process. Current models now tend to see the process of grief as a series of very individual processes or tasks (Rando, 1993; Stroebe & Schut, 1999; Worden, 2008).

While these reactions are generally common to all people, researchers and clinicians have identified particular manifestations of grief that may be found in individuals with IDD. Individuals with IDD often have limited or distorted emotional expressions (Todd & Hymes, 1999). One client, for illustration, would giggle whenever she was anxious. In recounting the story of her beloved father's death, she would giggle in this nervous fashion—sometimes confusing less empathic relatives. They also may have a positive bias—that is, a generally optimistic view of the world that may be inherent to the disability or a consequence of reinforcement (Todd & Hymes, 1999). This means that individuals with IDD may appear and report that they are happy. Such a perspective may mask the deep feelings of anxiety, dependency, ambivalence about the dependency and abandonment that may be generated by the loss (Kauffman, 2005).

Since the cognitive processes of these individuals are affected, individuals with IDD may have difficulty comprehending death. Lipe-Goodson and Goebel (1983) found that people in their sample of individuals with IDD were able to understand death. However, the ability to understand death was not dependent on level of intellectual functioning but rather chronological age, suggesting the critical importance of experiential learning. Because of these intellectual deficits, individuals with IDD may need to spend considerable time processing the implications of death and loss. Moreover, their limited coping repertoire might restrict their abilities to effectively respond to the loss (Lavin & Doka, 1999).

In addition, others may disenfranchise the experience of grief of individuals with IDD. *Disenfranchised grief* refers to situations in which an individual experiences a loss but that loss is not openly acknowledged, socially supported, or openly mourned (Doka, 2002a). In short, the person experiences a loss but has no socially sanctioned right to grieve.

The grief of individuals with IDD is often disenfranchised (Lavin, 2002). There may be many reasons why such grief is disenfranchised. Caregivers may feel inadequate in addressing grief in individuals with IDD and, hence, ignore their needs. Others may feel the pressure of time inhibits opening topics they feel ill equipped to handle. There may be a sense of overprotectiveness that creates a reluctance to upset individuals with IDD. This tendency to shelter the grieving person results in attempts to limit exposure or discussion of death, loss, and grief. In other situations, there may be erroneous conceptions that individuals with IDD are incapable of sustaining attachments, retaining attachment if the person is no longer present, or understanding grief (Duetsch, 1985; Lavin, 2002). Since individuals with IDD may manifest grief in distinct ways, others may not always recognize that grief. However, just because an individual's grief may not be understood by others does not mean that the individual does not understand and experience the loss.

This sense of disenfranchisement can often extend to families of individuals with IDD. There may be disenfranchisement of a family's own loss in having children with a disability. Since individuals with IDD may be less valued by the larger society, others may even disenfranchise the death of such a child. Clients who have had a child with IDD have often noted that others will often suggest that such a death should be perceived as a "blessing" or "relief" thus disenfranchising the parents' own sense of profound loss.

Counseling Individuals With IDD

Prior to discussing counseling individuals with IDD, it is important to reaffirm that individuals with IDD are not homogeneous. They share the same differences in terms of background as other groups. Levels of cognitive disability can vary from mild to severe. Living conditions can also vary: some may live independently, others with their families or in group homes, still others in institutions. Levels of social and psychological impairments can also differ, and these levels may not neatly correspond to cognitive impairments. Thus, the age of an individual with IDD may not be predictive of developmental level or behavior.

Lavin (2002) describes certain characteristics typical of individuals with IDD. They often have an external locus of control, lack confidence in their own ability to solve problems, find it difficult to think abstractly, have a limited ability to transfer skills from one level to another, and have poor short-term memory skills.

Because of these limitations, people with IDD may have a very difficult time coping with abstract concepts such as "disease," "dying," or "death." Some research has suggested that these concepts may be easier for people with these types of disabilities to master as they age. Chronological age—rather than cognitive level—may be a factor, since it provides a rough index of the person's level of experience with dying and death. Often family and staff may exacerbate these conceptual difficulties if they try to overprotect the person with IDD, effectively disenfranchising the person from any role in the treatment of their loss.

In providing grief counseling to people with IDD, Lavin (2002) makes a number of points that can be applied to counseling such individuals in any crisis. First, she emphasizes the need for caregivers to be patient and clear with their clients. Comfort and continued reassurance are particularly important throughout the crisis. Second, Lavin emphasizes that caregivers will have to teach coping skills throughout the crisis. This begins by analyzing what behaviors and skills will be necessary at each phase. Lavin then suggests that a four-step process can facilitate learning:

1. *Preparation*. Here, the goal is to prepare the person with IDD to be exposed to the experience. Counselors may wish to begin by talking about the individual's previous experiences with illness. This will provide an opportunity to draw upon these experiences in later times.

2. *Direct instruction*. The counselor can teach skills that may be useful to the person, providing constant reassurance and reinforcement. For example, he or she may have to go over circumstances in which the individual should notify an appropriate caregiver about changes in health, carefully explaining the symptoms the person might monitor.

3. *Modeling*. In this approach someone models the expected behavior for the individual. The counselor may help to interpret the event (e.g., "He is going to tell the nurse what's bothering him"). The person with IDD can then attempt to copy the behavior with the encouragement and support of the caregiver.

4. *Emotional support*. Throughout the crisis, people with IDD may have to be helped to understand and express their emotions. Directive questions such as, "Are you scared?" or "How do you feel when you are scared?" may help such individuals to recognize their emotions. Counselors may need to provide considerable support throughout the crisis of illness. Nonverbal behaviors, such as a reassuring touch, may provide that needed and welcome presence.

Counselors may find that counseling individuals with IDD requires considerable flexibility in approach. Depending on the level of disability, the present crisis, and the person's previous experiences, caregivers may have to continually adapt approaches to each person. But these clients still share the same needs as other individuals without disabilities, including the need for autonomy, control, and respect.

These basic approaches may be applied at any point in the illness process. Certainly intervention should begin as soon as one knows that a significant other is dying. There are two major reasons for this, especially in circumstances with individuals who have IDD. First, grieving begins with the illness. In recent years, Rando (2000) has redefined anticipatory mourning. Rando's redefinition emphasizes that anticipatory mourning is not simply a reaction to an event projected at some future time. Rather, it is a response to all the losses, encountered in the past, present, and future, within the illness experience. For example, the individual with IDD may already begin to grieve the losses associated with the illness, such as the parent visiting less or being less available for their child, or the client no longer is able to visit his or her parents. All these changes are secondary losses due to the illness and may generate grief within the client.

Second, the dying process can become a significant learning process. As stated earlier, individuals with IDD often benefit from experiential learning (Lipe-Goodson & Goebel, 1983). Involving the individual with IDD early in the illness experience can assist in helping the person eventually understand the fact that the other person is very sick, and perhaps this will even assist with eventually comprehending the death.

For these reasons, it is important to begin assisting individuals with IDD to cope with loss at the onset of the illness process. Rather than protecting individuals with IDD from the illness process, this should be an opportunity for supportive learning. Individuals with

IDD should have opportunities to visit relatives in hospitals, hospices, or home care so they can see the inevitable deterioration that the illness causes. Naturally, individuals with IDD need to retain a sense of control and choice as to what their role should be. Insuring that individuals with IDD are fully informed in an understandable way about what they are likely to observe works best. Such an educational approach should build on past experiences and may even include books or pictures illustrating what they might see, as many individuals with IDD learn visually. Second, individuals with IDD will need options. Do they wish to visit or would they rather call? Would they wish to go to the hospital or wait until the person returns home? Finally, individuals with IDD need support. There should be someone whose prime responsibility is to care for the individual with IDD—offering respite if the visit becomes uncomfortable and patently asking others (and soliciting from the individual with IDD) any questions or concerns that are likely to emerge.

Continued involvement with the illness allows individuals with IDD to comprehend it and avoid the shock of a death that is unexpected. Throughout the illness, questions should be answered in an honest yet supportive way. For example, early in the course of the disease when the prognosis is still unsettled, any question of whether the ill person might die should be answered in a way that allows for the possibility of death, even if the emphasis is on the ongoing medical care: "Momma is very sick, but the doctors are doing all they can to see if she gets better." Once the prognosis is terminal, an honest answer may be that "Momma may die, but her doctors are doing all they can to help her feel comfortable." Again, books and videos may be good adjuncts to the learning process. While involvement is essential, caregivers also need to respect that individuals with IDD, just like others, may choose moments to avoid or deny the illness. When one says, "I know Momma will get better," a response may be to say simply, "I hope so, too, but even if she does not, your brother and sisters will take care of you."

At the time of death, individuals with IDD should have the same opportunities for presence and involvement. Again, the rubrics of education, options in making choices, and support remain critical. At the time of death, it is also important to avoid, if possible, any rapid change. For example, if the individual with IDD is living at home but cannot remain there, it might be better if someone is able to stay with them for a short time or that the individual stay in a familiar and comfortable place of respite until an effective transition can be made. While effective permanency planning ought to have been complete prior to the death of a caregiver, if it is now necessary, care should be taken in assessment. Because grief is likely to be manifested in a range of dimensions including the cognitive and behavioral, any assessment done in the aftermath of the death is likely to significantly underestimate the capabilities of the individual with IDD. That fact should be taken into consideration. At the very least, placements ought to be considered tentative, and the individual with IDD should be reassessed at least 6 months later.

The question of whether individuals with IDD should attend funerals also needs to be addressed within the period immediately following the death. Funerals are therapeutic; they offer a time to be with others and to share memories and support. They allow opportunity to do *something* at a time that seems so disorganized and stressful. Funerals reaffirm the reality of death while providing an outlet for emotions. They even help individuals understand the death by allowing individuals to hear the ways that their own faith systems speak to the loss.

The value of the funeral does not cease simply because an individual has IDD. Funerals are liminal events: They touch individuals at the very edge, the threshold of consciousness. All can benefit from participation in meaningful ritual. Yet, individuals with IDD may need a little extra assistance as they prepare to participate in a funeral.

As before, it is critical that individuals retain choice regarding funerals. Often others may suggest that choices be made for the person. There may be a feeling that the event is too upsetting, or an individual may not be able to understand what is occurring. Rather than arbitrarily deciding whether or not an individual should attend, it is helpful to allow the person to make his or her own choices. Explain what the funeral will be like in words that an individual can understand. Sometimes, even books can help describe the setting or funeral directors can arrange a tour so the individual becomes familiar with the layout.

Sometimes individuals may choose to only attend part of the funeral. Most funerals have numerous parts: a visitation, a funeral service, a committal, and perhaps even a meal or gathering. A person may select to attend only some of the events. In such cases, the individual may be offered another meaningful role. One client attended the visitation but believed it would be too sad to be at the cemetery interment. Instead, he helped prepare food and set the table for a reception that would follow the cemetery ceremony.

One of the most valued aspects of a funeral is that it offers support. It is important that special efforts be made to provide support for all members of the family, as it is easy for the more vulnerable members of the family to get lost in the activity of the moment.

This offering of support can be done in a number of ways. For some it may mean allowing the individuals with IDD to invite their friends, such as other individuals with whom they work or reside. Staff and other caregivers have a useful role serving as a supportive other at the time of the funeral. This is especially important as immediate family members are likely to otherwise engage elsewhere and are unlikely to be as available as they might wish. In other cases, members of the extended family or family friends who are well known to the individual with IDD can play that role by answering questions and, if necessary, offering respite by allowing the individual with IDD the opportunity to leave for a while if the experience becomes overwhelming.

Training can also be a form of support. Many people pick up cues on how to behave by watching others. If one enters a room and sees everyone talking quietly and somberly, one behaves in similar fashion. Individuals with IDD may need specific instruction. For example, they may find it useful to "practice" what to say when people offer condolences. Providing that extra assistance is also a critical part of support.

Following the death, individuals with IDD will continue to need support. Staff should assess, on an ongoing basis over the next months, any manifestations of grief including anger, withdrawal, regressive behaviors including increased dependency and clinging behaviors, heightened compulsivity, or somatic distress. While somatic distress can be a manifestation of grief, any such physical symptoms should naturally be medically evaluated. Individuals often experience increased morbidity and mortality following a significant loss; hence health should always be monitored (Williams, 2002). Staff should be particularly observant around times that may trigger grief. This can include days of the week, times that the deceased individual would have visited or called, and significant dates such as birthdays, holidays, or the times around the anniversary of the death. Even with some individuals with IDD who may not remember or process dates, events around the date can trigger grief. One client with IDD, for example, would have anniversary reactions around Easter since he associated the time with his mother's death.

Expressive therapies often work very well with individuals with IDD since such persons are generally less verbal. Music, play, art, and even dance are among modalities that can be used. Therapeutic ritual also can be effective. Rituals can be created at different points within the grieving process to mark events such as anniversaries or to allow bereaved individuals to feel a sense of continuity, note transitions, affirm the relationship, or even create a reconciling act (Doka, 2002b). Rituals can be extremely useful in that they allow individuals with IDD the opportunity to take meaningful actions to express grief. Even a simple ritual like placing memorial ornaments on a Christmas tree can address the feelings of loss inevitably associated with the holidays. In another case, an individual client would take messages to his mother that he would play at appropriate times in the chapel. Luchterband and Murphy (1998), for example, offer multiple strategies for using expressive approaches and crafting therapeutic rituals.

Group support is often an effective mode of bereavement support. Grief support groups can offer a sense of validation in a shared community, thus easing the sense of isolation. They can help model and teach effective coping and can offer hope. Groups that utilize expressive approaches can be an especially effective modality with individuals with IDD. In one support group, it became the group practice to sing songs associated with the person who died. Each person would suggest a song and tell a story of how the song was associated with the individual who died. One young man, for example, suggested "Danny Boy," since his name was Danny, and his deceased mother would often sing that to him. Another member of the group insisted that the group join him in "Take Me Out to the Ballgame." He could not, though, verbalize a connection, leaving staff members wondering whether he was processing the exercise. Later, when a brother visited, they asked the brother if there was any connection to the death of his father. The brother recounted that his father was a baseball scout; he would often take the boys to games, especially his younger brother, since schools in the late 1940s had little to offer children with IDD. They would sing the song on every outing.

Another approach may be to create a memorial place, such as a wall or garden. This should be in a location that individuals can choose to go to rather than one that they will inevitably pass. Such a "sacred place" can be both an area for ongoing rituals as well as a spot for reflection and remembrance.

It is important to remember two things when working with grieving individuals with IDD. First, because of deficits in information processing, individuals with IDD may ask to have information continually repeated and reexplained. Such repetition is useful to assist them, as they comprehend the difficult and abstract realities of death and illness. Second, an experimental approach is necessary when assisting individuals with IDD in coping with loss. There is comparatively sparse research on this population that offers the possibility of evidence-based practice. One should continue to assess, even on an individual basis, the efficacy of varied approaches.

Beyond that, intervention strategies and grief support need to be crafted individually. Like other mourners, individuals with IDD will have their own unique issues and concerns as they cope with a particular loss.

Acknowledging Other Mourners

In discussing grief support for individuals with IDD, it is also important to acknowledge other mourners. Family members may need support. Often, the death of an individual with IDD can be disenfranchised by others. That is, the loss of an adult child with IDD may not always be acknowledged by others (Doka, 2002a). Memorial services at group homes or residences and at sheltered workshops can have much value. They can bring together a community of mourners that includes family members, staff, friends, fellow consumers, and coworkers. Such remembrances reaffirm the individual worth of the deceased and the inherent value of the deceased's life. This is particularly important when the larger community may view such a loss more ambivalently. Family members may also be invited to participate in subsequent memorialization at such facilities. In addition, it may be effective education to encourage the deceased's fellow consumers, coworkers, and residents to acknowledge the loss to the family through cards, drawings, or video tributes. Families often treasure such items.

Grief support should also be extended to staff members. Staff members can create strong bonds with individuals with IDD. In some cases these bonds can last years. These losses can be cumulative, especially as residents age. Moreover, the deaths of clients can result in numerous secondary losses. For example, meaningful contact with family members is likely to cease once a resident dies. The loss of a resident may have other complicating factors as well. Staff members, for example, may disagree with ethical decisions that have been made, or they may feel that end-of-life care was inappropriate or unsuited to the nature of the individual's disability. It is unrealistic to expect staff to develop close bonds with clients and to support other individuals with IDD at the time of the loss if their own needs for grief support are not met. The result of such unrealistic expectations is that staff members are either likely to experience a sense of occupational stress or burnout or likely to become wary of bonding to residents as closely in the future (Papadatou, 2000).

Effective grief support generally involves individual strategies of self-care. These include acknowledging and validating loss, finding effective methods of respite that allows one to manage stress, developing a personal and spiritual stance that allows a staff member to find an overarching framework for attributing meaning to life and death, and finding satisfaction in one's own work (Doka, 2006). However, research has also emphasized that organizations play a large role in effecting support. Effective organizations have both formal policies and informal procedures that validate loss. Formal policies can include time off to attend funerals or debriefings after death. Such policies can set a tone that creates an environment within the work setting where supervisors and other employees can be both validating and supportive of grief. In addition, some effective organizations offer both ongoing education and rituals that mark significant deaths (Vachon, 1987).

It is also important to acknowledge that not all losses involve death. Other losses, such as when residents or staff members leave, can also engender feelings of grief and ought to be marked by ritual.

Implications for Training and Education

The previous section emphasized the tasks inherent in offering grief support for individuals with IDD. Central to that process are implications for training and education.

Naturally, individuals with IDD would benefit from education about loss and grief. Life cycle education that emphasizes that living things are born, develop, and eventually die offers a basic foundation that may be useful when individuals face illness or loss. In addition, visits to hospitals, funeral homes, and cemeteries often are best done in a noncrisis atmosphere. Such field trips provide a basic familiarity that may very well be useful when such facilities need to be used. Resources that offer education about death and loss in simple ways—but with pictures of adults, especially individuals with IDD—can fill a present void. Often the only educational resources that are available (with the exception of some lifecycle books such as *Lifetimes* or *The Fall of Freddy the Leaf*) characterize children and are thus demeaning to adults with IDD.

Staff also should have opportunities for training on loss and grief. This type of educational process both assists in self-care and helps generate a sense of competence that might prepare staff receptiveness to reach out toward grieving individuals with IDD (Schwebach, 1992).

Moreover, organizations and systems of care for individuals with IDD should see their role not only in educating their clients and staff but in reaching out to other populations as well. Schwebach (1992), for example, found that parents and siblings of individuals with IDD often disenfranchised such individuals by trying to shield them from the illness or inhibiting such individuals from attending family rituals. Again, providing education about grieving processes in individuals with IDD in support groups or educational programs in communities can best be done in noncrisis situations and with open dialog between family, staff, and individuals with IDD about loss, illness, and grief.

Systems of care for individuals with IDD also may offer training to, or in collaboration with, other organizations. The philosophy of inclusion and normalization means that many individuals with IDD may end their lives in facilities such as hospices or nursing homes. Shared training can offer opportunities to open dialog and to mutually collaborate. Presently there is a program in New York State between the Young Adult Institute, a group established to assist individuals with IDD, and the New York Hospice Association to improve end-of-life care for individuals with IDD. In this training, the Young Adult Institute can offer education about IDD and the needs of their clients while they learn from the hospice staff about the general issues that face the dying.

Perhaps, though, this shows a larger need to revisit the ways individuals with IDD are educated. Often there is an emphasis on learning by rote and routine. Yet that same system contributes to a lack of flexibility that may impair coping. As caregivers in systems of care for individuals with IDD seriously consider ways to educate and to prepare clients to cope with illness, grief, and loss, they may find they need to reevaluate training and emphasize ways to train individuals with IDD to cope with the inevitable transitions that are a natural part of life.

CONCLUSION

Like other populations, individuals with IDD will inevitably have to cope with loss and grief as they age. While one cannot protect individuals from such loss, one can prepare and support individuals as they mourn. Such support begins even before the illness experience. People with IDD have the same needs as people without disabilities. Their emotional needs should be acknowledged, respected, and addressed. Their need to address issues regarding loss and grief is ongoing. It ends only with death.

REFERENCES

Bruce, E. J., & Schultz, C. L. (2001). *Nonfinite loss and grief: A psycho-educational approach.* Eastgardens, Australia: Maclennan Petty.

Doka, K. J. (Ed.). (2002a). *Disenfranchised grief: New directions, challenges, and strategies for practice.* Champaign, IL: Research Press.

Doka, K. J. (2002b). The role of ritual in the treatment of disenfranchised grief. In K. Doka (Ed.), *Disenfranchised grief: New directions, challenges, and strategies for practice* (pp. 135–149). Champaign, IL: Research Press.

Doka, K. J. (2006). Caring for the carer: The lessons of research. *Grief Matters: The Australian Journal of Grief and Bereavement, 9,* 4–7.

Duetsch, H. (1985). Grief counseling with the mentally retarded clients. *Psychiatric Aspects of Mental Retardation Reviews, 4*(5), 17–20.

Kauffman, J. (2005). *Guidebook on helping persons with mental retardation mourn.* Amityville, NY: Baywood.

Lavin, C. (2002). Disenfranchised grief and individuals with developmental disabilities. In K. J. Doka (Ed.), *Disenfranchised grief: New directions, challenges, and strategies for practice* (pp. 307–322). Champaign, IL: Research Press.

Lavin, C., & Doka, K. J. (1999). *Older adults with developmental disabilities.* Amityville, NY: Baywood.

Lipe-Goodson, P. S., & Goebel, B. L. (1983). Perception of age and death in mentally retarded adults. *Mental Retardation, 21,* 68–75.

Luchterband, C., & Murphy, N. (1998). *Helping adults with mental retardation grieve a death loss.* Philadelphia: Taylor & Francis.

Papadatou, D. (2000). A proposed model of health professionals' grieving process. *Omega: Journal of Death and Dying, 41,* 59–77.

Rando, T. A. (1993). *The treatment of complicated mourning.* Champaign, IL: Research Press.

Rando, T. A. (2000). *Clinical dimensions of anticipatory mourning: Theory and practice in working with the dying, their loved ones, and their caregivers.* Champaign, IL: Research Press.

Roos, S. (2002). *Chronic sorrow: A living loss.* New York: Brunner-Routledge.

Schwebach, I. A. (1992). *Disenfranchised grief in mentally ill and mentally retarded populations.* Unpublished doctoral dissertation, Indiana University, Indiana, PA.

Stroebe, M., & Schut, H. (1999). The dual process model of coping with bereavement: Rationale and description. *Death Studies, 21,* 197–224.

Todd, J., & Hymes, J. (1999, March). *Celebration of love: Bereavement support for the mentally challenged.* Paper presented to the 21st Annual Conference of the Association of Death Education and Counseling, San Antonio, TX.

Vachon, M. (1987). *Occupational stress in the care of the dying and the bereaved.* New York: Hemisphere.

Williams, J. R. (2002). Effects of grief on a survivor's health. In K. Doka (Ed.), *Living with grief: Loss in late life* (pp. 191–206). Washington, DC: The Hospice Foundation of America.

Worden, J. W. (2008). *Grief counseling and grief therapy* (4th ed.). New York: Springer.

PART V

Supports and Resources

CHAPTER 17

Use of Person-Centered Planning for End-of-Life Decision Making

LEIGH ANN C. KINGSBURY

A BRIEF HISTORY

The intent of this chapter is to look at the role person-centered planning can play in helping people with intellectual and developmental disabilities (IDD) specifically have more control over their health care decision making and their end-of-life choices. If we are doing good planning with people; if we are mindful of the person's needs, interests and values; and if we are required by the system from which the person receives services to "have a plan," why would that plan not include information about health care decision making such as surrogacy and wishes about end-of-life care? There is no getting around it; people we provide services for will die and service providers will be faced more and more with the challenge of caring for someone at the end of life. Just to be clear, this chapter is *not* about passive or active euthanasia of people with disabilities. It is about the fact that people with disabilities develop critical, chronic, and/or terminal illnesses just like people without disabilities. Therefore, just like people without disabilities, people with disabilities should be supported in planning their health care and end-of-life wishes. Where better to accomplish this planning than in an already-existing process that when done properly seeks to honor, value, and share control and responsibility with the person whose life is at the center of the process? Why would we not do this as part of a respectful person-centered planning process?

We have documented and planned some of the most intimate and private issues in people's lives. Why is it that we have avoided planning around the end of life? There are numerous reasons, most notably that as Americans the majority of us do not develop advance care plans for the end of our own lives, and, anecdotally, it is reported that advance care planning is almost never a routine part of planning with people who have IDD.

Additionally, it appears that our hesitancy to have conversations about the end of life is similar to our comfort level in talking about sex with people who have disabilities. In many places sex is a taboo subject for people who use services and their having intimate relationships is either not permitted or essentially ignored. Similarly, it is our experience that in more instances we are not talking with people about health care decision making and wishes regarding end-of-life care. These are topics that make people uncomfortable. These are subjects in which many people do not always feel well versed. These are matters easily avoided but which could be meaningfully addressed through a thoughtful person-centered plan, especially when we consider that many plans are rules driven and must be updated on an annual basis. Person-centered planning is an ideal "place" to bring people together and to focus on the express wishes of the person with whom the plan is being done.

According to Mount (1992), the term person-centered planning had become common by 1985. No matter what method one is using, it is person-centered planning when it shares four characteristics: (a) the use of people-first language that helps to identify the person with whom planning is being done as a person and not a set of diagnoses, (b) the use of everyday language and images that work to move away from professional jargon, (c) the search for and identification of the person's strengths and gifts (not "strengths and needs") within the context of the person's community, and (d) the strengthening of the voice of the person with whom the plan is being done and those who know and love the person. Thus, it validates the person's experiences and helps to define changes the person's wishes to see in his or her life (Mount, 1992).

There was a time when person-centered planning was so new and innovative that many people viewed it as a fad or the next trend. It was occasionally difficult for people who provided training ("trainers") to help participants understand why and how it was so different and why those committed trainers believed it was *not* a fad or a trend. Unfortunately, in too many places person-centered planning is not different; it does not feel or look any different than what was done before. The process is called "person centered" and the "forms" being used say "person-centered plan," but in reality nothing has changed. The person with IDD with or for whom the planning is being done still has no voice and still has no control. The process has been given lip service; the people implementing it have tried to figure out how to do it faster instead of being mindful that this is someone's *life* they are addressing. As O'Brien and O'Brien (1997) note, "Everyone is doing PCP." The process must have arrived at some status; in true human service fashion, we now have an acronym for it.

Essential Lifestyle Planning (ELP), Planning Alternative Tomorrows With Hope (PATH), Making Action Plans (MAPS), Personal Futures Planning: All of these represent a model of person-centered planning. Each was developed with a purpose and for a reason: Each grew out of the realization that traditional planning methods were no longer meeting the needs and desires of people with disabilities.

There is and should be a distinct difference between traditional planning methods (e.g., Individual Service Plans and Individual Habilitation Plans) and person-centered planning, whatever model is being used. The difference is about controlling one's health care decisions, making meaningful choices, and having a real voice. The difference is about who is in charge—who decides how and where the process occurs; the difference is that the process neither looks nor feels the same as it always has before.

The strength of a good plan lies not in its words (although those words matter a great deal) but rather in its ability to affect change in the owner's life. A poorly done person-centered plan is no better than a mediocre systems-driven support plan. In fact, it may be worse because by calling it a person-centered plan we have created some assumption that this plan will be different. If it is not—if in the end the person still has no positive control and no opportunities for decision making—we have clearly done an injustice to the person and the process. Smull et al. (2006) says, "Person-centered planning is an implicit set of promises to act on what we hear." If we do not act properly, we are breaking our promise. As end of life nears, if we cannot listen at that point—if we cannot support control and choice for individuals with IDD when time is sorely limited—when can we?

A plan that is implemented and used on a routine basis and that lives and grows with the person is one of person-centered planning's great strengths. Good person-centered plans are not just done at an annual review; they are shaped and molded over time as the person's life changes. Historically, good person-centered planning has made a strong effort to move people and planning away from the traditional medical, or deficit-based, models of support. Unfortunately, if the person's life changes dramatically from a medical standpoint such that the person is diagnosed with a critical or a terminal illness, it is all too easy to fall back into the medical model. This is especially true when there is likely to be an increase in traditional medical system involvement upon the initial diagnosis.

Logic would dictate that the thing to do would be to include the new information about diagnosis, goals for treatment, or prognosis in the individual's current person-centered plan. The problem, however, is that systems are often not logical, and we miss this opportunity. We may well add the diagnostic information to the plan (there are actually utilization review systems that will not let a plan get through the system without the *International Classification of Diseases 10th Revision* codes), but we fail to incorporate what it means to the person to now be *living with this diagnosis*. We most often fail to communicate what the person's goals for treatment are and how the person's values influence his or her decisions about future treatment. By applying the same values and approaches of good person-centered planning at the time of a critical or terminal diagnosis, we strengthen our commitment to the person to see the situation through to the end (even if that "end" is death). We demonstrate that we are still listening, and we bring the planning process full circle in the person's life, rather than leaving out significant pieces of information.

ADVANCE CARE AND PERSON-CENTERED PLANNING

In the community of people and professionals who deal with death, dying, and end of life, the process of planning ahead specifically around health care decision making and end of life is referred to as "advance care planning." Where the two processes of advance care planning and person-centered planning intersect will be addressed later in this chapter.

There are many reasons why we need to be doing advance care planning with people with IDD. First, people with disabilities are living longer and are experiencing the same age-related illnesses and conditions as people without disabilities. Thus, we are being presented with both the opportunity and necessity to have these conversations on a regular basis. Second, the concept of self-determination should encompass one's entire life. There are only five principles of self-determination, according to the Center for Self-Determination (2007)*; there is *not* a sixth principle that says, "The right to be in control and have authority over

---

* The five principles are (a) freedom, (b) authority, (c) support, (d) responsibility, and (e) confirmation.

one's life stops when one becomes critically or terminally ill or when one reaches a certain age." Third, from a purely logical standpoint, it makes sense to plan, and it really makes no sense to wait until it is necessary because of circumstances. "Eleventh hour" planning is not good planning. Decisions about health care treatment and end of life are almost never easy nor quick decisions. It is difficult and sometimes impossible to try and make such decisions during a time of stress, fear, and uncertainty.

For most people who do not receive services from a "disability system," doing advance care planning and sharing the necessary information means ensuring that family members, the closest of friends, and (hopefully) one's physicians know ahead of time one's values and wishes. For these individuals, it is not until the time that one's wishes need to be honored that there is the involvement of larger systems.

For people with disabilities who receive funding, supports, and/or services from a "system" (such as a community services board or a local managing authority), doing advance care planning helps inform the system, too. There are too many stories of people's dying wishes being honored (e.g., dying at their home with family and staff present) where the end result is an investigation that did not consider what the person and family wanted but rather presumed that because the person died at home and not in a medical setting, something must have been done wrong. Clearly, there are tragic situations in which people die because something *was* done wrong, but it is not those situations that are being referred to here.

Additionally, advance care planning with people with IDD can help bring to the surface any issues that need to be addressed while there is time. In particular, advance care planning through a person-centered planning process provides a structured means of identifying cultural, spiritual, and family rituals that may need to be addressed.

In 2005, we facilitated a planning session with a woman, Lydia, with severe intellectual disabilities who had been diagnosed with colon cancer and was dying. Due to an existing lawsuit, there was a regulation in place from the funding authority where Lydia lived that required an autopsy to be performed on anyone who died while receiving services from that funding authority. In the course of a simple conversation with her team as part of her advance care planning, it was learned that Lydia was Jewish. None of Lydia's team members present was aware of the religious issues surrounding Jewish law and autopsies. Thankfully, because planning was being done well in advance of needing the information, the team and family were able to work together to ensure that Lydia and her family's religious wishes were honored. Ultimately, the family had to go to court to ensure their wishes were respected. However, had the team not engaged in advance care planning with Lydia and her family, it is possible that the autopsy may have been completed before anyone was aware that it was a violation of her and her family's religious preferences.

Person-Centered Planning and Advance Care Planning Intersect

There are several places where the processes of person-centered planning and advance care planning meet. In at least five ways they are similar and have complimentary features. These include the following, which will be discussed in the following pages: (a) living well and quality of life,

(b) autonomy and control, (c) recognized and respected models for planning, (d) trust and promises, and (e) natural supports.

Living Well and Quality of Life

One of the issues that disability advocates are frequently faced with is addressing the concept of quality of life. Professionals often use this phrase in the context of identifying the supports and services a person needs to have to maintain a certain quality of life; from that, clearly a judgment is being made about what the quality of life for that person is. Of course, the biggest issue is that quality of life must be addressed by and with the person with the disability, not just those who are called professionals. Smull (1995) notes that quality of life is directly connected to support and accommodation for rituals in one's life and choice around those rituals. Rituals around health care and end of life are often significant and hold great meaning to the person with and for whom we are planning. Rituals can bring comfort, solace, and a sense of familiarity and consistency; they deserve the attention of planners and must be addressed in planning.

Choice is defined by Smull (1993) as the opportunity for "preferences, opportunities and control." For people who do not use oral language or any kind of augmented form of communication—and for the many people who are reliant on loved ones, friends, or paid staff to communicate information for them about their preferences—professionals often do have to make judgments about quality of life. It is critical we communicate with professionals who provide support and care by incorporating what we know is important to the person and where that person's values lie.

For people with disabilities who live with a chronic illness or are faced with a critical or terminal illness, judgments are also routinely made about treatment the person should or should not receive based on the notion of quality of life. As Diane Coleman, president of Not Dead Yet and someone with a physical disability requiring a motorized chair and respiratory support, reported to Congress (2006), "A number of my . . . friends have been pressured by hospital employees to sign do-not-resuscitate orders and other advance directives to forego treatment, coupled with negative statements about how bad it would be if they [the person] became more disabled."

The fact that these judgments continue to be made is yet another reason to record one's wishes ahead of time through advance care and person-centered planning. Although there are certainly still examples of people's wishes not being honored with such planning, having conversations about one's wishes, writing them down, and identifying someone to honor those wishes seemingly increases the chances that one's wishes will be recognized.

In the *Respecting Choices* (2002) curriculum of advance care planning, facilitators are taught to ask, "What does living well mean to the person?" By "person," they mean the person with whom planning is being done. Perhaps asking the question "What does living well mean *for this person*?" would be a clearer way to capture the information that we are looking for when we talk about quality of life. Many people live every single day with all sorts of disabilities and would describe themselves as "living well." Living well for people with disabilities may very well mean being healthy and having a quality of life as defined by that person, all within the context of living with a severe disability.

If the person can answer the question "What does living well mean?" or if others who know and love the person can put words to "what living well means" for those not able to articulate it themselves, it would seem that as planners we have the core value needed to start a person-centered planning process. If we assume that "living well" is equal to "quality of life" (obviously defined by each individual person), we have therefore identified one the first places that person-centered planning and advance care planning intersect.

Once planners know what living well means or how quality of life is defined by the person, we can then begin to gather additional information for the plan. In using the person-centered planning model of PATH, planners start with identifying the "north star" with the person for whom they are planning. The north star is the vision the person has for his or her life or the specific outcome he or she is aiming for and for which the PATH is being done. If we were doing a PATH with someone, having identified what "living well" means would mean we had created at least part of the vision for the north star. We now know the intended outcome; we just have to figure out how to get there. If we were doing Essential Lifestyle Planning and we knew what living well meant, we would have answered one of the core questions about "what is important to and what is important for the person" allowing the rest of the plan to be built around that information.

Autonomy and Control

The second place that person-centered planning and advance care planning intersect is around the ideas of autonomy and control. Person-centered planning is designed to help people who have little to no control over their lives regain that positive control and achieve a balance between what is important *to* them and what is important *for* them (Smull, et al., 2006). Advance care planning is designed to essentially do the same thing: to help people have control. In this case it is control over their health care decisions and the ability to communicate that information in a way that others can hear and honor it.

Especially for people who are critically or terminally ill, where there may be a multitude of decisions being made *about* the person and *without* the person, advance care planning is designed as a means for the person to be able say, "Listen to me. This is what I want and this is what I expect." Person-centered planning is no different, as it allows individuals to say, "Here is what matters to me. Here is the support I need. Here is what I expect from people who support me." In the language of the self-advocacy movement, "nothing about me without me."

Recognized and Respectful Planning Methods

The third place that person-centered planning and advance care planning intersect is that they are both recognized and respected methods of planning within their own arenas. Both represent best practice and both are intended to communicate critical information that someone wants others to know, respect, and honor. The efficacy of both practices has been demonstrated (Hammes & Briggs, 2002; Holburn & Vietze, 2002). Both expect that people will communicate information with loved ones and others in their lives. Both require that action be taken at certain times, and both identify who is responsible for those actions. Action planning is a critical piece of both good person-centered planning and advance care planning. Though not usually defined as "action planning," in advance care planning, one of the essential elements is the identification of the surrogate decision maker, or the person who is trusted to "act" when the individual cannot.

Trust and Promises

The fourth intersection of person-centered planning and advance care planning is around the issue of trust. If we believe that person-centered planning is an implicit set of promises (Smull, et al., 2006), then we also must trust that the people involved will act on those promises. Advance care planning implies that there is trust between the person doing the planning and the person chosen to carry out the plans. In both cases, assuming that trust is present, the person with or for whom planning is done believes that the trusted soul will act in accordance with one's values, goals for one's life, and one's wishes.

Natural Supports

Finally, the fifth area where person-centered planning and advance care planning meet is that of "natural supports." This meeting point is also a window into one of the biggest challenges facing the disability community today and in the near future. Advance care planning relies on family and friends. In fact, in many states where there are statutory requirements for advance care planning, the legislation includes language that specifically prohibits paid caregivers or employees of one's health care provider from being one's surrogate decision maker. Advance care planning is unfortunately yet another place where we are reminded how disconnected from friends and community people with disabilities can be. In structured systems of support we have found that many people with disabilities are surrounded by paid staff and have few, if any, "nonpaid" supports in their lives. In the lives of people without disabilities, those "nonpaid" supports would be loved ones, family, and friends. Relative to advance care planning, not having family and friends available to help make and honor health care decisions leaves many people in limbo, and it means people will die in ways they do not wish, in places they do not know, and surrounded by people who are unfamiliar to them.

WHERE AND HOW DO WE START?

One of the things that is known about advance care planning is that people will change their minds about their wishes over time. In addition, most people who are young and healthy have little to no context for making complex health care decisions such as whether they want cardiopulmonary resuscitation (CPR) or intubation. It therefore follows that we need to figure out who it is we are planning with or for and what is the purpose of that planning. Not everyone needs end-of-life planning. For many people, surrogate decision making may be the key issue. Through a person-centered process, we have the ability to bring planning full circle but in differing degrees. As adapted with permission from the Respecting Choices (Hammes & Briggs, 2002) facilitator training curriculum, it is helpful to consider when doing advance care planning that there are three "groups" of people with whom one may be planning, and each of these three groups has a slightly different need or focus that can then be addressed through one's person-centered plan. This is a broad generalization, with the intent of helping planners identify what the critical issues around planning may be; clearly not everyone falls neatly into one of these "categories" and the notion of "categorizing" people is obviously not in line with the values of person-centered planning. These groups are the following:

- People who are young and healthy, for whom the issue is surrogate decision making. For this group of people, the critical issue is identifying who the person trusts to help make health care decisions, if the person him/herself were to be unable to do so.
- People whose age and/or health is the defining factor and for whom the issues of age or health will impact on health care decisions and future treatment. Therefore, the key issues in planning with people in this category are understanding what the person wants from his or her health care and treatment and who will be the surrogate decision maker. People with critical and chronic illnesses and progressive disabilities fall into this category. People in this group do not have terminal illnesses.
- People who have a terminal illness and who (using the Medicare criteria) have been told they have 6 months or less to live. For people in this category, the issues are similar to those identified for the second group—"What does the person desire from his or her health care or treatment and who will be the surrogate decision maker?"—but given the potential time frames that exist, there is a sense of urgency.

The question routinely asked when helping others learn about health care decision making and end of life is "When do we start?" or "How old should someone be?" There are those who will answer those questions with "start immediately." For people with IDD, the experiences gained so far in planning have taught us that starting as soon as one can definitely makes sense, but we also must recognize that many people, many families, and many guardians are not comfortable with these conversations. Starting the conversation around decision making, rather than "end of life," is a much easier and gentler means of beginning to gather the necessary information.

Given that in most structured systems of support for people with disabilities there is a requirement that an "annual" plan be done, we also know that we are presented with an opportunity for advanced planning at least once a year. This is not to suggest however, that one can just add to the agenda for the annual meeting end-of-life planning. For most people, that tag line is a conversation stopper, and we have learned that for many people with and without IDD, the topic is very frightening and requires a great deal of time, thought, and sensitivity.

Vignette 1: Louise's Story

Several years ago while helping a program coordinator learn about advance care planning, we met with a woman and several of her support staff in order to begin talking about health care decisions and surrogate decision making. Louise is in her early 60s and has moderate intellectual disabilities. She has often said that when she gets old, she wants to stay in her apartment and, very specifically, "does not want to move to a nursing home." The agency supporting Louise is very committed to honoring her wishes and wanted to start planning in order to ensure that she was able to remain in her apartment for as long as she could.

Although we thought Louise understood why we were meeting with her—and with the exception of me as the guide, she had trusted relationships with everyone who was present—the process very quickly became upsetting to her. We did not start out immediately with the end-of-life conversation, but nonetheless Louise began crying and telling us, "I don't want to go to a nursing home." It was evident she did not understand why we were meeting. In fact, she was convinced we were there to talk about "moving her to a nursing home." Based on Louise's reaction, we changed our course of action and spent much more time on learning what was important to Louise about staying in her apartment and her daily life. The question of surrogate decision making naturally followed once we know who and what was important in Louise's life.

Louise's experience reminds us of at least two things that need to be present when planning well. First, "start where the person is," not where you want them to be or where you need to be. Louise's supporters really wanted to make sure she had a surrogate decision maker as she aged. That is where "they" were. Louise was in a different place—she needed reassurance that she was not moving to a nursing home—and it was critical for the success of the planning to start from that point. Second, there has to be a means for support after the conversation ends and the planners leave. Louise helped reinforce for us that conversations about the unknown can be frightening. It is likely these conversations will be unfamiliar to people. We must provide support after the conversation for the person in case additional questions or fears arise.

One of the occasionally still heard criticisms of person-centered planning is "it takes too long." That can be true in some circumstances, and it is understood that we need to find a balance between what can be a time-consuming process and the need for efficiency in moving plans forward involving large groups of people. However, when we speed things up, we may fail to be sensitive to the fact that we are helping *plan someone's life*. What audacity it takes to tell someone who has had little to no opportunity for real life experiences that "we do not have time" to help him or her figure it out. Again, if we cannot support someone to have authority and be in control at the end of his or her life—and furthermore if we cannot offer someone the time he or she needs given the limited time available—we are clearly doing an injustice to the person and others involved in the planning process. If the issue is literally "end of life," frankly, we may be out of time.

ISSUES FACING THE DISABILITY COMMUNITY, MODELS FOR DECISION MAKING, AND PERSON-CENTERED PLANNING COME TOGETHER

In *What Should We Do for Jay? The Edges of Life and Cognitive Disability*, Turnbull (2005) proposed five models of decision making, each of which has bearing on health care and end-of-life decisions. Each model reflects a key issue that needs to be considered when planning, and person-centered planning provides a means of addressing those issues in a concrete manner. The five models are the following:

- The human capacity model
- The public law model
- The cultural model
- The technological model
- The theological/ethical model

The human capacity model helps guide us as we plan with people and consider whether each person has, does not have, or can acquire the capacity to make a health care decision. As Turnbull (2005) says, "When we decide whether to intervene at the 'edges of life,' we take into account (the person's) ability to have increased capacity and our ability to contribute to that capacity" (p. 15).

Distinguishing between and establishing competency and capacity is one of the first critical issues that must be addressed in health care decision making and end-of-life planning with people with IDD. Through person-centered planning, one can gather much of the information needed to determine if a person with IDD is capable of making a health care decision.

Competency is a legal term and a legal process. Capacity on the other hand, "is a state, not a trait" (Lyden, 2006) for which there is no standardized assessment for people with IDD. Lack of standardized assessments is not necessarily something to be changed (one can easily debate the perils of standardized testing). However, in the absence of standardized assessments, individuals with IDD are routinely thought to be "incompetent" and wrongly considered to not have the capacity to make health care decisions when, in fact, many times the person is perfectly capable of making the decision at hand.

Shortly after Louise and her team made their way through the person-centered planning and health care decision-making process, by coincidence she needed emergency surgery. In preparation for the surgery, a physician performed what was referred to as a "capacity assessment." Louise was asked who the president of the United States was, what her address was, what the date was, and so on. As Louise and her coordinator reported it, Louise was not feeling well, she was somewhat frightened (as most any of us would be), and she was afraid of giving the wrong answers to the doctor, which in fact she did given the pressure she was under. Under less stressful circumstances, it was reported that Louise would have been able to answer all the questions correctly with no problems, though we should be skeptical of the questions asked as "determining capacity," as compared to a more traditional assessment of reality orientation. Based on her incorrect answers and the fact that she had a diagnosis of intellectual disabilities, the surgeon deemed her to be incapable of consenting for surgery. Louise needed surgery quickly and there was no time to argue that she was able to consent. The good news in this case was that since Louise and her team had gone through a health care decision-planning process and Louise had identified a surrogate decision maker (a health care power of attorney), she was able to have a conversation with her surrogate and the surrogate was able to consent for surgery.

Although no standardized assessment for people with IDD is currently in use, there is literature that exists on evaluating the capacity of people without intellectual disabilities that can be used as a guideline for assessing capability for people with IDD. Applebaum (2007) describes four criteria that should be considered in evaluating an individual's ability to give informed consent. The person must be able to (a) communicate a choice (not necessarily verbally); (b) understand information that is relevant to the decision being made; (c) "appreciate the situation and its consequences"—that is, understand the issue at hand for which the decision needs to be made and the "likely consequences of treatment options"; and (d) be able to "reason" about the available options and choices. In addition to these four criteria, Grisso (1986) proposed an additional criterion: to "make a decision that is *voluntary*, free from coercion or other forms of undue influence."

A second set of criteria that is very useful, though also not specific to individuals with intellectual disabilities comes from the Respecting Choices (Hammes & Briggs, 2002) facilitator curriculum. It also lists four criteria for evaluating one's capacity for making a health care decision: (a) the ability to understand that one has authority and that there is a choice to be made, (b) the ability to understand information and understand the benefits and consequences of the decision to be made, (c) the ability to communicate a decision and the rationale for it, and (d) the ability to make a decision that is consistent with one's values and goals and that remains consistent over time.

At a minimum, these criteria provide a foundation for and a parameter within which planners can help evaluate one's capacity for making a health care decision and that can guide planners in helping to determine where and when surrogate decision making may be necessary.

Unfortunately, the issues of competency and capacity continue to be unclear within the medical community. Ganzini, Volicer, Nelson, Fox, and Derse reported in 2004 that 2 of the 10 myths around decision-making capacity were that "competency and capacity are the same thing," and that "a cognitive impairment is equal to lack of decision making capacity." Clearly, competency and capacity are *not* the same and we must be explicit about the differences and be clear about what the issue truly is relative to the person with or for whom we are planning. A good person-centered planning process will do several things to support the knowledge that the person is *capable* of making certain decisions:

- It will identify allies in the person's life who can attest to the person's capabilities, including family, friends, and clinicians.
- It should outline how the person communicates, how the person makes decisions, and what decisions the person routinely makes.
- It should provide structure for the supports the person needs to make decisions; that is, it can define how best to clearly communicate with the person in such a way that informed consent is present.

Turnbull's (2005) second model of decision making, the public law model, is reflected when decisions are made based on the person's "legal rights." The challenge in planning with people who have IDD is that many people are legally competent but in fact, may not have the capacity to make the decision at hand. Planners may feel caught between what the person "should" be supported to do (more often described as "allowed" to do) given that the person is legally competent and what the person is "capable" of doing. Everyone makes bad decisions in their lives and everyone makes choices they sometimes regret. Certainly everyone with or without a disability deserves the opportunity to make mistakes; everyone deserves the "dignity of risk." Supporting someone to make a decision just because "it is his or her right," however, without considering the potential ramifications and without considering if the person has the support or capability needed to make the decision, is dangerous.

The public law model of decision making includes two core values of person-centered planning: empowerment and participatory decision making. As reflected in this model, a good person-centered planning process being used to help facilitate advance care planning will thus empower the person to be in control of the decisions being made, even if the decision is simply "Who can make a health care decision for me? Whom do I trust to be my surrogate decision maker?" Second, it should provide the forum for participatory decision making. A good person-centered planning process will always include the person (in a way that makes sense for the person) along with the people who know and care about the person—in the case of health care and/or end-of-life decision making, those who can speak to the medical issues at hand and whom the person wishes to have present. In a similar fashion, Martyn (1994) espouses the concept of "Best respect": "best respect . . . identifies a group of persons best able to collect the most relevant information concerning objective medical facts and subjective moral voice."

The third model of decision making, the cultural model, is reflected in health care and end-of-life decision making when we use a person-centered planning process to learn about, clearly communicate, and act upon the cultural and ethnic beliefs that guide the person and his or her family. Generally, there are several consistent events in people's lives where cultural rituals are significant: births, transitions from childhood to adulthood, marriages, and the end of life (there are certainly more, but these tend to stand out as significant). Planning with people with IDD has not historically been culturally sensitive; person-centered planning has taught us that it is critical to learn about, recognize, and honor one's culture. Rituals around the end of life are centuries old. Person-centered planning is a structured and respectful means for identifying the culture of the person with whom we are planning, the rituals that need to be honored, and the person's and family's expectations for the provider of services and supports during this time.

The fourth model of decision making, the technological model, expects us to consider the role of technology. Turnbull (2005) indicates it is for prevention, cure, or for changing the way people with disabilities live. For many people with disabilities, technology is neither prevention nor cure, but in fact it allows the person to continue living every day. Technology may be the means by which the person leads an ordinary life. For some people, feeding tubes and ventilators are ordinary parts of everyday life; they are not, in traditional medical language, "extraordinary treatment." It is absolutely imperative that when planning with someone who uses technology to live everyday, one takes into consideration the role that technology plays. It is imperative that planners communicate through the person-centered planning and advance care-planning processes that the technology the person uses is not "extraordinary" but, in fact, quite "ordinary" for that particular person. It is also important to capture in the planning process how the person feels about using technology if the issue is impending.

Vignette 2: José's story

José lived all of his life except for the previous 2 years in a state institution for people with IDD. He had significant physical disabilities, and his health was often compromised by the physical position of his body. It was very questionable whether José actually had an intellectual disability, though he spent at least 30 years in an institution and was clearly affected by that situation. A dear friend and advocate of José's had suggested we get together and discuss health care decision making and planning because José had recently experienced several bouts of pneumonia that had resulted in him being hospitalized and being on a ventilator while in the hospital. The advocate's concern was, "What if this happens again and you can't come off the ventilator successfully. What do you want to do?" In talking with José and his advocate, we learned that the advocate was pretty sure José would not wish to live on a ventilator, but he really did not know and was therefore encouraging José to do some planning. José uses very few words to communicate, so the planning process took a long time to be sure we understood exactly what he wanted to communicate with us. What we ultimately learned was that the ventilator was not the issue; the issue was where José lived. Through a series of questions around daily life, rituals, dreams, issues related to hospitalization, and we learned that as long as José could continue to live in the community and continue to spend time with his friends and advocate's family, then the ventilator was not the issue. But if in fact using it meant that José would need to go back to living in some sort of institutional facility, he would choose not to use the ventilator. "I grew up in an institution, I will not die in one," he told us.

Turnbull's (2005) last model of decision making is the theological/ethical model. This model views disability through its relationship with a higher power or deity. Turnbull asks us to consider "whose theology or ethic prevails if there is a conflict between what the person wants, the family wants and the public domain wants (courts, legislatures)?" As with issues of culture, traditional planning with people with disabilities has not often taken into consideration the role of religion, faith, and spirituality in people's lives. Again as with culture, it is often at the end of life that we see people and their families returning to their faith for guidance and comfort. Rituals of faith bring consistency and something that is "known" to an event that can be sad, scary, and emotional. Doing advance care planning within a person-centered planning process should first identify faith and spirituality rituals that the person and family wish to engage and that may need the system's support. Second, it should identify who within the system (e.g., health care provider, agency, or staff) can help support these rituals and how the system can offer the same support. Third, it should identify the processes the person and family wish to see carried out after the person has passed on.

What We Are Learning

Over the past several years of using person-centered planning to help support health care decision making and end-of-life conversations, we have captured our learning by using information gathering processes from *The Learning Community for Person Centered Practices*, specifically "The 4+1 Questions" format as developed by the Learning Community for Person Centered Practices (http://www.learningcommunity.us). Much of that learning is embedded in this chapter; much of it is not new information if one has been actively involved in person-centered planning for a long time. Still, there are other lessons we have learned that are important to keep in mind when planning. There are certainly more than 10 lessons we have learned, but the following lessons seem to be at the heart of good planning and should be helpful for all planners:

1. The emotion attached to this subject cannot be overestimated. There must always be follow-up support in place for people with whom we plan.
2. Like all good person-centered planning, advance care planning is a process, not an event. We have learned that it usually takes a minimum of two to three meetings with the person to capture the information needed. We also know that it is important to keep having this conversation even when we think we're finished. We must talk about it more than once if we want trust to develop and if we want to capture all the information we need.

3. The issue of surrogate decision making once again demonstrates that people are disconnected from their communities and nonpaid supports. One of the biggest hurdles we face is surrogate decision making for people who literally have no one but paid staff in their lives. This is a systems challenge that will need to be addressed. Planners must be prepared to help people address this issue in their own lives.

4. People are clearly confused about and do not understand the difference between competency and capacity. There are existing criteria to guide us through issues of capacity. Planners must be familiar with the criteria and must be able to involve people who know the person and the circumstances well in order to differentiate between competency and capacity.

5. People, staff, families, and other stakeholders are actually very interested in knowing how to have these conversations, but they are equally fearful of these conversations. People really want to know more but also need the opportunity to take their time and wade through the process at a pace that works for them. Always "start where the person is," not where you need them to be.

6. Almost 100% of the time that we brought people together to discuss surrogate decision making or to address end-of-life issues initially, a huge issue would surface that people had not talked about or were unsure of how to address (e.g., Lydia being Jewish). Be prepared!

7. We must get better at learning about, supporting, and addressing issues of faith, religion, and culture while people are alive and when they are dying. We must be able to weave this information into the person-centered and advance care planning process.

8. As a new planner, do not start your learning with someone who is in a crisis if you can avoid it. Most planners are challenged by the advance care planning process; trying to learn the process while addressing a crisis can be immensely difficult and will likely be unsuccessful.

9. Unless the person you are planning with is dying, do not start the process with talking about end of life. Remember, "Who are you planning with?" Surrogate decision making may be where you need to begin.

10. As you start planning, you need to know where the plan will run into resistance. Are there people who need to be involved who are not present? Planners must recognize the importance of family history and culture on current decision making. Do people talk about end of life, death, and dying in the person's family and culture? What does the family's history and culture say about how people will or should behave? What does their culture dictate (e.g., some Native American tribes would not be supportive of having end-of-life conversations).

Person-centered planning thankfully is not a fad. Advance care planning is also not a fad. The two processes share many of the same values and underpinnings. Although engaging in conversation about health care decision making and the end of life may be challenging and uncomfortable at first, it is incumbent upon those of us who plan with and for people with IDD to move beyond our own discomfort and recognize that everyone deserves the opportunity to be in control of all parts of his or her life, including the end. It is our responsibility to bring our person-centered planning processes full circle and include health care and end-of-life decision making in the process in a respectful and sensitive way.

REFERENCES

Applebaum, P. (2007). Assessment of patient's competence to consent to treatment. *New England Journal of Medicine, 357,* 1834–1840.

Center for Self-Determination. (2007). Principles of self-determination. Retrieved July 27, 2009, from http://www.self-determination.com/principles/index.html

The Consequences of Legalized Assisted Suicide and Euthanasia. (2006). United States Senate Judiciary Subcommittee on the Constitution, Civil Rights and Property Rights (testimony of Diane Coleman).

Ganzini, L., Volicer, L., Nelson, W., Fox, E., & Derse, A. (2004, July/August). Ten myths about decision-making capacity. *Journal of the American Medical Directors Association, 5,* 263–267.

Grisso, T. (1986). *Evaluating competencies: Forensic assessments & instruments.* New York: Plenum Press.

Hammes, B. J., & Briggs, L. (2002). *Respecting Choices® advance care planning facilitator manual.* La Crosse, WI: Gundersen Lutheran Medical Foundation.

Holburn, S., & Vietze, P. M. (Eds.). (2002). *Person-centered planning: Research, practice, and future directions.* Baltimore: Paul H. Brookes.

Lyden, M. (2006). Capacity issues related to the healthcare proxy. *Mental Retardation, 44*(4), 272–282.

Martyn, S. R. (1994). Substituted judgment, best interests and the need for best respect. *Cambridge Quarterly of Healthcare Ethics, 3,* 195–208.

Mount, B. (1992). *Person-centered planning: A sourcebook of values, ideas and methodologies to encourage person-centered development.* New York: Graphic Futures.

O'Brien, J., & O'Brien C. L. (Eds.). (1997). *A little book about person centered planning.* Toronto: Inclusion Press.

Smull, M. (1993). *Positive rituals and quality of life.* Retrieved March 13, 2008, from http://www.learningcommunity.us/documents/RitualsandQOL.pdf

Smull, M. (1995). *Revisiting choice.* Retrieved March 13, 2008, from http://learningcommunity.us/documents/RevisitingChoiceParts1and2.pdf

Turnbull, H. R., III. (2005). What should we do for Jay? The edges of life and cognitive disability. In W. C. Gaventa & D. L. Coulter (Eds.), *End of life care: Bridging disability and aging with person-centered care* (pp. 1–25). Binghamton, NY: Haworth Press.

CHAPTER 18

Supports and Resources
for Families of Children With
Special Health Care Needs

LAUREN C. BERMAN AND SOYUN KWAN

INTRODUCTION

The world of children with special health care needs (CSHCN) has changed dramatically as life-sustaining medicine has given rise to a population of children who have numerous complex health problems (Graham & Robinson, 2005; Klick & Ballantine, 2007). Medical conditions with concomitant intellectual and developmental disabilities (IDD) can include progressive metabolic disorders, congenital and genetic anomalies, extreme prematurity, mucopolysaccharides/storage disorders, and infectious or other diseases with neurological consequences. Because chronic and life-threatening conditions are often episodic—mixing periods of stability and health with acute periods of crisis, exacerbation, and recovery—anticipating the course of an illness in a child with complex medical needs is extremely difficult (Davies et al., 2008; Graham & Robinson; Mack & Wolfe, 2006).

The rewards and challenges of raising CSHCN are different for every family. Although the diagnosis of a child with complex medical issues and/or developmental disabilities may initially be met with shock or fear, raising a child with special health care needs can be an opportunity for connection and growth, both spiritual and emotional. In this chapter we use a strengths-based approach to support families as they deal with medical complexities, uncertain outcomes, and decisions that involve life and death dilemmas. We also describe resources that families might find helpful in the various stages of their journey with their child. For the purpose of this chapter, we define CSHCN as children who are at risk for and/or require health and health-related services beyond those required by children who do not have such disabilities (McPherson et al., 1998). This definition underscores the fact that it is not the disability or illness that characterizes this population but the need for services within a social and cultural context.

Pediatric Palliative Care

The goals of pediatric palliative care are to improve the quality of life and to decrease suffering for children with life-threatening conditions (Rushton, 2004). A pediatric palliative care team is typically child focused, family oriented, and relationship centered with psychosocial support as a critical part of the work. Services can be integrated into various settings, including the home, a hospital, a hospice setting, and/or a nursing home. Most pediatric palliative care teams receive input from specialists in pediatric illness, pain management, child development, and mental health. The team will often include physicians, nurses, social workers, and psychologists, as well as medical subspecialists related to the care of a child's particular condition. Ideally, the interdisciplinary team coordinates care among different specialties and across all delivery sites (Himelstein, 2005).

The death of a child is devastating to a family, as it violates a core belief in the natural order of life. In the United States alone, approximately 55,000 children under the age of 18 die each year (Field & Behrman, 2003; Meyer & Tunick, 2009). An estimated one third of childhood deaths are caused by injuries, while the remaining two thirds are related to underlying conditions, such as prematurity, congenital abnormalities, metabolic disorders, and malignancies (Arias, MacDorman, Strobino, & Guyer, 2003; Mack & Wolfe, 2006). A retrospective study from 1980 to 1998 by Feudtner, Silverira, and Christakis (2002) found that of the 31,455 deaths in children and adolescents ages 0 to 24 years, 52% died in the hospital, 17.2% died at home, 8.5% died in the emergency department or in transport, 0.4% died in nursing homes, and 21.7% died in other locations. The majority of children younger than 1 year died in the hospital (Himelstein, 2005).

Although many children have conditions that are life threatening, the possibility of death is rarely discussed during times of medical stability (Mack & Wolfe, 2006). Of the 55,000 children who die annually in the United States, less than 3,000 receive palliative care services (Levetown, 2001); however, estimates show that more than 8,600 children could benefit from such services (Field & Berhman, 2003; Rushton, 2004). Medical providers typically recognize the lack of curative interventions and the limited chances for recovery long before families have any awareness of the situation. A study at a leading pediatric hospital revealed that 78% of childhood deaths are experienced by families as unexpected, leaving them little time to grapple with the challenges involved (Mack & Wolfe).

Ethnicity, race, and religion are significant factors in shaping a family's beliefs, values, and approaches to end-of-life planning, as also discussed in chapter 14. While attitudes about death and dying vary greatly by culture, invasive and life-extending measures are generally considered appropriate only when there is hope for improvement of symptoms or sustained quality of life. Families, however, often feel compelled to pursue all medical options for their child because to do otherwise may be considered "giving up" on their son or daughter (Klick & Ballantine, 2007). The hope for medical breakthroughs and miracle recoveries may make families believe that they should prolong life rather than focus efforts on promoting comfort, at least until death is clearly imminent (Levetown, 2001). The tendency to deny the reality of childhood death, coupled with the challenges of medical prognostication, may lead families to believe that their child will still have a normal life expectancy (Graham & Robinson, 2005; Klick & Ballantine).

The desire for a peaceful death, symptom control, comfort, and lack of suffering may get lost in the hope for survival at any cost, particularly in an ICU setting, where trauma and acuity are high and circumstances often call for aggressive and life-prolonging interventions. Because there is a misconception that palliative care and curative treatment are mutually exclusive, with palliative care as an option only after all other interventions have failed, misunderstandings about the concepts of palliative care and the degree to which life-extending therapies can be beneficial may further create barriers to the integration of palliative care services (Himelstein, 2005; Rushton, 2004). Palliative care does not, in fact, preclude curative treatments, as the goal of managing symptoms and quality of life can coexist and complement each other (Mack & Wolfe, 2006; Rushton). A study of deaths in a neonatal intensive care unit found that when palliative care services were initiated proactively, there were fewer aggressive treatments and increased psychosocial supports during the last 48 hours of life (Pierucci, Kirby, & Leuthner, 2001).

Without the integration of palliative services, parents and professionals may unwittingly subject children to therapies that are not beneficial and may in fact increase and prolong their child's pain and suffering (Mack & Wolfe, 2006; Meyer & Tunick, 2009). Results of a retrospective study of parents whose children died in the intensive care unit revealed that more than half of the parents reported that they had little control during their child's final days (Meyer, Burns, Griffith, & Troug, 2002). One fourth of the parents reported that if they had another chance, they would have made different decisions. Furthermore, it was the physician (90% of the time) who initiated discussions about withdrawal of life support, although nearly half of the parents had considered it before the conversation was ever formally raised. By remaining silent about end-of-life issues, providers may inadvertently give families the message that these conversations are unspeakable, contributing to stigma and leaving families fearful of discussing or raising these issues themselves.

If providers initiate and engage with families in discussions about preferences for end-of-life care prior to the onset of a crisis, families may become empowered to set goals for care and to determine the location of care in accordance with choices they feel are right for their child and family (Mack & Wolfe, 2006; Smith, 2001). Despite many families' preferences for their child to die at home, lack of advanced planning results in a majority of children with chronic illness dying in the hospital (Berger & Levetown, 2009). Parents struggle for hope in these situations, and the way professionals present and share information requires an understanding of the family's emotional process and level of readiness. When talking with families, attention to details—such as offering a private setting and using culturally sensitive language—can make all the difference in their receptiveness to painful conversations. It can also be helpful to remind families that they are not choosing their child's death (in that they do not have a choice) but are making informed choices about how their child will live until death (Rushton, 2004). Conversely, by avoiding these conversations, professionals may exclude parents from an opportunity to demonstrate their love and deep commitment to their child until the very end.

STIGMA AND DISABILITIES

Although attitudes about caring for children with IDD have changed over time, there has been a tendency in the health care field to judge such children and their families based on preconceptions or incomplete information (Burns et al., 2000; Kirschner, Brashler, & Savage, 2007). Stienstra and Chochinov (2006) contend that because medical providers make inaccurate assumptions about decision making and other capacity in a person with disabilities, there is a special vulnerability in disability populations when facing end-of-life issues. Because professionals often see families when they are most stressed or in crisis, they may not be aware of or may not witness the mutual and reciprocal nature of family connections and relationships (Berman, Freeman, & Helm, 2006; Klick & Ballantine, 2007). Even in the most innovative settings, it is not unusual to hear care providers ascribe such characteristics as "unloving" or "uninvolved" to families that place their child in a long-term care facility, while simultaneously considering those who care for their child at home to be enmeshed, overinvolved, or out of touch with reality (Kirschner et al.).

As such, families with CSHCN who interact with health care professionals may feel stigmatized and misunderstood. Such attitudes may cause parents to fear that their child's life is not valued in the same way as a child without special health care needs (SHCN). Thus, they may come to question the intentions of their child's medical providers and feel threatened by those who initiate end-of-life discussions, even in the most dire of situations. Disparities in access to health care, quality of care, and delivery of services for those with disabilities can intensify feelings of distrust (Linton & Feudtner, 2008; Stienstra & Chochinov, 2006). Consequently, parents need ready access to information and some sense of having control, particularly in settings where providers are unfamiliar with their child.

ATTACHMENT

Family members form attachments in the seeking and giving of comfort in response to threat or distress (Hill, Fonagy, Safier, & Sargent, 2003). In families where children have SHCN, attachments can be intense and deeply interdependent. Like families with very young children, parents of CSHCN become immersed in the nuances of their child's gestures, movements, expressions, and sounds in order to understand and interpret their child's needs and underlying meanings. For families whose children do not have impairments, the intensity of this experience gradually lessens as their child grows older, developing skills that allow him or her to become independent. For families with CSHCN, however, the unpredictably and complexity of their child's developmental and cognitive abilities can further magnify the intensity of the attachment.

Because families experience increased distress if developmental milestones are not fully reached within culturally expected time frames, parents may reexperience the grieving process at each new developmental stage (Berman et al., 2006). With few normative guidelines in assessing and meeting their child's varied and unpredictable developmental needs, families may feel "out of sync" with others who would normally be their peers (Mack & Berman, 1988; Neugarten, 1979). The multiple challenges these parents can face in connecting with others may result in their withdrawal from their community while simultaneously intensifying their relationships with their children. Consequently, family lives can become drastically reconfigured and relationships become increasingly interwoven.

The level of commitment for parents of CSHCN is extraordinary. Most families struggle to manage their child at home, regardless of the physical, emotional, and financial stresses involved. Parents' responsibilities may range from the day-to-day challenges of managing tube feeding, tracheal suctioning and tube care, changing colostomy bags, ostomy care, and dialysis and ventilator troubleshooting, to the external tasks of analyzing and modifying the setup of one's home. Families must prepare for any type of emergency that could compromise their child's health, including loss of electricity and heat, or disconnection of phone service. They must also learn the medical skills necessary to respond to health emergencies when professionals are not available. These considerations become a routine part of a family's daily life (Lash & Kahn, 1998).

While some families strive to function independently, most require some degree of outside help. Families must balance the life of their child, their other children, and the entire family constellation within a complex system of care and services. They need to continually reevaluate their child's needs and care strategies based on the severity of their child's health issues, his or her development, family dynamics, financial limitations, and the availability of resources and supports—all of which change over the course of a child's life (Lash & Kahn, 1998). Parents must become knowledgeable and effective advocates within a complex maze of providers and services. Because family life is so deeply interdependent, the very thought of life without their child can be unimaginable, as the death of their child compounds the loss of the family's natural way of life and existence (Graham & Robinson, 2005).

APPROACHES TO WORKING WITH FAMILIES WITH CSHCN

We have outlined several approaches that are helpful when working with families of children with SHCN (see Table 18.1).

Table 18.1
Approaches to Working With Families With CSHCN

- *Build relationships.* Initiate conversations with the family. Assess their unique needs for communication and support. Create a working relationship and establish trust and rapport.

- *Understand families.* Listen to family members. Take the time to hear their stories and to understand their experience.

- *Collaborate with families.* Join with the family and maintain relationships. Provide support and empathy. Acknowledge the efforts of the family and the challenges they face.

- *Coordinate care.* Identify continuity care physicians and consistent interdisciplinary care team members. Arrange frequent family meetings. Set goals for care.

- *Communicate with families.* Be honest. Share information, options, and prognoses.

- *Include the child.* Acknowledge the child and communicate directly with him or her whenever possible. Assess pain and treat accordingly. Also encourage parents' open communication with the child.

- *Involve siblings.* Recognize the needs of siblings. Invite opportunities for them to visit, to have their questions addressed, and help guide their parents in how to best communicate with them.

Build Relationships With Families

Families are the center of a child's social, emotional, and spiritual life. Understanding the relational environment within a family is a vital part of communicating and connecting with families. Work with families should always begin with a comprehensive, psychosocial assessment. The family unit is complex; not only is it a subsystem of the community and greater society, but it contains its own inherent dynamic systems, such as siblings, grandparents, spousal relationships, and parent-child connections. Providers need to increase their awareness of the mental health status and emotional state of family members through identification of risk factors such as depression, substance abuse, child maltreatment, and trauma. A full assessment will also explore past, present, and future resources and available supports. Social workers or other mental health professionals skilled in assessment and formulation can serve to evaluate the family's strengths, vulnerabilities, cultural and environmental context, social and systems level concerns, as well as to assess their needs and preferences for communication and building relationships.

It is important that providers expand their definition of family to extend beyond that of the traditional nuclear family. For families from other cultures, factors such as level of acculturation, the immigration/migration experience, the impact of culture of origin, and information about the family and community that has been left behind should be included in the assessment. Issues of language, cultural identity, perspectives on cultural causes of illness, accepted help-seeking behaviors, cultural rituals, and how the family shows distress are also important considerations (Kleinman, 1988). When working with gay, lesbian, bisexual, or transgender (GLBT) families, providers should use gender-neutral language and not make assumptions about who is included in the family. Because of issues of stigma, prejudice, and custody laws, GLBT families may be afraid to reveal the true nature of their relationships (Ariel & McPherson, 2000; Martin, 1998).

Understand Family Perspectives

In order to honor a family's wishes, the medical team needs to be aware of the family's worldviews and values as well as how their own personal and professional beliefs color their perspective. If they are not aware, they are apt to be critical of difference rather than explore creative and complimentary ways to incorporate the family's views into their child's medical care. Like an anthropologist who lives with and understands people while participating in their culture, providers must strive to engage in side-by-side relationships with families, to advocate for participation of the child and family in decision-making processes, and to ensure that care is consistent with the family's beliefs and values.

The way that parents perceive their child's illness is central to understanding the family perspective. The stories people tell reveal the events and evaluation of their experience, and these stories are revised as people transition from one moment to another (Berger & Luckman, 1996). Both the content and subtext of the story are helpful in understanding the central theme of the narrative, which acts as a filter guiding the family's interpretation of events (Young & Rodriguez, 2006). Working from a perspective that uses language and cognitive restructuring to highlight families' strengths, one can address issues of stigma and social oppression as well as learn about natural support systems. Understanding the family's values and experiences enables providers to empower families and diminishes isolation. Themes of quality of life, physical and emotional cost of treatment, and spirituality are important when working with families as they deal with end-of-life issues (Robinson, Thiel, Backus, & Meyer, 2006). Romanoff and Thompson (2006) found that deciphering people's stories provides insight to values and perceptions when working with spiritual and existential issues.

Collaborate With Families

Professionals must take responsibility to set the tone for collaboration by building respectful, reciprocal relationships with families early in the course of a child's care. Shared decision making among the family, the child, and the medical team is the goal. Even when disagreements arise between the family and the medical team, providers can validate the family's experience by acknowledging their effort, sense of caring, and good intentions. Doing so fosters trust, while minimizing the potential for the family to feel threatened or judged. Simple tasks—such as taking opportunities to listen to a family's needs and expressing compassion for their situation—can build trust over time (Clarke & Quin, 2007; Contro, Larson, Scofield, Sourkes, & Cohen, 2004; Meyer, Ritholz, Burns, & Truog, 2006).

While medical providers attend to multifaceted medical issues, social workers can advocate and support the family by checking in with parents about their concerns and exploring their interpretations of medical information. Social workers support families during periods of crisis, hospitalization, and new diagnoses. As such, they are in an ideal position to maintain therapeutic relationships over time and can act as a bridge to the medical team to ensure that the family's current and historical viewpoint is understood. It is important for physicians to consult with nurses and social workers to get the most recent information relative to the child's care needs as well as the family's resources, capabilities, and the mental status and emotional state of various family members, before necessarily offering medical options.

Coordinate Medical Care

Because children with SHCN see multiple care providers, chances for miscommunication between specialties are inevitable. Assignment of a continuity health care provider who can offer family meetings and maintain ongoing communication between providers can help ensure that families and subspecialists are updated and have the most recent and accurate information. Helpful structures include daily interdisciplinary team rounds, regularly scheduled patient care conferences, joint team and family meetings, and ethics consultations as appropriate (Rushton, 2009). Care providers should also work with families to reevaluate the child's health status, the team's plans, and the family's goals on a regular basis. These opportunities can help families feel increasingly secure, well cared for by their team, and less overwhelmed when making decisions during times of crisis.

Because local pediatricians are often limited in their ability to manage the complex nature of children with SHCN, they commonly refer children to emergency hospital services for assessment and admission to the hospital. However, if parents have direct contact with a physician who specializes in the care of children with complex medical needs, they can consult with that provider in advance to assess the need to even come into the hospital, thereby eliminating the stress and waiting time in the emergency room. Offering long-term (continuity) providers allows families to address acute concerns as they arise and potentially maximizes the opportunities for these children to remain at home, thereby avoiding unnecessary hospital visits.

Communicate and Share Information

Families vary in their preferences for receiving information, but most will benefit from clear communication about their child's prognosis and discussions around goals of care. According to Levetown (2001), the treatment of symptoms, prevention of unnecessary pain, psychosocial support around the effect of illness on the family, assistance with concrete needs, and financial assistance are critical for families. A study by McDonagh, Elliot, and Engelberg (2004) on end-of-life care in the intensive care unit found that allowing families more time to speak during family conferences was significantly associated with increased family satisfaction and improved communication.

Most parents want honest and complete information even if they feel overwhelmed with the severity of their child's condition. Providers need to be empathetic yet truthful when they communicate with families. Sometimes, in an attempt to protect parents, professionals convey prognoses in an unclear or idealistic way. This can result in confusion for families and may interfere with setting established goals of care, as families may misconstrue the information and intentions of the medical team. By offering treatments unlikely to bring a long-term positive outcome, parents may feel obligated to pursue a path they might not otherwise consider.

Include Children in Decisions

The management of pain in children is central to families and is the principal goal of pediatric palliative care. While self-reporting is the usual standard for pain management, children with SHCN cannot always verbally communicate their experience of pain. Instead they may display or express pain via changes in their heart rate or blood pressure, grimacing, crying or moaning, tensing of their muscles or body, or through presentations of irritability, inconsolability, inactivity/lack of energy, or disturbed sleep patterns (Hunt, Mastroyannopoulou, Goldman, & Seers, 2002). Because pain can be difficult to adequately assess, caregivers need to be aware of and learn from families the many ways that each child signals discomfort.

Whenever possible, age-appropriate communication with children about death and dying is helpful. Studies of pediatric patients with cancer have revealed that children often realize the severity of their illness and prefer open exchanges of information about their condition and prognosis. Such communication can provide anticipatory guidance to help minimize children's fears about what is to come, while fostering trust in their family and their care team (Beale, Baile, & Aaron, 2005; Hilden, Watterson, & Chrastek, 2003; Stillion & Papadatou, 2002). Even when children are unable to communicate verbally, their experiences, hopes, and fears may be expressed through body language or play (Himelstein, 2005). Results of a retrospective study of parents who lost a child to cancer in Sweden revealed that of the 147 parents who talked with their child about death, none of them were regretful about their discussion. Meanwhile, 27% of the 258 parents who did not talk to their child about death were sorry they missed the opportunity. Additionally, parents who sensed that their child was aware of his or her impending death were more likely to regret not having had such a conversation. The parents who did not discuss death with their child also showed higher levels of anxiety long after their child's death (Himelstein; Kreicbergs, Valdimarsdottir, Onelov, Henter, & Steineck, 2004).

Involve Siblings

Both professionals and families may underestimate the importance of involving siblings in the hospital and illness experience. Acute and chronic illness and hospitalization affects all members of a family, including the often forgotten siblings. It was once thought that young children were unaware or unaffected by their brother's or sister's illness or death due to their age or developmental stage and that parents were protecting their other children by minimizing their exposure to the hospital, the dying experience, and their sick brother or sister. However, siblings recognize changes within their family, their environment, and their routine.

Children of all ages grieve, and siblings may have unique emotional needs that require specific attention. Because so much attention is focused on the child who is ill, siblings may feel anxious, confused, abandoned, jealous, or angry at times (Gursky, 2007; Meyer & Tunick, 2009). They may have less access to their parents, have extra responsibilities, feel the need to act as a bridge between their brother or sister and the outside world, attempt to protect their parents by remaining silent about their questions, thoughts, and fears (Berman et al., 2006). Open exchange and discussion about the effects of the illness and encouragement of siblings' emotional expression are important (Craft, 1993; Kleiber, Montgomery, & Craft-Rosenberg, 1995). Silence and lack of communication from parents can increase fear and foster uncertainties for siblings, who may assign inaccurate interpretations to the circumstances of their brother or sister's illness. This is especially true for young children who are prone to magical thinking and may believe that they are somehow responsible for the family's pain and suffering (Gursky; Meyer & Tunick).

Siblings need to feel both welcomed and cared for by their brother's or sister's medical team (Meyer & Tunick, 2009). Siblings bear witness to their brother's or sister's illness at home but are often left with extended family or friends during hospitalizations. Parental stress and denial may result in failure to accurately assess siblings' coping, and parents can feel intimidated and overwhelmed as to how to best share and communicate information (Craft, 1993; Gursky, 2007). Providers can help families by creating opportunities to meet with brothers and sisters, offering age-appropriate information, and assisting parents in reassuring all their children by planning for the future (Meyer & Vadasy, 1994). A team of social work, psychology, and child life providers can assist in identifying the unique coping styles of brothers and sisters; provide support, including individual, family, or group counseling; and help to guide families during times of great stress.

END-OF-LIFE DECISIONS

The aforementioned approaches can help improve the death experience for families and create lasting impressions for them during a time that most parents identify as the most difficult they have experienced in their lives. Team members can also help to decrease anxiety, depression, and traumatic responses in families by demonstrating the commitment to ensuring dignity for the child and family throughout the dying process (Meyer et al., 2006; Meyer & Tunick, 2009). When making end-of-life decisions on behalf of their children, quality of life, expected recovery and improvement, and the perception of the child's pain and suffering are most important to parents (Meyer et al., 2002). Honest and clear communication, ready access to staff, coordination of care, empathy and support from staff, preservation of the integrity of the parent-child relationship, and respect for spiritual meaning and connections are critical (Meyer et al., 2006; Robinson, Thiel, Backus, & Meyer, 2006).

Making end-of-life decisions may be extraordinarily difficult for families, but medical providers can help the process by encouraging more communication. Parents who are unable to specify exact care decisions, such as Do Not Intubate or Do Not Resuscitate (DNI/DNR) or no chest compressions, may still be able to identify overarching goals for their child ("We just want him to be comfortable"). Conversations about what a family does not want for their child ("Nothing invasive or prolonged") as well as what they want ("We want everything done") are also helpful. Eliciting general goals allows for clarification over time while eliminating the pressure for parents to make immediate decisions. Ongoing conversations and transparency are important. A study by Friedman (2006) of a pediatric skilled-nursing facility population showed that by simply providing written information about current resuscitation options, 43% of families changed their directives from full resuscitation to DNR.

DEATH AND BEREAVEMENT

Anticipatory guidance and support are essential during the end-of-life process (see Table 18.2). Families need assistance in knowing how and when things will happen and what to expect (Meyer & Tunick, 2009).

Providers should ensure the involvement of team members—including social workers, psychologists, child life specialists, and chaplains—not only for the immediate family, but also for extended family members and friends who may wish to say good-bye. Comprehensive and collaborative psychosocial support services are important for all individuals affected by the child's death, for providing attendance to the specific needs of multiple

---

Table 18.2
Guidance and Support for Families at the End of Life

- Allow private time for the child and family members, with minimal interruptions. Encourage families to engage in favorite pastimes or to bring in comforts from home for their child.
- Provide opportunities for parents' participation in their child's care.
- Assist the family in creating lasting memories. Offer mementos for families to take home with them.
- Provide bereavement materials, books, and referrals for all family members.
- Follow up with families after their child's death. Attend memorial services, send cards, and make phone calls. Recognize their child's birthday and the anniversary of their child's death.
- Maintain connections. Encourage families to stay connected with the team. Invite families back to the hospital for memorial services and/or other events.

family members, for assistance with funeral service planning, for assessment of the family's safety upon leaving the hospital, for coordination of strategies to help ease the family's transition home, and for evaluation of any necessary mental health/bereavement referrals for the family. Families may also benefit from bereavement materials and books, which can help to normalize their reactions and also help to guide them in ways to support their other children through the loss of their brother or sister.

At the end of life, parents need to spend time with their child, both alone and as a family (Meyer & Tunick, 2009). This may include simply lying in bed with their child or helping to bathe him or her. In the case described at the end of this chapter, the mother sat with her child for hours, just watching their favorite movies together and not wanting to be interrupted. Parents should also be provided with the opportunity to make memories with their child (Meyer & Tunick). This may include making handprint and footprint impressions, cutting locks of hair, or taking photographs with their child (Duncan, Joselow, & Hilden, 2006). Such opportunities can be invaluable for a family, yet they can easily be missed if the team does not let the family know that they are available or does not underscore their importance.

Bereavement support does not end after a child dies. Children with SHCN are often followed in the same setting their entire lives; many parents feel closely connected with their care teams and can suffer a compounded loss when they simultaneously lose contact with their child's care providers. After a child's death, parents continue to benefit from ongoing support. Simple tasks such as team members making follow-up calls, attending the child's wake or funeral service, and sending condolence cards are meaningful to families (Meyer et al., 2006; Meyer & Tunick, 2009). Inviting families to hospital-sponsored memorial services, allowing them the opportunity to return to visit the pediatric intensive care unit (PICU), or having them meet with the team to address any lingering questions can also be important, as some families may wish to remain connected to hospital staff that knew and cared for their child. In a support group for families whose children had terminal illnesses, parents were allowed to continue to meet with the group after their child's death. One of the fathers who chose to continue beyond his son's death said, "Even [my son's] death is better than being alone" (Mack & Berman, 1988).

INTERDISCIPLINARY COLLABORATION

The following vignette illustrates the impact of interdisciplinary collaboration, both within the team and with a family. Although the care described is in a setting with multiple resources, the concepts can be applied to settings when fewer resources are available.

Jane's Story

Jane, age 13 years and an only child, was never predicted to live past infancy. Born with a chromosomal anomaly, Jane was diagnosed with cognitive and developmental delays. She was nonverbal and ambulated with a wheelchair. Whenever death was imminent, she surpassed the expectations of her doctors. She was admitted to the PICU following a car accident in which her mother was driving. While her mother acquired only minor injuries from the accident, Jane suffered a serious spinal cord injury and permanent quadriplegia. She ultimately required a colostomy and tracheostomy and became dependent on a ventilator. She was not expected to regain the ability to use her wheelchair or breathe independently. Social workers, psychologists, and chaplains were immediately consulted for family assessment and support around this acute trauma.

Jane was described by her parents as always being "medically fragile" and had required numerous surgeries throughout her life. She had been in continuous good health for 2 years prior to the accident, and her mother had been diligent in learning all of the required home care practices in order to avoid the need for home nursing. Both parents were devoted to her. After the accident, Jane's mother was clear about her desire to take Jane home rather than sending her to an inpatient rehabilitation facility. The team worked diligently with her parents to help them understand the new demands of her care as well as to provide culturally sensitive support services.

Despite being eligible for a significant amount of home nursing hours, Jane's mother used minimal outside assistance and maintained Jane's care at home with the help of Jane's father, neighbors, and several extended family members. She emphasized, "My house is a home, not a nursing home. I'm not doing this to prove a point; I'm doing it so that I can keep my daughter at home." Despite her commitment, the stress of Jane's illness and continuous medical management was overwhelming, particularly since Jane's father needed to return to work outside the home. During night shifts, Jane's parents would alternate turns sleeping on the floor of the living room, which had become Jane's bedroom. The degree of sleep deprivation her mother experienced led to her own extensive worry about her ability to awaken to machine alarms.

Jane had six PICU admissions following her accident for concerns of recurrent fevers, infections, and abdominal distensions, which required further surgeries; some hospital stays lasted several weeks while others lasted a few months. Approximately a year after Jane's injury, the PICU team raised concerns around Jane's growing discomfort and continued medical decline. Her parents agreed that Jane had not been anywhere close to her baseline, and that at best, she averaged one "good" day out of the entire week. They both expressed that their daughter's "spirit" seemed absent and felt that she was suffering despite their best efforts. Jane's parents ultimately decided to withdraw care, and with the assistance of the PICU team, removed her ventilator support.

Jane's story illustrates the journey, commitment, and struggles of one family with a child with SHCN. Driven partly by guilt, Jane's mother exhausted herself in caring for Jane at home. Despite all of her parents' efforts, Jane's condition continued to deteriorate, as her underlying medical issues further complicated her acute trauma. Her mother could not initially bring herself to recognize Jane's decline and the irreversibility of her condition. She had two miscarriages prior to getting pregnant with Jane and she had dealt with each loss by planning for and investing in the next pregnancy. The couple did not plan to have any more children. Being a parent was central to this mother's core identity, and she prided herself in how well she cared for her daughter. Up until the accident, Jane's course of illness had been unpredictable, with unanticipated medical improvements that resulted in many years of good health. These factors, coupled with mother's hope for Jane's recovery, led to a physical and emotional roller coaster that involved months of surgeries and repeated PICU hospitalizations.

Jane's story highlights the significance of interdisciplinary teamwork and collaboration in assisting families with complex end-of-life decision making. During her first admission (the longest of all Jane's hospitalizations), the PICU team was able to establish a strong bond with Jane's parents. An interdisciplinary team of PICU physicians and nursing staff, respiratory therapists, social workers, psychologists, child life specialists, chaplains, and case management staff met collaboratively to discuss care options based on Jane's medical needs, the available resources, and the capabilities of her parents. The team also met with the family to establish goals of care. Jane's parents wanted her to be as comfortable as possible for as long as possible at home. The PICU team supported the family's choices and found ways to help the family manage Jane's care at home.

A pediatric palliative care team was also consulted and maintained involvement with the family in collaboration with the PICU team. Together, the interdisciplinary team met with the parents during each of Jane's subsequent admissions; the conversations were focused on reevaluating their goals, reassessing the need for more home-based services, and, conversely, discussing if Jane's care had exceeded her parents' capabilities. Through these purposeful efforts, the strength of the team's relationship with Jane's parents continued to grow, and they became increasingly trustful of the team's guidance. The family was assigned a PICU attending physician who made home visits following her discharges from the hospital. In addition, a complex care physician was enlisted to triage urgent needs and to assist with determining the medical necessity of Jane returning to the hospital.

Despite these efforts, concerns emerged regarding Jane's level of pain and discomfort, which was becoming unmanageable. When team members initiated a conversation with Jane's parents about end-of-life care, both parents acknowledged the growing severity of Jane's condition while simultaneously expressing the unimaginable difficulty in saying good-bye to their only child. It was only with careful guidance and support of the interdisciplinary health care team—a group of medical and psychosocial professionals whom the parents knew and trusted—that they could see that Jane was suffering and ultimately decided to refocus their goal from prolonging her life to making her as comfortable as possible.

When the goals of prolonging life and providing comfort are in conflict, there may be instances where the family's preferences and the medical team's recommendations diverge. Referral to a hospital ethics committee may be helpful to care providers who are experiencing ethical distress around conflicting care goals of the family and the team. An ethics consultation can be initiated by any member of a child's care team and may provide guidance as to how to mediate these complicated situations.

It may also be helpful for medical providers to encourage parents to spend time at the bedside with their child, especially during resuscitation efforts (Twibell et al., 2008). The process of witnessing invasive and prolonged resuscitation procedures may reassure families that the medical team is committed to all the efforts on behalf of their child. In a situation of a teenage boy with SHCN, his father was adamant that the medical team "do everything" for his son despite multiorgan failure and limited possible interventions. An overnight stay by the father helped him to understand the impact of his decision. After witnessing several hours of nurses providing repeated rounds of epinephrine to try to stabilize his son's blood pressure, with the growing likelihood of needing cardiopulmonary resuscitation (CPR), he finally asked the care team to stop, stating, "I think I'm ready to let him go. I don't want him to suffer anymore."

Table 18.3 provides suggestions for partnering with families during the course of a child's illness.

Table 18.3

Recommendations for Partnering With Families Around End-of-Life Decisions

- Collaborate and communicate as an interdisciplinary team. Include psychosocial providers and pediatric palliative care teams and request ethics consultations when necessary.

- Set goals of care with families and meet often to review/revisit changing goals.

- Provide frequent and ongoing support for the entire family. Provide opportunities for home visits, follow-up calls, and home care services.

- Be truthful. Make culturally sensitive recommendations and provide guidance and support for what to expect at the end of life.

- Encourage families to spend time at their child's bedside.

RESOURCES FOR FAMILIES

The increasing lifespan of children with SHCN has led to the growing complexity for parents in managing their children independently. For families of children with SHCN, community resources may be insufficient, and limits on insurance coverage and public benefits can strain already tight budgets (Lash & Kahn, 1998). A study by Freedman and Boyer (2000) found that families of children with disabilities want services that are proactive and preventive, not simply crisis oriented. Because the experience of many families with CSHCN can be one of isolation, high levels of interagency collaboration and coordination and increased access to case management and counseling services are important. Referrals to social workers and case managers are appropriate for assistance in accessing specific resources based on a family's unique needs.

FINANCIAL ISSUES

Compared to families of children without disabilities, families of children with SHCN face significant financial burdens. Parents must often reduce their work hours or even discontinue working altogether in order to stay home and provide care for their child. Out-of-pocket expenses for therapies, respite services, specialized day care, medical equipment, transportation, and home adaptation can drain family budgets. Parish, Rose, Grinstein-Weiss, Richman, and Andrews (2008) found that families of children with disabilities experienced significantly greater financial hardship (measured in terms of food insecurity, housing instability, health care access, and telephone disconnection) than families whose children did not have disabilities. In the sample study, results revealed that as family income rose above the federal poverty level, hardship declined sharply for families of children without disabilities, but not in families raising children with SHCN. Any disruption in financial security can put families at risk for homelessness, decreased access to medical care, and life-threatening circumstances. Among these families, single-parent and unmarried-partner families are at disproportionate risk for experiencing severe hardship relative to their married counterparts (Himelstein, 2005; Parish et al., 2008). Even when local communities provide necessary services, there can be a rebound effect on families of children with SHCN, resulting in perceptions of resentment from others in the community for using so many of the neighborhood and school's scarce resources.

GOVERNMENT INSURANCE PROGRAMS

Supplemental Security Income (SSI)

SSI is a federal program that provides supplemental income to families of children who meet criteria for a physical or mental condition or a combination that results in "marked and severe functional limitations." To qualify, the condition must either last or be expected to last at least 12 months, or result in death or severe disability (U.S. Social Security Administration, 2009). Most states provide Medicaid coverage in conjunction with SSI. The income and resources of the child's family are considered in the determination of eligibility. Sometimes children are initially refused SSI benefits based on incomplete information, and in most instances the family should file an appeal. Medical providers should be aware that a physician's letter that includes the child's medical history, the results of diagnostic tests, the medications and treatments that were tried and failed, as well as the prognosis and reasons for certain treatments is critical to winning an appeal (Jaff, 2005).

Medicaid

Medicaid is a federal health care program for people with low incomes and limited resources (U.S. Social Security Administration, 2009). Some children can qualify for Medicaid even if they do not qualify for SSI. In situations when families already have private coverage but also qualify for Medicaid, it can be used as a secondary insurance, providing coverage for costs the family might otherwise incur if their primary insurance benefits reach or exceed their maximum allowance. When income levels of families exceed the eligibility levels of Medicaid, families can also explore the possibility of purchasing state insurance for a premium. In many cases, the coverage the state insurance provides can make the extra cost worthwhile for families.

Special Insurance Programs

In many states there are specific programs that provide insurance for disabled children when parental income would otherwise render these families ineligible. For example, the Kaleigh Mulligan program in Massachusetts is a Medicaid program that covers home-based medical services for children with severe disabilities so that they can receive care in their home instead of in a hospital or other institutional setting. This program helps families who would be otherwise ineligible for other government-sponsored programs. It typically serves children who have tracheostomies, are ventilator dependent, and/or need other specialized care that must otherwise be provided in a pediatric nursing home or other specialized setting (Boston Public Health Commission, 2008).

CASE MANAGEMENT AND COORDINATION OF HOME HEALTH CARE

Case managers can help to identify medical community resources, to explain the full range of available public benefits related to a child's diagnosis, and to plan for health care supports and challenges. Most states have hospital case managers or care coordinators who work with insurance companies to assist families in accessing appropriate posthospital care and services for their child. These services include, but are not limited to, facilitation of home health care, skilled nursing services, personal care assistance, and the acquisition of durable medical equipment. The services offered and the allocation of hours depends on the child's degree of medical need, the family's health insurance coverage, and the ability to access appropriate care providers within the community. Case managers also work with rehabilitation hospitals and long-term care facilities to make referrals and arrange for transfers following discharge from inpatient hospitalizations. They can provide consultation to parents, educators, and medical and social service providers by providing assessment, coordination, education, and referral for discharge planning purposes. Care coordinators can further help a family navigate medical, social, and educational systems; access referral information about specific programs; and become more effective in advocacy for their child.

HOSPITAL RESOURCES

When a child is hospitalized, families are often unaware of the many resources that may be available to them. Social workers can assess the child and family's needs and facilitate connections to resources within the hospital and in the community. Many hospitals have family resource centers that have Internet access and medical libraries, as well as resource staff who can help provide a range of information and referrals to families for support groups and can also facilitate parent-to-parent networking. Additional hospital support and resource personnel include bilingual/bicultural interpreters who can facilitate communication by helping families understand medical issues and helping medical staff become more aware of important cultural/social factors. Pastoral counseling and spiritual support are also often available on site. In addition, child life specialists work with patients and their siblings, often using play therapy to help children better understand and adapt to the demands of their condition. Speech-language pathologists are also available to help bridge communication gaps with children who are intubated or have limited communication means by facilitating use of augmentative communication devices and techniques.

EDUCATIONAL RESOURCES

For children who are medically fragile and attend school, parents need to inform the district and school personnel of DNR orders. It is important that school health care providers, teachers, emergency response teams, primary health care providers, local hospital staff, and families work together to develop a collaborative plan. The identified team should be up to date on its state's guidelines, laws, court decisions, and rulings of the state's medical and nursing board on DNR orders in schools (Porter, Haynie, Bierle, Heintz-Caldwell, & Palfrey, 1997).

Early Intervention

Most states have early intervention programs that provide integrated developmental services for families of medically fragile children between birth and 3 years of age. Some states provide early intervention services until the age of 5. All children referred to early intervention services receive a comprehensive developmental evaluation to determine eligibility and the child's strengths and needs.

The Individuals With Disabilities Education Act and the Individualized Education Plan

The Individuals With Disabilities Education Act (IDEA) is a statute that protects educational rights for children in schools at the state and local level. IDEA entitles any child with a disability who requires special education services to a "free appropriate public education" (Jaff, 2005). After verifying that the child meets established criteria, each child receives an individualized education plan (IEP) that includes an assessment of the child's present level of educational performance, a statement of goals, and an evaluation of services and aids that are necessary for the child. Funding is provided at the state level (but allocated by the federal government) to cover at least a portion of the related costs. According to law, the IEP must be in effect for all eligible children by the beginning of every school year, with reevaluations conducted no less than every 3 years. Parental permission is required for evaluations to take place (Jaff).

Section 504

The second statute aimed at protecting educational rights of children with disabilities is Section 504 of the Rehabilitation Act of 1973, which promotes "inclusion and integration into the mainstream" via accommodations (Jaff). Any and all assistance must be provided at no cost to the family. Section 504 covers medically fragile children and children with IDD. It is applicable at the federal level and at all educational levels (elementary through graduate school) with the premise that "disabled children cannot be denied any of the benefits of any program that receives federal financial assistance" (Jaff). The definition of disability is broader for Section 504 than it is for IDEA; in some instances, a child may qualify for Section 504, but not for IDEA. Section 504 further provides that students with disabilities will be educated with other students whenever possible (Jaff).

Hospice Resources

Hospice provides spiritual and psychological support, as well as symptom management for children at the end of life (Himelstein, 2005). Hospice care can be provided either in the home or in a hospice setting. Compared to emergency personnel, hospice providers have extensive experience in palliative care and bereavement. It should be noted that eligibility for hospice usually requires that all curative treatments be stopped. Additionally, because a survival prognosis of 6 months or less is required for hospice admission, many children with SHCN do not get access to hospice services (Schmidt, 2003).

Bereavement Resources

The grief process may be overwhelming, particularly for families with CSHCN that have sacrificed so much to care for their children and who have established a way of life that can never be recreated. For many, the desire to protect their children from death conflicts with the realization that their child is dying. Palliative care should be integrated into the ongoing medical management of the child, regardless of the curative intent of therapy. Available bereavement resources include parent-to-parent networks that connect families to others who have lost a child with a similar diagnosis or under similar circumstances, as well as hospital and community support groups for parents and siblings. Community, state, and national resources will vary. Online searches and social work referrals will help to identify possible bereavement resources for families.

SUMMARY

In an ideal world, all children would be accepted and cherished for who they are; families would have access to resources for their child's optimal health, development, and physical comfort; and the concept of palliative care would be integrated early into the treatment of any child who is at risk for an untimely death. Families of children with SHCN are especially vulnerable when dealing with end-of-life issues. Families require anticipatory guidance and support throughout the lifespan of their child, starting from the point of diagnosis and continuing with bereavement and follow-up after the child's death. The psychological distress families can face may be overwhelming, and comprehensive psychosocial support is critical throughout the course of the child's illness. Families need support not only around decision making but also in handling the day-to-day experience of caring for their child, in dealing with isolation and emotional concerns, and especially in dealing with the process of death.

Interdisciplinary teams are essential to palliative care work, and medical professionals should be trained to work in an interdisciplinary manner. Just as psychosocial providers need to understand medical conditions and sequelae for patients and families, medical providers need to be cognizant of psychological and social factors that may inhibit or promote adaptive-coping skills within the family. Programs that bring medical providers as visitors into homes of families whose children have SHCN can provide opportunities for providers to bear witness to the unique gifts and relationships these children bring to their families. In one such program a participating physician reported, "I believe my eyes have been opened. I now understand the level of sacrifice, the value of the individual and the important influence on brothers and sisters." Another physician reported, "The boys made the biggest impression on me. It was great to see them smiling and comfortable in their familiar home, rather than their discomfort in my office." By monitoring and evaluating their own attitudes toward disability, medical professionals can tune into families and offer them a more meaningful experience.

Finally, health care frameworks need to evolve in order to improve support for families of children with SHCN. Not only does this require true interdisciplinary collaboration, but it also requires innovation in the types of services offered to families. The availability of pediatric palliative care teams and the increasing development of home care teams to manage and monitor children at home are also beneficial for families and may help to increase collaboration with community hospice services.

REFERENCES

Arias, E., MacDorman, M. F., Strobino, D. M., & Guyer, B. (2003). Annual summary of vital statistics—2002. *Pediatrics, 112*, 1215–1230.

Ariel, J., & McPherson, D. W. (2000). Therapy with lesbian and gay parents and their children. *Journal of Marital and Family Therapy, 26*(4), 421–432.

Beale, E., Baile, W. F., & Aaron, J. (2005). Silence is not golden: Communicating with children dying from cancer. *Journal of Clinical Oncology, 23*(15), 3629–3631.

Berger, K., & Levetown, M. (2009). Hospice and special services. In T. D. Walsh, K. M. Foley, P. Glare, M. Lloyd-Williams, & A. T. Caraceni (Eds.), *Palliative medicine* (pp. 1105–1109). Philadelphia: Saunders.

Berger, P., & Luckman, T. (1996). *The social construction of reality: A treatise in the sociology of knowledge.* Garden City, NY: Doubleday.

Berman, L., Freeman, L., & Helm, D. (2006). People and programs. In I. L. Rubin & A. C. Crocker (Eds.), *Medical care for children and adults with developmental disabilities* (2nd ed., pp. 43–56). Baltimore, MD: Paul H. Brookes.

Boston Public Health Commission. (2008). *Information and referral resources.* Retrieved July 6, 2009, from http://www.bphc.org/programs/cib/civicengagement/mhl/accessinghealthinsurance/informationandreferral/pages/home.aspx

Burns, J. P., Mitchell, C., Outwater, K. M., Geller, M., Griffith, J. L., Trodres, I. D., et al. (2000). End of life care in the pediatric intensive care unit after forgoing intensive life-sustaining treatment. *Critical Care Medicine, 28,* 3060–3066.

Clark, J., & Quin, S. (2007). Professional carers' experiences of providing a pediatric palliative care service in Ireland. *Qualitative Health Research, 17*(9), 1219–1231.

Contro, N. A., Larson, J., Scofield, S., Sourkes, B., & Cohen, H. J. (2004). Hospital, staff, and family perspectives regarding quality of pediatric palliative care. *Pediatrics, 114,* 1248–1252.

Craft, M. J. (1993). Siblings of hospitalized children: Assessment and intervention. *Journal of Pediatric Nursing, 8*(5), 289–297.

Davies, B., Sehring, S. A., Partridge, J. C., Cooper, B. A., Hughes, A., Philip, J. C., et al. (2008). Barriers to palliative care for children: Perceptions of pediatric health care providers, *Pediatrics, 121,* 282–288.

Duncan, J., Joselow, M., & Hilden, J. (2006). Program interventions for children at the end-of-life and their siblings. *Child and Adolescent Psychiatric Clinics of North America, 15,* 739–758.

Feudtner, C., Silverira, M. J., & Christakis, D. A. (2002). Where do children with complex chronic conditions die? Patterns in Washington State, 1980–1998. *Pediatrics, 109*(4), 656–660.

Field, M. J., & Behrman, R. E. (Eds.). (2003). *When children die: Improving palliative and end-of-life care for children and their families.* Report of the Institute of Medicine, Washington, DC: National Academic Press.

Freedman, R., & Boyer, N. (2000). The power to choose: Supports for families caring for individuals with developmental disabilities. *Health and Social Work, 25,* 59–68.

Friedman, S. L. (2006). Parent resuscitation preferences for young people with severe developmental disabilities. *Journal of the America Medical Directors Association, 7*(2), 67–72.

Godfrey, K., Haddock, S., Fisher, A., & Lund, L. (2006). Essential components of curricula for preparing therapists to work effectively with lesbian, gay and bisexual clients: A Delphi Study. *Journal of Marital and Family Therapy, 32*(4), 491–504.

Graham, R. J., & Robinson, W. M. (2005). Commentary: Integrating palliative care into chronic care for children with severe neurodevelopmental disabilities. *Journal of Developmental & Behavioral Pediatrics, 26*(5), 361–365.

Gursky, B. (2007). The effect of educational interventions with siblings of hospitalized children. *Journal of Developmental & Behavioral Pediatrics, 28,* 392–398.

Hilden, J., Watterson, J., & Chrastek, J. (2003). Tell the children. *Journal of Clinical Oncology, 21*(9S), 37s–39s.

Hill, J., Fonagy, P., Safier, E., & Sargent, J. (2003). The ecology of attachment in the family. *Family Process, 41,* 455–476.

Himelstein, B. P. (2005). Palliative care in pediatrics. *Anesthesiology Clinics of North America, 23,* 837–856.

Hunt, A., Mastroyannopoulou, K., Goldman, A., & Seers, K. (2002). Not knowing—the problem of pain in children with severe neurological impairment. *Journal of Nursing Studies, 40,* 171–183.

Jaff, J. C. (2005). *Know your rights: A handbook for patients with chronic illness.* Farmington, CT: Advocacy for Patients With Chronic Illness.

Kirschner, K. L., Brashler, R., & Savage T. A. (2007). Ashley X. *American Journal of Physical Medicine & Rehabilitation, 86*(12), 1023–1029.

Kleiber, C., Montgomery, L. A., & Craft-Rosenberg M. (1995). Information needs of the siblings of critically ill children. *Children's Health Care, 24*(1), 47–60.

Kleinman, A. (1988). *The illness narrative: Suffering, healing and the human condition.* New York: Basic Books.

Klick, J. C., & Ballantine, A. (2007). Providing care in chronic disease: The ever-changing balance of integrating palliative and restorative medicine. *Pediatric Clinics of North America, 54,* 799–812.

Kreicbergs, U., Valdimarsdottir, U., Onelov, E., Henter, J. I., & Steineck, G. (2004). Talking about death with children who have severe malignant disease. *New England Journal of Medicine, 351,* 1175–1186.

Lash, M., & Kahn, P. (1998). *Choosing home or residential care: A guide for families of children with severe physical disabilities.* Wake Forest, NC: Lash and Associates.

Levetown, M. (2001). New programs for children living with life threatening conditions. *Texas Medicine, 97*(8), 60–63.

Linton, J. M., & Feudtner, C. (2008). What accounts for differences of disparities in pediatric palliative and end of life care? A systemic review focusing on possible multilevel mechanisms. *Pediatrics, 122,* 574–582.

Mack, S., & Berman, L. (1988). A group for parents of children with fatal genetic illnesses. *American Journal of Orthopsychiatry, 58*(3), 397–404.

Mack, J. W., & Wolfe, J. (2006). Early integration of pediatric palliative care: For some children, palliative care starts at diagnosis. *Current Opinion in Pediatrics, 18,* 10–14.

Martin, A. (1998). Clinical issues in psychotherapy with lesbian, gay and bisexual parented families. In C. J. Patterson & A. R. D'Augelli (Eds.), *Lesbian, gay, and bisexual identities in families: Psychological perspectives* (pp. 270–291). New York: Oxford University Press.

McDonagh, J. R., Elliot, T. B., & Engelberg, R. A. (2004). Family satisfaction with family conferences about end of life care in the intensive care unit: Increase proportion of family speech is associated with increased satisfaction. *Critical Care Medicine, 32*(7), 1484–1488.

McPherson, M., Arango, P., Fox, H., Laurer, C., McManus, M., Newacheck, P. W., et al. (1998). A new definition of children with special health care needs. *Pediatrics, 102*(1), 137–139.

Meyer, D., & Vadasy, P. F. (1994). *Sib-shops: Workshops for siblings of children with special needs.* Baltimore, MD: Paul H. Brookes.

Meyer, E. C., Burns, J. P., Griffith, J. L., & Troug, R. D. (2002). Parental perspectives on end-of-life care in the medical intensive care unit. *Critical Care Medicine, 30,* 226–231.

Meyer, E. C., Ritholz, M. D., Burns, J. P., & Truog, R. D. (2006). Improving the quality of end-of-life care in the pediatric intensive unit: Parents' priorities and recommendations. *Pediatrics, 117,* 649–657.

Meyer, E. C., & Tunick, R. A. (2009). Family adjustment and support. In T. D. Walsh, K. M. Foley, P. Glare, M. Lloyd-Williams, & A. T. Caraceni (Eds.), *Palliative medicine* (pp. 23–27). Philadelphia: Saunders.

Neugarten, B. (1979). Time, age, and the lifecycle. *American Journal of Psychiatry, 183*(7), 887–893.

Parish, S., Rose, R., Grinstein-Weiss, M., Richman, E., & Andrews, M. (2008). Material hardship in U.S. families raising children with disabilities. *Counsel for Exceptional Children, 75*(1), 71–92.

Pierucci, R. L., Kirby, R. S., & Leuthner, S. R. (2001). End-of-life for neonates and infants: The experience and effects of a palliative care consultation service. *Pediatrics, 108,* 653–660.

Porter, S., Haynie, M., Bierle, T., Heintz-Caldwell, T., & Palfrey, J. (1997). *Children and youth assisted by medical technology in educational setting: Guidelines for care* (2nd ed.). Baltimore: Paul H. Brookes.

Robinson, M. R., Thiel, M. M., Backus, M. M., & Meyer, E. C. (2006). Matters of spirituality at the end of life in the pediatric intensive care unit. *Pediatrics, 118*(3), 719–729.

Romanoff, B. D., & Thompson, B. E. (2006). Meaning construction in palliative care: The use of narrative, ritual, and the expressive arts. *American Journal of Hospice and Palliative Medicine, 23*(4), 309–316.

Rushton, C. H. (2004). Ethics and palliative care in pediatrics: When should parents agree to withdraw life-sustaining therapy for children? *American Journal of Nursing, 104*(4) 54–64.

Rushton, C. H. (2009). Pediatric palliative care: Interdisciplinary support. In T. D. Walsh, K. M. Foley, P. Glare, M. Lloyd-Williams, & A. T. Caraceni (Eds.), *Palliative medicine* (pp. 1110–1114). Philadelphia: Saunders.

Schmidt, L. M. (2003). Pediatric end-of-life care: Coming of age? *Caring: National Association for Home Care Magazine, 22*(5), 20–22.

Smith, E. D. (2001). Alleviating suffering in the face of death: Insights form constructivism and a transpersonal narrative approach. *Social Thought, 20*(1/2), 45–61.

Stienstra, D., & Chochinov, H. M. (2006). Vulnerability, disability, and palliative end-of-life care. *Journal of Palliative Care, 22*(3), 166–174.

Stillion, J., & Papadatou, D. (2002). Suffer the children: An examination of psychosocial issues in children and adolescents with terminal illness. *American Behavioral Scientist, 46*(2), 299–315.

Twibell, R. S., Siela, D., Riwiis, C., Wheatley, J., Riegle, T., Bousman, D., et al. (2008). Nurses' perceptions of their self-confidence and the benefits and risks of family presence during resuscitation. *American Journal of Critical Care, 17*(2), 101–111.

U.S. Social Security Administration. (2009). *Disability programs.* Retrieved September 22, 2008, from http://ssa.gov/disability/disability_starter_kits_child_factsheet.htm#disability

Young, A. J., & Rodriguez, K. L. (2006). The role of narrative in discussing end of life care: Eliciting values and goals from text, context and subtext. *Health Communication, 19*(1), 49–59.

Chapter 19

Supports and Resources for Adults

Teresa A. Savage, Katherine Ast, Reva Bess,
Marykay Castrogiovanni, and Patricia Conway

Background

Life expectancy for people with intellectual and developmental disabilities (IDD) is nearly the same as for the general population (Bittles et al., 2002; Janicki, Dalton, Henderson, & Davidson, 1999; Patja, Iivanainen, Vesala, Oksanen, & Ruoppila, 2000). As people with IDD age, they face all of the issues of those in the general population, with some unique additions. Everyone may encounter declining health, retirement from employment or other structured activities, the deaths of loved ones, or a necessary change in living arrangements. However, a unique issue for individuals with IDD is that they previously did not make major life decisions or at least did not have a family member, close friend, or paid caregiver to assist them. They may not have experience in expressing their preferences in medical treatment, living arrangements, or life goals. This chapter will discuss the challenges in providing end-of-life care to people with IDD and will provide resources to assist people with IDD, their families, and caregivers.

End-of-Life Care for the General Population

Since the Quinlan case in 1976 (In re Quinlan, 1976), there has been a growing movement to exert control over the dying process. The use of advance directives, such as a living will or durable power of attorney for health care, was promoted as a way to control one's end of life. The Patient Self-Determination Act of 1990 (Omnibus Budget Reconciliation Act of 1990, P. L. 101-508), in response to the Nancy Cruzan case (*Cruzan v. Director, Missouri Department of Health,* 1990), was a milestone. This act mandates that each patient be educated about advance directives. A decade after the act was passed, only 15% of adults had written advance directives (Tilden, 2000). In order to complete an advance directive, one needs to understand very basic concepts of death, the dying process, palliative and hospice care, and postdeath arrangements. The statutory language contained in the advanced directive forms can sometimes be a challenge for anyone to complete.

Most people have some experience with death at various points in their lives. It may be the loss of a pet, a grandparent, or the sudden, unexpected loss of a friend or parent.

One might attend a wake or funeral, see the deceased person in the casket, and/or visit the burial plot in the cemetery or vault in a mausoleum. Fewer people have had close-up experience with the dying process. For the majority of Americans who die in the hospital, a multitude of decisions regarding curative and/or life-sustaining treatment, pain and symptom management, and observance of important family rituals must be made at the end of life. Advance directives permit people to indicate preferences if they are incapable of communicating at a time in which decisions need to be made or to name a surrogate to make those decisions for them. Some states have statutes that assist in identifying a surrogate should a person require one and not have an advance directive. That surrogate is then expected to make decisions using substituted judgment, that is, to make decisions that the surrogate believes the person would make, if capable. In instances in which the person's wishes are not known, the surrogate is expected to make decisions in the best interests of the person. People with IDD may not have participated in medical decision making for themselves or have only done so on a limited basis. They often lack experience in decision making and expressing preferences. These issues related to decision making are expanded in greater detail in chapter 8.

Their experiences with managing money, finding resources, and seeking assistance also may have been limited. People with IDD may have little exposure to death except what they see in movies and on television. Often families try to protect them from the emotional impact of death with simplistic explanations and may not include them in experiences related to death and dying. Specifically, they may have been kept away from sick loved ones, or they may not have been allowed to attend rituals such as wakes or funerals.

The determination of the site of care and the management of pain and symptoms are other issues that need to be addressed at the end of life. Although more and more people die in hospitals, it may not be their choice but rather a default decision if they cannot receive comparable quality care in their home. Pain and symptom management often require a specialized depth of knowledge, great technical skill, superb communication, compassion, and resourcefulness. Family members, even those in the health professions, often find the situation overwhelming and may seek assistance.

Bereavement and grief previously may not have been adequately addressed or understood. People with IDD may have felt grief but may have not understood it well, or they may not have been able to articulate the feelings associated with loss. Issues related to loss, bereavement, and grief are also addressed in chapter 16. Individuals with IDD may not be adequately prepared to address their own or a family member's terminal illness. A host of resources are available and may be helpful in shepherding the person with IDD through end-of-life care. Before addressing the barriers and resources, it is important to review the issue of skepticism of end-of-life care that is held by some activists and some of the associated obstacles to providing this type of care to people with IDD (Not Dead Yet, 2007).

Skepticism About End-of-Life Care

One of the ironies of promoting access to end-of-life care is that people with disabilities sometimes have difficulty accessing life-sustaining treatment. This is more of a systemic problem than an issue for individuals with IDD directly, but it has impact on the societal attitudes on end-of-life care. The Sandra Jensen case is an example in which a 34-year-old woman with Down syndrome was denied a heart-lung transplant because of her intellectual disability. The medical director of the institution's heart and lung transplant center was quoted in the *New York Times* as saying, "We rejected her out of hand, based on a label. That was wrong, and I'm willing to admit that" (Stolberg, 1998). The institution has since changed its policy and does not summarily reject people with IDD. In a review of the literature on organ transplantation in people with "mental retardation," Martens, Jones and Reiss (2006) found that people with IDD have some access to organs, primarily kidneys, but they concluded that is it unclear if people with IDD have equal access.

In that same study, the authors found that people with IDD could be candidates for organ transplantation, but the issue of informed consent complicated the cases. Although some courts allowed guardians to give consent to the organ donation, a number of ethicists argued against having people with IDD as organ donors unless they can give informed consent themselves (Martens, Jones, & Reiss, 2006).

More recently there was the case of Ruben Navarro, a 25-year-old man who had adrenal leukodystrophy, a neurodegenerative disorder, diagnosed at age 10 (McKinley, 2008). Because of physical and cognitive deterioration, he was placed in a skilled-nursing facility at age 25. One evening he was found without a pulse; he was resuscitated and transferred to a medical center. He was placed on a ventilator. Accounts vary on the details of what happened, but 5 days after admission, in accordance with the hospital's futility policy, Mr. Navarro was removed from the ventilator. Futility policies were created to permit the hospital to decide unilaterally to remove life-sustaining treatment in instances where the physicians believed continued treatment was futile. Mr. Navarro's mother was informed of this policy. She could not afford to stay in the city where her son was hospitalized, so she went home and when reached by phone, gave telephone consent for his organs to be donated. Since he was not brain dead, the "donation after cardiac death" protocol was implemented. Death is expected to ensue within 30 to 60 minutes after life support is withdrawn, and then the organs are harvested. Additional information about donation after cardiac death is provided in chapter 12.

The transplant surgeon entered the operating suite, which was in violation of hospital policy and state law, and ordered morphine and Ativan (medications for pain and sedation) to be administered. The exact amounts are disputed; the transplant coordinator told the court that the records had been lost. The transplant surgeon inserted a nasogastric tube and inserted Betadine, an external antiseptic agent that is inserted into the stomach of a donor after death. Mr. Navarro died approximately 8 hours later; his organs were not suitable for donation. The transplant surgeon was charged with felony counts of dependent adult abuse but was acquitted at trial in December 2008. A civil suit brought by Mr. Navarro's mother, and complaints filed by the California Medical Board are still pending (Parrilla, 2008). Charges of unlawful controlled substance prescription were dismissed (Associated Press, 2008; McKinley, 2008). Disability rights activists offer this case as an example of failed efforts to obtain life-sustaining treatment for a person with a disability. They warn that people with disabilities should be skeptical of "futility" policies like the one used in the Navarro case.

DISPARATE QUALITY-OF-LIFE PERSPECTIVES

Well-educated and medically sophisticated consumers who are accustomed to exerting control over most things in their lives have been at the forefront of the "death with dignity" movement. They desire to control the dying process and fear losing control (Ganzini, Goy, & Dobscha, 2007). The experience of people with disabilities has been very different. In some situations, it has been noted that people with disabilities have had to fight to obtain treatment, so their families, direct care providers, and disability activists may be skeptical of end-of-life care (Gallagher, 1995; Gething, 1992; Longmore, 1995; Savage, 1998). Extra effort should be demonstrated to ensure that people with disabilities are not "fast tracked" into end-of-life care because of health care provider biases.

Some health care providers assume that the quality of life of people with disabilities is so poor that they would choose to forgo life-sustaining treatment (Gerhart, Koziol-McLain, Lowenstein, & Whiteneck, 1994). Health care providers may also identify with the caregivers and assume they are fatigued and ready to agree to withhold or withdraw treatment. If people with disabilities are unable to communicate their preferences—either because of physical disability or intellectual disability—health care providers may assume that the people with disabilities would rather forgo treatment. Yet there are studies to show that people with disabilities rate their quality of life as high as the general popula-tion rates theirs—a phenomenon labeled "the disability paradox" (Albrecht & Devlieger, 1999; Ubel, Loewenstein, Schwarz, & Smith, 2005).

When persons with disabilities are diagnosed with a terminal condition, there should not be an automatic assumption that treatment will be refused. As with anyone with a terminal condition, the benefits and burdens should be weighed. The decision to transi-tion to end-of-life care should be based on a realistic prognosis for cure; knowledge of the preferences of the people with disabilities or if those preferences are not known, the pref-erences of the family, close friends, or direct care staff; and a balance of the benefits and burdens to the people with disabilities. Kaufert and Koch (2003) point out the disparity in perspectives on the use of ventilators between health care providers and persons who live with chronic, life-limiting, disabling conditions: "For the clinicians, 'normalcy' was the standard against which deviant physical conditions are to be measured. They assisted the patient to make what was, implicitly in their presentation, the 'correct decision' [to forgo treatment]" (p. 465).

As King, Janicki, Kissinger, and Lash state,

> Decisions must be made with a pro-disability attitude. We must be clear in our advocacy for individuals with developmental disabilities that each person has the right to life, despite the level of their disability. Every person has the right to choose curative care, even in the face of a dismal prognosis. The right to high-quality palliative care should also be fully extended to individuals with develop-mental disabilities who choose this end of life treatment option. (2005, p. e3)

Advance Directives and Capacity

The use of advance directives is not without problems, although people with disabilities have not been able to access advance directives easily. Freedman (1998) explored the use of advance directives as a communication process to facilitate decision making between adults with IDD and their families. She recognized the thorny problem of wanting to honor the person's autonomy but lacking guidelines for assessing decision-making capac-ity. In order to construct an advance directive, one must be able to understand informa-tion, to contemplate how the information and options will impact the person, and to express a choice (Grisso & Appelbaum, 1998).

Although there are no instruments specifically for people with IDD, two instruments may be adaptable. The MacArthur Competence Assessment Tool for Treatment (MacCAT-T) was developed by Grisso and Appelbaum (1998) based on their research into decision-making capacity. They also have a version for use in determining capacity to consent to research. Information is provided to the person whose capacity is being assessed (disclosure); the assessor then asks questions (probes) and will repeat or further explain the information and assess understanding (redisclosure and reinquiry; Grisso & Appelbaum, 1998, p. 177). A score of 0, 1, or 2 is given for each category with a total score ranging between 0 and 8. The authors cautioned that there is no "passing" score where capacity is above a certain number. The assessor is still required to exercise clinical judgment in the determination of capacity, but the instrument assists in structuring the interviews. Keywood and Flynn (n.d.) first maintained that health care providers should assume capacity unless it is demonstrated through careful assessment that the person lacks the ability to understand the specific information relative to the health care issues or is unable to use the information to make a decision. They endorse the use of the MacCAT-T by the National Health Service in the UK.

The other instrument is the Aid to Capacity Evaluation (ACE), developed by Etchells and colleagues from the University of Toronto Joint Centre for Bioethics (1999). The ACE has been adapted by the Henrico Area Mental Health & Retardation Services of Henrico County, Virginia, for use with people with IDD whose capacity is in question.* Patient capacity has been evaluated in medical practices with use of the ACE (Tunzi, 2001). Regardless of the instrument used, the person assessing capacity should have the skills to tailor the assessment to various levels of health literacy. Ideally, the assessor should also have familiarity with people with IDD and, ideally, the person being evaluated in particular. People with IDD may be accustomed to relying on family, friends, or staff to support them in the decision-making process. The assessor should be respectful of supported decision making but mindful of coercion. Discussions about the end of life are fraught with emotion. The assessor needs the ability to share emotionally laden content and therapeutically support the person in the conversation or to have another person, family, friend, or professional, available to support the person.

Many older people with IDD have legal guardians who provide consent, or consent may be provided by the legally determined next of kin. Direct care providers sometimes find this frustrating when they believe the person with IDD is capable of making a decision but is not asked. Well-meaning family or guardians may wish to protect the person from difficult decisions or upsetting information, or they may not want or be able to take the time to include him or her in the decision-making process. Currently, there is a trend toward supported decision making, which is how most people make their decisions. In this process, issues are discussed with family or close friends in order to gather opinions and use others as sounding boards. People with IDD may require more time to gather and understand information, more assistance in thinking about the impact of the options on their life situation, and more help in understanding the process and finality of certain choices. Although another person is legally empowered to make decisions, people with IDD should not abrogate their right to participate. State law may dictate who gives the

---

* See Resources section for Web site address.

legal consent, but advocates for the person with IDD may argue that assent, or the affirmative agreement, should be obtained.

If supported decision making cannot be demonstrated for a specific decision, or the people closest to the person with IDD believe it is not in his or her best interests to be involved in the discussion, then consent from the legally authorized person should be obtained. The presumption, however, should be that the person has capacity unless proved otherwise. Paternalism, while well-meaning, erodes autonomy, and persons with IDD deserve the dignity of risk in experiencing all of life's ups and downs. Conflicts between family or guardians, the person with IDD, and caregivers can occur, and although wide latitude is usually given to family or guardians, referral to an ethics committee or an ethics consultant may help in resolving the conflict. Judicial review may be necessary as a last resort.

Death Education

The goal in having a conversation around advance directives may not be to draft a document, but to educate and explore feelings on this important, difficult topic. Before initiating the conversation, though, it would be ideal for the person with IDD to have had preparation about death, dying, and end-of-life care.

Heller, Miller, Hsieh, and Sterns (2000) advocate a later-life training program that educates persons with IDD on retirement, healthy behaviors, living arrangements, and leisure activities. They developed and tested a curriculum based on person-centered planning with objectives to increase knowledge, facilitate choices and decision-making participation, set goals, and increase life satisfaction. Based on their study, they conclude that adults with IDD can continue to learn later in life and can improve their decision-making skills. Information about the process of person-centered planning is provided in chapter 17.

Botsford (2000) proposes an integration of end-of-life care into other services that people with IDD receive. She sees death education belonging in a life cycle approach and advocates an experiential-learning process including field trips to funeral homes and cemeteries, for example. Staff education is critical to the success of both the later-life training programs and integration of end-of-life care. Ideally, collaboration between experts in hospice/palliative care and providers and families of persons with IDD will help in improving knowledge and decision-making abilities in end-of-life care for people with IDD. However, even with increasing knowledge and decision-making skills, there remain barriers to end-of-life care.

A number of obstacles can interfere with good end-of-life care. For instance, health care provider assumptions about the quality of life of people with disabilities can result in premature death by the withholding or withdrawal of desired life-sustaining treatment. There may be a lack of knowledge about end-of-life care in people with expertise in working with people with IDD. Similarly, there may be lack of familiarity with care of people with disabilities by experts in hospice and palliative care. Each of these issues may create barriers to good end-of-life care and will be discussed in greater detail.

Barriers to End-of-Life Care

Direct care staff and family caregivers often lack the preparation to provide end-of-life care to people with disabilities (Botsford, 2004; Peters-Beumer, Dexter, & Johnson, 2008). Volunteers of America conducted a survey of directors of agencies to gather baseline information on the current state of end-of-life for people with IDD and their families. Results confirmed that there is a need for end-of-life care in these organizations, but there are inadequate resources. Guidelines are needed, as is additional staff training and policies that are supportive of end-of-life care (Botsford, 2004).

Peters-Beumer, Dexter, and Johnson (2008) informally polled Easter Seals Adult Day-care Services as they developed a proposal to enhance community-based options for end-of-life care. They learned that over a third of the programs serve older adults with IDD. In these programs, the staff received 2.2 hours of training in end-of-life care annually. The daycare staff describe the challenges of having clients with extensive medical needs, confusion about reimbursement and funding mechanisms, and resistance from family or others client regarding hospice. In the delivery of end-of-life care, they identify barriers such as the lack of education about pain management, lack of appropriate staff, lack of private space, lack of time for individual care, and lack of awareness in recognizing pain symptoms. Community hospice program staff were also polled. They identified reasons why they would not refer a hospice patient to an adult daycare program, which included a lack of knowledge about adult daycare services, including their locations, cost, and available transportation; the belief that their patients were too ill or required too much care and medication; or the idea that clients could not participate in adult daycare if they had a Do-Not-Resuscitate (DNR) order.

In piloting their revised later-life training program curriculum, Heller et al. (2000) found that persons with IDD sometimes had inadequate support from family or staff who felt they had no time, did not think the curriculum was important, or did not see it as their job to participate in the later-life training. As with all people, whether with or without IDD, it is useful to have knowledge of the dying process, what to expect as far as pain and symptoms and how those are managed, and the grieving process and bereavement rituals. Direct care staff have the skills to educate people with IDD, but they may not have the knowledge of how palliative care and hospice care are delivered. Table 19.1 summarizes these findings.

End-of-Life Care of Family Members and Loved Ones

Another area of need is one where direct care providers support a person with IDD whose loved one is dying or has died. This type of crisis may precipitate out-of-home placement for the person with IDD. The direct care staff may not be prepared to support the person through the crisis and grieving process. It is not expected that all staff will be capable and eager to provide support around death and dying. This type of circumstance requires a person with expertise or experience in supporting a grieving person and understanding issues related to end-of-life care. At times, a consultant may need to be sought who can offer suggestions to guide the care or join the team for the period of time that end-of-life care is needed.

Vignette 1

Frederick was a 29-year-old man with cerebral palsy, microcephaly, intellectual disability, seizures, gastroesophageal reflux, a gastrostomy tube, severe scoliosis, reactive airway disease, and multiple episodes of aspiration pneumonia. He resided in a residential facility since age 2. Despite adjustments to his medication, he usually was asleep and was difficult to arouse. He had more "sick" days than well days and he did not return to his previous baseline of functioning

Table 19.1
Expertise Needed for Provision of Optimal End-of-Life Care to People With IDD

Palliative care and hospice

- Knowledge of philosophy about death and dying
- Acceptance of inevitability of death
- Ability to talk about death and dying
- Skill in providing psychological and spiritual support
- Skill in managing symptoms, especially pain
- Skill in managing resources in the health care environment with complex funding protocols for palliative care and hospice
- Knowledge and facilitation of grief, loss, and bereavement
- Appreciation of the importance of rituals

Intellectual and developmental disabilities

- Knowledge of client's unique needs and range of abilities
- Knowledge of client's responses to change
- Ability to assess client's needs and preferences
- Ability to communicate with client and read his or her cues
- Knowledge of case-management skills in coordinating care
- Familiarity with funding sources, rules, and regulations
- Long-term relationships with client and family
- Familiarity with surrogate decision making and decision-making capacity assessments

---

after each illness. He was no longer taken to therapy sessions because of his lack of alertness. His parents, who visited weekly, no longer took him home for holidays as he was medically fragile and became ill after any outing. His parents had been called to the facility on several occasions when Frederick's condition worsened and death was thought to be imminent.

He had a Life Care Plan, a care plan describing the actions to be taken should he need resuscitation or other treatments. This plan was developed a numbers of years ago and revisited every 6 months and after any change in his medical condition. His plan included aggressive treatments, such as nebulizations; oxygen; intermittent medications for reactive airway disease, seizures, gastroesophageal reflux, constipation, spasticity, fevers, or infection; continuous feedings; and other nursing measures to provide comfort. He would not receive artificial respiration, intubation, external cardiac massage, intravenous medication, or resuscitative medications through oral, inhalation, osseous, or rectal routes. He would not be transferred out of the facility or receive emergency medical treatment.

His parents were called to the facility 3 times in the last week. The medical director said that Frederick was receiving maximum support at the facility. It was her opinion that if he were transferred to an intensive care unit (ICU), he might recover from this episode, but would likely need to remain on a ventilator for the rest of his life. She also believed it was highly likely that the ICU physicians would suggest that the ventilator be withdrawn if Frederick was unable to be weaned. In analyzing the benefits and burdens to Frederick, she asked the parents to consider the experience of an ICU admission. The parents decided not to have Frederick transferred to ICU, but they wanted all other treatments to be continued.

After further deterioration, when Frederick appeared near death, the nursing and respiratory staff recommended limiting treatments. They believed treatment was prolonging the dying process and causing discomfort to Frederick. The parents agreed and Frederick was moved into a room where they could stay and other family members could visit. He received one-to-one nursing care, the staff played music that he enjoyed in the past, and he was given medication to treat hunger, increased spasticity, and pain. His parents planned his funeral, the clothing he would wear, the music to be played, and the passages of scripture to be read. His siblings wrote letters they wanted read at his funeral service and then placed in the casket with Frederick. Over the next 3 days, his medication was increased whenever he showed any discomfort. He displayed a pattern of slowed breathing for 10 to 12 hours with brief periods of apnea, then had longer periods of apnea until his heart stopped. His parents and the staff who had cared for him for 27 years were present. Services were held as the parents had planned in the chapel adjacent to the facility. Many of the family members of other residents at the facility attended the services.

Commentary: Frederick's caregivers gave him the best care they could give under the circumstances. They made the decision to redirect goals of care from aggressive treatment to comfort measures, rather than transfer him to an ICU. They modified his routine and their staffing patterns in order to provide more intensive nursing care and permit his family greater access and privacy. They addressed the grief of the direct care staff, family, other residents and their families. Pursuant to regulation, a death review was required for any death in the facility. Intended to monitor any possibility of death by abuse or neglect, the investigation casts a pall on the integrity of the end-of-life care given by this staff in accordance with family wishes. It treats death as a critical incident instead of a natural passage.

Frederick received medication via the gastrostomy tube; would intravenous (IV) medication have been a better alternative? The facility did not have the staff or license to provide IV therapy. The staff and family believed that it would have been more stressful for all parties involved to have Frederick transferred to an acute care facility, such as the local hospital or tertiary medical center, where he had been treated previously. They feared losing control of the situation. They knew Frederick had his best interests at heart and believed it was better to manage him in his current setting than to transfer him to another setting.

Suppose Frederick had been living at home, though, as most people with IDD do, or in a small group home. Would there be skilled workers familiar with IDD and hospice or palliative care? Would Frederick have to go to an inpatient facility? With the level of care that Frederick required, it is possible that a general floor in the hospital or ICU may not have staff prepared to provide palliative care. It is unlikely that he would be admitted to an Intermediate Care Facility for hospice. These types of situations pose challenges to providers of end-of-life care.

Vignette 2

Clifford lived in a Community Independent Living Arrangement (CILA) for almost a decade. He was in his 50s; his diagnosis was autism. A diehard baseball fan, Clifford would listen to his favorite teams on the radio. He shared his room with Floyd, who was in the room when Clifford collapsed from a massive stroke. Floyd was very upset, especially when he was asked to move Clifford so that the paramedics could get into the room. Clifford was taken to the hospital and died later that day. Clifford's parents, who were deceased, had made prearrangements for Clifford's funeral but those plans were lost; however, Clifford had bought a burial plot, casket, and made funeral arrangements with assistance from the CILA staff. Thinking that Clifford had no family or friends, Clifford's next of kin, a distant relative, did not want a wake or funeral. The CILA manager explained that he indeed had many friends and the staff felt like his family, and so they wanted to honor his wishes for the wake and funeral. The relative was unaware of these relationships and agreed to go forward with the plans as Clifford had made them.

Clifford's death was a shock, especially to his roommate, Floyd. The CILA staff arranged for Floyd to see a grief counselor from a local hospice. Approximately 1 year after Clifford's death, the staff at the CILA decided to hold another memorial service for Clifford. The staff of the CILA used the opportunity of the memorial service for Clifford to discuss death and grief since another client, Wally, had been diagnosed with colon cancer. The staff struggled with how to talk with clients about death, grief, and coping. A number of staff had experienced deaths in their own families and found the prospect of having these discussions very emotionally difficult. Knowing this, the administrators developed a plan to obtain assistance for staff to discuss death and dying with clients in the CILA. The staff was encouraged to break down concepts in simple language. When possible, they were to gently introduce the idea about Wally's condition and anticipated outcome.

At the memorial service for Clifford, clients made comments like "Clifford is with God now," "He is better off now. . . . At least he's not suffering anymore," and "I'm real sorry he's gone. I'm sad."

Commentary. The CILA staff wanted to honor Clifford's wishes regarding his funeral and burial and advocated for him when a legal authority for those decisions fell to a distant relative. They also addressed the traumatic experience of his roommate witnessing Clifford's collapse by contacting a counselor at a local hospice. In working together, the hospice counselor and CILA staff supported Floyd in his loss and grief for Clifford. In anticipation of Wally's death, they also identified the situation as a teaching opportunity for other clients and an entrée for broaching the subject.

Vignette 3

The CILA staff wanted to keep Wally in the CILA for as long as possible. They were able to get his state guardian to approve a DNR order when his physician indicated he was in the final stages of colon cancer. Hospice referral was initiated, and a member of their staff assessed Wally, did interviews with the CILA staff, and arranged regular sessions for the staff and clients to discuss their feelings. The hospice sent certified nursing assistants to assist regular staff with Wally's care in the CILA. The hospice provided music therapy, written resources, information about stages of grief and loss, and stressed the normalization of the processes that everyone was experiencing. His condition had rapidly deteriorated; he curled up into a fetal position, did not recognize staff, and had become incontinent. At this point, he required more care than he could receive at the CILA. A few days prior to his death, Wally was transferred to the inpatient hospice.

After Wally's death, the hospice chaplain presided over his funeral and the music therapist provided the music, which were all of Wally's favorite songs. Two clients had deaths in their families, which complicated the grief they had for Wally's death. Hospice provided a bereavement counselor who worked with the clients for a year about Wally's death. Other hospice staff met with the CILA staff and clients monthly for a while, and maintained contact for the year after Wally's death. Additionally, students doing an internship at the CILA's agency developed material for remembrance activities, education on grief and loss, coping skills development, art and "letting go" activities. The CILA manager was able to access Wally's bank account to pay for a portion of his funeral. The funeral home used funds from the state funeral directors' association to cover the rest of the costs.

Commentary: In this situation, a death provided the impetus for death education. The CILA staff, together with hospice staff, tailored their care and teaching to clients who were most affected by Clifford's sudden death and Wally's impending death. Wally's care was managed in the CILA up to the point at which he required more care than he could receive in his usual setting. Medicaid waivers are the source of funding for clients in CILAs. If a client requires a personal care attendant (PCA), they are not usually eligible to live in the CILA. Hospice, paid by Medicaid or Medicare, is averaged per diem and all hospice services must be covered by the per diem amount. It is sometimes difficult to access all the necessary services while complying with local, state, and federal regulations regarding CILAs, Medicaid waivers, and hospice eligibility.

The goals in Wally's case were to provide appropriate, person-centered, end-of-life care in the least restrictive setting. Collaboration between IDD and hospice experts is essential in planning and providing this type of end-of-life care. These case examples demonstrate the complementary collaboration between experts in specialty care and the resourcefulness of both groups—staff in the CILA and hospice staff—in supporting and educating the client in the CILA.

Vignette 4

Violet, 55, who had an intellectual disability of unknown etiology, lived at home with her parents, age 76 and 78. Her parents, who were her legal guardians, made arrangements for her to move to a small group home upon their deaths or if they needed to enter a skilled-nursing facility. Violet was diagnosed with breast cancer. With enormous effort on the part of her parents and health care providers, Violet underwent surgery, radiation, and chemotherapy. She was identified as having metastasis to her bone 6 months later. Although she enjoyed adult day care, she stopped participating when she began treatment for breast cancer. Her parents made all the decisions and informed Violet but did not discuss the extent of her condition. They did not want her told of the metastasis. They also decided not to pursue any further curative treatment. The oncology team recommended home hospice.

Violet's parents contacted the hospice program but required that they agree not to tell Violet she was dying. The hospice had not cared for a person with IDD before and would have preferred to be free to talk with Violet, especially if she asked any questions. However, they believed the parents, Violet's legal guardians, were acting in Violet's best interests, and therefore they agreed to enroll her in home hospice. Staff from the adult day care program kept in touch and occasionally sent cards. Over the next 3 months, Violet's behavior changed, becoming agitated and combative. Her parents did not want her to be given narcotics for fear that she would become an "addict." Despite the hospice nurse's explanation, they did not want her to get anything stronger than oral codeine, which frequently made her vomit.

Violet lay in bed and moaned; the hospice nurse explained to her parents that she thought Violet was in severe pain that was not relieved with her current medications. Violet's IV access had been removed when her parents decided not to pursue further curative treatment, so the hospice nurse suggested subcutaneous administration of morphine. The nurse obtained an order from the hospice physician and started a morphine infusion. Within 4 hours of the start of the infusion, Violet stopped moaning and appeared less agitated. She died two days later.

Commentary: One wonders that if Violet did not have an intellectual disability, (a) whether her breast cancer would have been discovered earlier; (b) whether she would have been allowed to participate in treatment decisions or, at a minimum, been informed about what was happening to her; and (c) whether she would have had better relief from pain medication if the hospice nurse was free to be more aggressive in pain management. Perhaps her parents could have been better informed that their concern about addiction to narcotics is not relevant when providing palliative pain control, particularly when death is imminent. There were missed opportunities to devise a comprehensive end-of-life care plan by her parents, the adult daycare staff who knew Violet well and in a different context, and the hospice staff.

Would Violet have been able to understand her situation? An assessment of her capacity may have demonstrated if and at what level she could have understood her condition and prognosis. Would she have wanted to know she was dying, made any plans, or said any good-byes? Perhaps hospice and the adult day care staff could have collaborated to assist the parents, hospice nurse, or day care staff to have a conversation with Violet about these matters. Would it have been possible to discuss how pain is assessed and managed, especially pain associated with metastatic bone cancer?

Had Violet known she was dying and had some preparation, she may have had some "unfinished business" to complete. Awareness, mobilization of resources, and collaboration may have limited the time that Violet had unrelieved pain.

One resource for the hospice nurse might have been an ethics consultant or ethics committee. The hospice may have an ethics committee or an ethics consultant available to them to help the nurse strategize on how she might resolve the conflict over adequate pain relief. The nurse might also contact the daycare program or another agency serving people with IDD to obtain advice. The nurse would, of course, keep identifiable information confidential or get the guardians' permission to discuss the situation.

Conclusion

Consistent with the American Association on Intellectual and Developmental Disabilities's position statement "Caring at the End of Life" (2007), there is much work to be done in improving end-of-life care for everyone and especially for people with IDD. There are challenges in determining the point at which transition to end-of-life care is appropriate, learning the preferences of persons with IDD and their families, and accessing palliative care and hospice personnel who are familiar with or willing to learn about the unique needs of people with IDD and their families.

Areas for further investigation are the use of current instruments to assess capacity in people with IDD and the use of advance care planning including advance directives. Issues related to guardianship and legal authority need a closer look in relation to end-of-life care. Resources such as ethics committee, ethics consultants, guardianship and advocacy commissions, or other human rights organizations may be useful when conflict occurs between the person and guardian, the person and other caregivers, or the guardian and caregivers.

Institutional policies, usually based on regulatory requirements, should be examined in relation to standards of end-of-life care. Can death reviews be categorized and conducted in a way that doesn't pathologize end-of-life care? Would the transition to hospice care serve as a signal that a death review is not needed, or does it invite abuse? Regulations regarding funding streams may need to be revised in order to keep a person in the appropriate setting and obtain all the necessary services without having to change settings because of funding restrictions or conflicts.

As with the general population, the biggest step in improving end-of-life care is to educate the public and health care providers about palliative care and the dying process. Public and health care provider education has been the focus for a number of groups, such as the Robert Wood Johnson Foundation and Volunteers of America. Some excellent resources have been developed through the collaboration of groups focused on end-of-life care and groups serving people with IDD. The following is a listing of those resources.

RESOURCES

Books and Journal Articles

Beltran, J. E. (1996). Shared decision making: The ethics of caring and best respect. *Bioethics Forum, 12*(3), 17–25.

Friedman, S., & Gilmore, D. (2007). Factors that impact resuscitation preferences for young people with severe developmental disabilities. *Intellectual and Developmental Disabilities, 45*(2), 90–97.

Gaventa, W. C., & Coulter, D. I. (2005). *EOL care: Bridging disability and aging with person-centered care.* Binghamton, NY: Haworth Press (now distributed by Routledge Press). Simultaneously copublished in *Journal of Religion, Disability, and Health, 9*(2), 2005.

Midwest Bioethics Center, Task Force on Health Care for Adults With Developmental Disabilities. (1996). Health care treatment decision-making guidelines for adults with developmental disabilities. *Bioethics Forum, 12*(3), S1–S8.

Reynolds, D. F. (1999). Project BRIDGE—People with disabilities participate in their health care decisions. *Bioethics Forum, 15*(2), 36–45.

St. Clair, B. (1996). People with developmental disabilities focusing on their own health care. *Bioethics Forum, 12*(3), 27–36.

Capacity Evaluation Aids

Aid to Capacity Evaluation: http://www.jointcentreforbioethics.ca/tools/ace.shtClifford

Glossary of terms in end-of-life care: http://www.caringinfo.org/Resources/Glossary.htm

Henrico Area Mental Health & Retardation Services: Aid to Capacity Evaluation adapted from http://www.piedmontcsb.org/qmc/AR%20Aid%20to%20Capacity%20Evaluation.pdf

MacArthur Competence Assessment Test—Treatment: MacCAT-T. Available from PRPress at http://www.prpress.com/books/mact-sctfr.html

Practical Guidelines for Clinical Assessment and Care Management of Alzheimer and Other Dementias Among Adults With Mental Retardation: http://www.aamr.org/Reading_Room/Practical/practical_guidelines.pdf

Newsletters

Developmental Disabilities Hospice & Palliative Care E-Newsletter—requires subscription through Developmental Disabilities and Palliative Care Forum: http://www.ddhospicepalliativecare.org/register.cfm

Ethics and Intellectual Disability: Newsletter of the Network on Ethics and Intellectual Disability: published twice yearly by Network. Contact Robert M. Veatch, Joseph P. Kennedy, and Rose F. Kennedy Institute of Ethics, Georgetown University, Washington, DC 20057-1065, USA, veatchr@georgetown.edu or Professor de Johannes S. Reinders, Institute for Ethics, Free University, Amsterdam, The Netherlands, J.S.Reinders@esau.th.vu.nl.

Training Manuals

Abbatiello, G., Faulkner, L. R., Shenise, C., & O'Brien, M. J. (20007). *Hospice and palliative care & developmental disabilities: Making the connection*. Delaware, NY: New York State ARC.

Botsford, A. L., & Force, L. T. (2004). *End-of-life care: A guide for supporting older people with intellectual disabilities and their families* (2nd ed.). Albany, NY: NYSARC.

Botsford, A. L., & Force, L. T. (2004). *End-of-life care: A guide for supporting older people with intellectual disabilities and their families* (2nd Ed.). Resource supplement. Albany, NY: NYSARC.

Force, L. T., Abbatiello, G., Doka, K., & Faulkner, L. R. (2004). *Trainer's guide: EOL care: Supporting older people with intellectual disabilities and their families*. Delaware, NY: NYSRC.

Web Sites

5 Wishes: From the Aging With Dignity Organization; Web site has documents available for purchase online intended to facilitate discussions about a person's wishes. It has a booklet for children titled "My Wishes," which uses simpler language and concepts and may be useful in conversations with people with IDD: http://www.agingwithoutdignity.org/5wishes.htClifford

Agreement for Hospice Care: http://www.albany.edu/aging/lastpassages/docs/Agreement%20for%20Hospice%20Care.pdf

Caring Connections: Brochures and links to resources on advance care planning legal issues, advance directives, planning ahead, caregiving, end-of-life care, grief, pain, pediatric, planning for long-term care, professional resources, serious illness spirituality, and resources in Spanish: http://www.caringinfo.org/resources

End-of-Life Care Training, based on Volunteers of America training curriculum: http://www.uic.edu/orgs/rrtcamr/End_of_life_care_training.html

General aging with developmental disabilities: http://www.uic.edu/orgs/rrtcamr/pubslist.html#general_aging

Last Passages: This Web site has a large number of links, including a library of resources with special attention to end-of-life care for people with developmental disabilities. It includes links for advance planning, facts about developmental disabilities, papers by Gaventa and Coulter on controversial issues in end-of-life care for people with disabilities, sample individual service plans, palliative care, sample agreement for hospice care, and many more relevant links. Available at http://www.albany.edu/aging/lastpassages/endoflifeissues.htm

Rehabilitation Research and Training Center on Aging With Developmental Disabilities, Department of Disability and Human Development, University of Illinois at Chicago: http://www.uic.edu/orgs/rrtcamr

Sample Addendum to Individual Service Plan for Hospice and Palliative Care: http://www.albany.edu/aging/lastpassages/docs/Addendum%20to%20ISP%20Hospice%20and%20Palliative%20Care.pdf

Local Resources to Investigate

- Support groups at agencies serving people with IDD
- Local hospices: community and volunteer services including educational programs
- Network of pastors: spiritual support, as well as resources for referrals for palliative care services
- Funeral homes: community education, advance care planning, and sources of funding for funeral services
- Ethics committees or ethics consultants at academic medical centers, universities, agencies, or other programs serving people with disabilities

ACKNOWLEDGMENTS

The authors would like to acknowledge the contributions in editing and coordination from Teresa T. Moro, AM, LSW; Amy Bowers, LCSW; and Kristi L. Kirschner, MD.

REFERENCES

Albrecht, G. L., & Devlieger, P. J. (1999). The disability paradox: High quality of life against all odds. *Social Science & Medicine, 48*, 977–988.

Associated Press. (2008). *Transplant doctor ordered to trial.* Retrieved on March 21, 2008, from http://today.msnbc.msn.com/i/23743238

Bittles, A. H., Petterson, B. A., Sullivan, S. G., Hussain, R., Glasson, E. J., & Montgomery, P. D. (2002). The influence of intellectual disability on life expectancy. *Journal of Gerontology Series A: Biological Science and Medical Science, 57A*(7), M470–M472.

Botsford, A. L. (2000). Integrating end of life care into services for people with an intellectual disability. *Social Work in Health Care, 31*(1), 35–48.

Botsford, A. L. (2004). Status of end of life care in organizations providing services for older people with a developmental disability. *American Journal on Mental Retardation, 109*(5), 421–428.

Cruzan v. Director, Missouri Department of Health, 110S. Ct. 2841 (1990).

Etchells, E., Darzins, P., Silberfeld, M., Singer, P. A., McKenny, J., Naglie, G., et al. (1999). Assessment of patient capacity to consent to treatment. *Journal of General Internal Medicine, 14*, 27–34.

Freedman, R. I. (1998). Use of advance directives: Facilitating health care decisions by adults with mental retardation and their families. *Mental Retardation, 36*(6), 444–456.

Gallagher, H. G. (1995). "Slapping up spastics": The persistence of social attitudes toward people with disabilities. *Issues in Law & Medicine, 10*(4), 401–414.

Ganzini, L., Goy, E. R., & Dobscha, S. K. (2007). Why Oregon patients request assisted death: Family members' views. *Journal of General Internal Medicine, 23*(2), 154–157.

Gerhart, K. A., Koziol-McLain, J., Lowenstein, S. R., & Whiteneck, G. G. (1994). Quality of life following spinal cord injury: Knowledge and attitudes of emergency care providers. *Annals of Emergency Medicine, 23*(4), 807–812.

Gething, L. (1992). Judgments by health professionals of personal characteristics of people with a visible physical disability. *Social Science & Medicine 34*(7), 809–815.

Grisso, T., & Appelbaum, P. S. (1998). *Assessing competence to consent to treatment: A guide for physicians and other health professionals.* New York: Oxford University Press.

Heller, T., Miller, A. B., Hsieh, K., & Sterns, H. (2000). Later-life planning: Promoting knowledge of options and choice-making. *Mental Retardation, 38*(5), 395–406.

In re Quinlan, 70 N. J. 10, 355 A.2d 647, *cert. denied*, 429 U.S. 922 (1976).

Janicki, M. P., Dalton, A. J., Henderson, C., & Davidson, P. (1999). Mortality and morbidity among older adults with intellectual disability: Health services considerations. *Disability and Rehabilitation, 21*(5/6), 284–294.

Kaufert, J., & Koch, T. (2003). Disability or EOL? Competing narratives in bioethics. *Theoretical Medicine, 24*, 459–469.

Keywood, K., & Flynn, M. (n.d.). *Healthcare decision-making by adults with intellectual disabilities: Some levers to changing practice.* Retrieved June 1, 2008, from http://www.intellectualdisability .info/values/P_decision_kk.htClifford

King, A., Janicki, M., Kissinger, K., & Lash, S. (2005). *End of life care for people with developmental disabilities: Philosophy and recommendations.* Retrieved May 26, 2008, from http://www.albany .edu/aging.lastpassages/lp-philosophy.htm

Longmore, P. (1995). Medical decision-making and people with disabilities: A clash of cultures. *Journal of Law, Medicine, & Ethics, 23*, 82–87.

Martens, M. A., Jones, L., & Reiss, S. (2006). Organ transplantation, organ donation and mental retardation. *Pediatric Transplantation, 10*, 658–664.

McKinley, J. (2008, February 27). Surgeon accused of speeding a death to get organs. *New York Times.* Retrieved July 27, 2009, from http://www.nytimes.com/2008/02/27/ us/27transplant.html?pagewanted=2&_r=1&sq=Surgeon%20accused%20of%20speeding%20 a%20death&st=cse&scp=1

Not Dead Yet. (2007, October 6). *"End of Life" questions and suggested responses for disability advocates.* Retrieved July 27, 2009, from http://notdeadyetnewscommentary.blogspot.com/search/ label/life-ending%20decisions

Omnibus Budget Reconciliation Act of 1990, P. L. 101-508, sec. 4206 and 4751, 104 Stat. 1388, 1388-115, and 1388-204 (classified respectively at 42 U. S. C. 1395cc(f) (Medicare) and 1396a (w) (Medicaid).

Parrilla, L. (2008). *Transplant surgeon Hootan Roozrokh acquitted in Sierra Vista organ harvest case.* Retrieved February 21, 2009, from http://www.sanluisobispo.com/news/local/v-print/ story/564066.html

Patja, K., Iivanainen, M., Vesala, H., Oksanen, H., & Ruoppila, I. (2000). Life expectancy of people with intellectual disability: A 35 year follow-up study. *Journal of Intellectual Disability Research, 44*, 591–599.

Peters-Beumer, L., Dexter, J., & Johnson, J. (2008). Enhancing community-based options for EOL care. Unpublished survey results of adult daycare services and hospice services presented at meeting. Chicago: Easter Seals Headquarters.

Savage, T. A. (1998). Children with severe and profound disabilities and the issue of social justice. *Advanced Practice Nursing Quarterly, 4*(2), 53–58.

Stolberg, S. G. (1998, April 5). Ideas & trends: The unlisted; live and let die over transplants. *New York Times*, section 4, p. 3.

Tilden, V. P. (2000). Advance directives. *American Journal of Nursing, 100*(12), 49–51.

Tunzi, M. (2001). Can the patient decide? Evaluating patient capacity in practice. *American Family Physician, 64*(2), 299–306. Retrieved May 30, 2008, from http://www.aafp.org/ afp.20010715/299.pdf

Ubel, P. A., Loewenstein, G., Schwarz, N., & Smith, D. (2005). Misimagining the unimaginable: The disability paradox and health care decisions making. *Health Psychology, 24*(4), S57–S62.

CHAPTER 20

Palliative Care and Pain Management

Resources for Direct Care Providers

AMY C. STEVENS, ANNE-MARIE BARRON, AND PATRICIA N. RISSMILLER

Providing excellent end-of-life care is challenging under most circumstances. Issues surrounding end-of-life care for people with intellectual and developmental disabilities (IDD) are particularly complex. The purpose of this chapter is to describe resources that may be helpful for those providing direct care during this important time of life for people with IDD and their families.

Best practice palliative care and pain management are based on interdisciplinary assessment and treatment (National Consensus Project for Quality Palliative Care, 2004). Direct care providers take pivotal roles within the interdisciplinary team when caring for a person with IDD at the end of life. Each discipline supports and advises other team members in the provision of person-centered, culturally competent, comprehensive, and coordinated care. Registered nurses develop, coordinate, and execute plans of care in collaboration with physicians and other providers. Nursing assistants may provide up to 90% of assistance with activities of daily living for people residing in long-term care facilities and in the community (Hospice and Palliative Nurses Association [HPNA], 2005). The relationships between nursing assistants and the people they care for are intimate and sustaining, and their work at end of life must be valued and supported. Physical, occupational, and respiratory therapists apply their skills across the continuum of care to assist people with IDD at end of life, as do physical and occupational therapy assistants. Direct mental health care is provided by psychiatrists, psychologists, psychiatric nurses, and social workers. People with IDD are cared for, supported by, and touched by nonclinical service workers, certified medication aides, physician assistants, licensed practical nurses, dieticians, advanced practice nurses, and members of the clergy. It is our hope that each direct care provider who turns to this chapter will find discipline-relevant resources within the context of a larger shared frame of reference.

Two cases will be presented in the chapter. One vignette illustrates the complex needs of an older woman with mild IDD and highlights the importance of offering care in a situation in which there is a question about her capacity for informed consent, as well as limited family and social supports. The second case presents a situation in which a child with profound IDD has the loving, committed involvement of his family. That example highlights ethical considerations related to redirecting care to intensive comfort measures and the importance of education and values clarification with all members of the team.

There is an emphasis in this chapter on pain management resources for people with IDD—both because comfort is a central goal for end-of-life care and because there is a well-developed evidence base for pain management that is just beginning to address the needs of people with IDD. Pain management serves as one important way to explore the needs and resources for people with IDD at the end of life. Much is known about best practice palliative care and pain management. Health care of people with IDD exists as an established subspecialty. The blending of these practice domains and the development of research-based evidence has only recently begun (American Association on Intellectual and Developmental Disabilities [AAIDD], 2007; King, Janicki, Kissinger, & Lash, 2004; Oberlander & Symonds, 2006b).

How do we assess pain in a nonverbal person? What models, guidelines, and systems of care are available? How do we facilitate person-centered discussions and identify end-of-life wishes and priorities of people with IDD and their loved ones? What policy initiatives shape our current practice of end-of-life care with people with IDD? How do we translate knowledge into practice across the continuum of care and across the life span? Resources are available to assist with clinical decision making; many are included in the tables throughout the chapter. Table 20.1 provides selected basic topical references to the general issues pertaining to end-of-life care for individuals with IDD.

Table 20.1
Basic References

- American Association on Intellectual and Developmental Disabilities. (2007, July 5). *AAIDD position statement: Caring at the end of life.* Retrieved March 3, 2008, from http://www.aamr.org/content_170.cfm?navID=31

- King, A., Janicki, M., Kissinger, K., & Lash, S. (2004). *End of life care for people with developmental disabilities: The Last Passages project philosophy and recommendations.* Retrieved December 27, 2007, from http://www.albany.edu/aging/lastpassages

- National Hospice and Palliative Care Organization. (2005, February). *End of life care for people with developmental disabilities bibliography.* Retrieved December 27, 2007, from http://www.nhpco.org

- Oberlander, T., & Symonds, F. (Eds.). (2006). *Pain in children and adults with developmental disabilities.* Baltimore, MD: Paul H Brookes.

- Rubin, L., & Crocker, A. (Eds.). (2006). *Medical care for children and adults with developmental disabilities* (2nd ed.). Baltimore, MD: Paul H. Brookes.

- Symonds, F., Shinde, S., & Gilles, E. (2008). Perspectives on pain and intellectual disability. *Intellectual Disability Research, 52*(4), 275–286.

- Tuffrey-Wijne, I. (2003). The palliative care needs of people with intellectual disabilities: A literature review. *Palliative Medicine, 17*(1), 55–62.

Vignette 1

Mrs. Johnson, a 68-year-old married woman with a history of major depressive episodes and mild intellectual disability, was admitted to the inpatient oncology unit with a serious cancer diagnosis. Her husband accompanied her. He also had mild intellectual disability and a severe anxiety disorder and was visibly distraught and extremely anxious. In contrast, Mrs. Johnson had a calm and pleasant demeanor and expressed concern about her husband's distress. Mr. and Mrs. Johnson live independently in a local apartment complex. The couple reported they had no family support but identified several professional and community agencies to which they felt connected. Mrs. Johnson did not have a designated guardian, nor did she have an advance directive or health care proxy.

During the course of her hospitalization, it was important to evaluate Mrs. Johnson's capacity for consent, as well as the supports needed and available to her during her hospitalization and after her hospital discharge. A number of resources were mobilized. The psychiatric clinical nurse specialist provided consultation to the nursing staff with regard to gathering specific information about her history and baseline circumstance. Mrs. Johnson's primary care physician (PCP) provided information about the couple's prior ability to function well in the community and support each other. He also provided information about her psychiatric disorder that had been well managed with medications prescribed by her psychiatrist. In addition, a release was obtained from Mr. Johnson to speak to his medical and psychiatric providers to assess his capacity to provide ongoing support during this stressful time.

The medical oncology team provided information and management pertaining to the cancer. Consultation was also provided by the hospital psychiatrist to determine Mrs. Johnson's ability to consent to care and management of her psychiatric disorder. The psychiatrist met with Mrs. Johnson, who requested that her husband, therapist, and PCP be present to serve as advocates. She was able to understand the information and communicate her understanding of her cancer diagnosis, prognosis, and the consequences of her treatment options. She also was able to communicate her choices and explain the reason for her decisions.

Over the next couple of days, Mrs. Johnson decided to forgo chemotherapy because of the low likelihood of extending her life and high likelihood that it would negatively impact the quality of her remaining months of life. Mrs. Johnson's medical providers, nursing staff, oncology social worker, and hospital chaplain provided support to the couple. Mr. Johnson's medical and psychiatric providers were also involved in providing support. The palliative care team was consulted to assure that optimal symptom management strategies, support, and discharge planning were in place. The nurse case manager coordinated discharge planning with the visiting nurse's organization in the couple's hometown. Mrs. Johnson was discharged on a "bridge to hospice" plan of care.

In an environment of caring and support, Mr. and Mrs. Johnson do extraordinarily well from a psychosocial perspective. They both exhibit very clear strengths in coping with a difficult, complex, and profoundly sad situation. They make use of the many resources in the hospital setting and stay connected to their usual providers of care. While there is no family support for them, there is a team of familiar professionals available and prepared to support them.

Frameworks of Care

Palliative care improves quality of life through the prevention and relief of suffering and the treatment of pain and other physical, psychological, and spiritual problems (World

Health Organization [WHO], 2009). Hospice is a philosophy-driven system of care that is focused on noncurative services provided in the last 6 months of life. Hospice provides continuous palliative and supportive services to dying people and their families, through physical, psychological, social, and spiritual care given in the home or in freestanding centers (Lynn, Shuster, & Kabcenell, 2000). Hospice reimbursement requires physician certification and explicit redirection of care from curative to palliative treatment (National Consensus Project for Quality Palliative Care, 2004). "End of life" may be seen as the last 6 months of life, reflecting the standard for hospice care (AAIDD, 2007). Alternately, end-of-life care can be seen as that which is provided when death is a probable outcome (Friedman, 2006). Increasingly, palliative and hospice care are seen as existing along a continuum of care that rejects the 6 month timeline as arbitrary and acknowledges the palliative effects of treatments that may be classified as curative. Complex reimbursement issues are imbedded in creating a palliative and hospice care continuum (National Consensus Project, 2004).

For some people who have lived their entire lives with serious chronic medical conditions that are intertwined with cognitive and functional disability, anticipating the end-of-life time frame is less relevant than recognizing a likely nonreversible change or deterioration of condition. For others with an intellectual disability, like Mrs. Johnson, a recognized life-limiting disease is newly imposed upon a person's baseline level of functioning. In both cases, intensive support and relief of suffering are required. Regardless of circumstance, the presence of IDD does not make life any less valuable; it is not in and of itself a cause of suffering. The end-of-life needs of people with IDD may be complex and may require different skill sets from providers, but they are fundamentally no different from the end-of-life needs of people without IDD. Most importantly, unique needs must not limit access to excellent end-of-life care (AAIDD, 2007).

ETHICAL FOUNDATIONS

Direct care providers and their professional organizations have developed codes of ethics, systems, guidelines, position papers, and standards of care to articulate best practice when providing care to people with IDD throughout the life span, including the end of life. Ethics provides a moral foundation for professional practice and a helpful framework for caregiving where clinical situations appear unique, uncertain, complex, or without a clear evidence base.

Professional codes of ethics (American Association of Respiratory Care, 2007; American Physical Therapy Association [APTA], 2000; American Nurses Association [ANA], 2008; American Occupational Therapy Association Commission on Standards and Ethics [AOTA], 2005) mandate respect for human rights and human dignity. Further ethical principles of clinical practice relevant to the care of people with IDD at end of life include autonomy, or the right to self-determination; justice; nonmaleficence, or the principle of doing no harm; and beneficence, the principle of doing good. Professional codes of ethics are available for many of the professions that provide direct care to patients (AARC, 2007; ANA, 2008; AOTA, 2005; APTA, 2000).

The principles of autonomy and self-determination require that direct care providers include the person with IDD in decision-making processes (ANA and Nursing Division of the American Association on Mental Retardation, 2004). The ability to provide informed consent is deemed "competency," whereas the clinical ability to give informed consent is deemed "capacity" (Applebaum, 2007). Laws are conflicting and vary by state (King et al., 2004). Once people reach the age of 18, they are presumed to be competent to make their own medical decisions. In cases when competency is challenged, the court may appoint a guardian. Appointment of guardianship, however, may compromise dignity (Emmerich, 2006) as well as autonomy. People with IDD will have varying decision-making capacity and may have the capacity to express preferences even when competence has been challenged. These preferences should be respected (AAIDD, 2007). In situations in which a person does not have the capacity or competency to give consent, agreement with treatment, or assent, should be sought. It is always preferable to determine ability to provide consent before an acute clinical situation occurs; physicians and care teams frequently are presented with questions of capacity and competence when medical emergencies arise (Applebaum, 2007; Emmerich, 2006).

Scope and Standards of Practice

Direct care providers must function within their scope and standards of practice, as determined by state licensing boards, national credentialing boards, and professional governing bodies (ANA, 2004; ANA, 2005; ANA, 2007; APTA, 2003). Standards of practice for nurses who specialize in the care of people with IDD include providing care that is collaborative, comprehensive, coordinated, culturally competent, developmentally appropriate, person centered, inclusive, and supportive of normalization (ANA and Nursing Division of the American Association on Mental Retardation, 2004). Providers must understand clearly the scope of practice and standards of care of their chosen profession. They also are responsible for communicating explicitly their role and qualifications to individuals and families. In some states, nursing assistants may administer medications in long-term care, while certified medication aides and nonlicensed nurses may administer medications in community settings (*Texas Administrative Code*, 2008). Nurse practitioner and physician assistant prescription privileges, especially with regard to controlled substances, vary by state. Best interdisciplinary care is achieved when roles are clearly defined.

Position statements from professional governing bodies also provide guidance for care in specific clinical situations. Membership associations will articulate a position on an issue of importance to their members. This position may be in favor of a practice, may be against it, or may describe the scope of the issue without making recommendations (HPNA, n.d.). Position statements reflect current best scholarship on the issue and are important resources for direct care providers. The position statement references noted in Table 20.2 relate to end-of-life and pain management issues.

Pain Management

A wealth of resources exists for the direct care provider managing pain at end of life; however, fewer pain management resources are designed specifically to alleviate suffering of people with IDD at end of life. Until recently, little—if any—research focused on pain, its expression, and its treatment for people with IDD (Oberlander & Symonds, 2006a), severely limiting access to evidence-based pain management practice. The fundamental

---

Table 20.2
Position Statement References

- American Academy of Pain Medicine and American Pain Society. (1996, August 20). *The use of opioids for the treatment of chronic pain.* Retrieved April 21, 2008, from http://www.ampainsoc.org/advocacy/opioids.htm

- American Geriatrics Society Panel on Persistent Pain in Older Persons. (2002). AGS panel on persistent pain in older adults. *Journal of the American Geriatric Society, 50*(6), S205–S224.

- American Society for Pain Management Nursing. (2003). *ASPMN position statement on pain management at end of life.* Retrieved March 3, 2008, from http://www.aspmn.org/Organization/documents/EndofLifeCare.pdf

- American Society for Pain Management Nursing. (2006, June). *Authorized and unauthorized ("PCA by proxy") dosing of analgesic infusion pumps.* Retrieved March 3, 2008, from http://www.aspmn.org/Organization/documents/PCAbyProxy -final-EW_004.pdf

- Gorman, L., Beach, P., Ersek, M., Montana, B., Bartel, J. (2003, October). *HPNA position statement on pain.* Retrieved February 23, 2009, from http://www.hpna.org/ DisplayPage.aspx?Title=Position%20Statements

- Hospice and Palliative Nurses Association (HPNA). (n.d.). *Hospice and Palliative Nurses Association: HPNA Position Statements: 13 position statements addressing topics such as pain, palliative sedation at end of life, and the value of the a nursing assistant in end of life care.* Retrieved February 23, 2009, from http://www.hpna.org/ DisplayPage.aspx?Title=Position%20Statements

---

tenets of end-of-life pain management need not be rewritten to be relevant to the care of people with IDD. People of all ages with IDD must have their pain recognized and treated, and it is imperative to apply bedrock principles of palliation, pain assessment, and pain management to their care at end of life.

The challenges are to identify current knowledge and translate it into effective clinical practice. Direct care providers may not be aware of resources that have been developed specifically for people with IDD, and they may not be aware of important clinical considerations relevant to pain management for people with IDD. Another challenge is to individualize this knowledge and practice. Children and adults with IDD are a heterogeneous group, with each person embodying unique abilities, capacities, and health status. Best practice pain management requires a skilled blending of knowledge obtained from the person with pain, his or her loved ones, and care providers; the knowledge of pain management in people with IDD; and the best pain management practices in general.

PAIN IN IDD

McCaffery's iconic definition of pain states that "pain is what the experiencing person says it is, existing whenever he says it does" (McCaffery, 1968). The International Association for the Study of Pain (IASP) definition of pain states that pain is an "unpleasant sensory and emotional experience associated with actual or potential tissue damage, or described in terms of such damage" (IASP, 1994, p. 210). These definitions have been recognized to exclude pain felt by people who cannot speak or describe their pain experience (Kennedy & O'Reilly, 2006, Symonds, Shinde, & Gilles, 2008). Current conceptions of pain describe a subjective, multidimensional phenomenon with emotional and sensory attributes (Kennedy & O'Reilly, 2006). In 2002, the IASP annotated their definition of pain to acknowledge that "the inability to communicate verbally does not negate the possibility that an individual is experiencing pain and is in need of appropriate pain relieving treatment" (IASP, 2002).

There are long-held and inaccurate assumptions about the pain experience of people with IDD. Historically, people with IDD have been thought to be less sensitive, or indifferent to pain (Symonds et al., 2008). However, people with IDD often live with chronic medical conditions that put them at higher risk for pain and painful medical procedures than the general population. Adults with cerebral palsy report substantial musculoskeletal pain (Bottos & Chambers, 2006; Hodgkinson et al., 2001; Winter & Kiely, 2006). Gastroesophageal reflux disease (GERD) and its associated discomfort are found in 70%–75% of children with neurodevelopmental disability (Fishman & Bousvaros, 2006). Studies of pain response and perception in adults with IDD indicate that, while a person's response time to stimulus may be delayed, sensation of pain may be greater (Breau, McGrath, & Zabalia, 2006). Nurses and physicians have been observed to underestimate pain experienced by a person with IDD (Colatarci & Nehring, 2002). Parents and family caregivers may be best at identifying pain in a child with IDD, but even they have been seen to underestimate a child's pain (Stallard, Williams, Lenton, & Vellman, 2001). Pain may be misconstrued as "behavior" to be managed (Bodfish, Harper, Deacon, Deacon, & Symons, 2006). We may conclude that people with IDD are at higher risk for both pain and the nonidentification of that pain.

VIGNETTE 2

Aaron, a 15-year-old Asian American adolescent, had profound intellectual disability, spastic quadriplegic cerebral palsy, severe kyphoscoliosis, epilepsy, recurrent aspiration pneumonia, and reactive airway disease. Neuropsychological testing indicated that he functioned within the 6- to 9-month developmental age range. He was born at 27 weeks gestation and required a prolonged hospital course with a number of complications. Soon after hospital discharge, he experienced a respiratory arrest that was later determined to be secondary to aspiration. He subsequently required tracheostomy for upper airway obstruction and placement of a feeding tube for failure to thrive. Soon after, he experienced the first of many difficult-to-control seizures. At 15, he continued to require supplemental oxygen.

Aaron resided at home with his parents and his 17-year-old sister. When he was in good health, he was described as being socially responsive and happy. He enjoyed being included in family activities, often protesting loudly if left alone. He showed particular pleasure in close face-to-face interaction with family members, especially his sister. He attended school and received home services from registered nurses, licensed practical nurses, and nursing assistants who assisted the family in his care.

Over the years, however, his chronic lung disease worsened, the frequency of his hospitalizations increased, and his recovery time began to lengthen. Aaron became withdrawn and appeared sad when in the hospital. His parents worried that he did not understand what was occurring in this unfamiliar place and that he was unable to communicate all but the worst pain to caregivers who did not know him well.

At his last hospitalization, his health care team discussed with his family the significant deterioration of his medical condition, with anticipation of continued worsening. This discussion led to the decision for a Do-Not-Resuscitate (DNR) order. This decision was consistent with their desire to protect him from further hospitalizations and painful treatments that would detract from his quality of life without changing the progression of his disease. When he was discharged from the hospital, his community primary care provider signed a community DNR/comfort care order.

Aaron's sister became withdrawn and moody when he returned from the hospital. His direct care staff also had a mixed reaction to the change in his resuscitation status. While the home health agency did provide general end-of-life training, additional support was accessed from the agency's palliative care team. Emphasis was placed on how to best translate philosophy of care into practice: palliation to provide comfort and relief of symptoms. Family counseling and spiritual needs were evaluated. It was reiterated that the DNR order does not preclude active and responsive treatment of pain and reversible illness, and every effort was made to identify ways to improve symptom management and quality of life. A pain and symptom management plan was developed with Aaron's physician and nurse practitioner in consultation with the hospital pain specialist. The nurses identified a validated pain-assessment tool and reviewed its use with direct care staff and family members. In keeping with the hospice model, care and support were available to Aaron and his family at all times of day and night. The family and team agreed to give antibiotics by feeding tube and to provide pulmonary toilet but to avoid rehospitalization.

Within a month, Aaron developed another lower respiratory tract infection and his medical condition deteriorated further. His family and nurses arranged a home visit from his primary care provider to assess Aaron's illness and to discuss ongoing care. Aaron's pediatrician informed the family that Aaron was gravely ill. In spite of their previous decision to avoid hospitalization, his parents were reassured that they could change their minds at any time. Options for Aaron's care were reviewed, and it was decided that hospice services could best be provided in Aaron's home setting. The decision not to transport Aaron to an acute care facility was reaffirmed.

In the next days, family and caregivers worked to assure pain relief and symptom control while acknowledging and processing grief and loss. The physical therapist reviewed positioning and mobility recommendations with the family and direct care providers. The respiratory therapist evaluated and revised the plan for Aaron's pulmonary toilet and suctioning needs. It was clearly communicated that Aaron's death was expected within days. Aaron's parents discussed family and cultural death practices that they wished to have observed. Pain and air hunger were treated with around-the-clock opioid analgesics. Blow-by oxygen and tracheal suction were provided for comfort. Aaron was monitored for constipation, urinary retention, nausea, and other side effects of opioids.

Aaron's periods of wakefulness decreased. Caregivers and family members understood that an actively dying person does not experience hunger or thirst. After a single episode of retching with a formula feeding, Aaron was transitioned to small amounts of clear liquid by tube. As bowel functions slowed, feedings were stopped altogether. Aaron died quietly in the family living room with his parents, sister, and direct care providers at his side.

PAIN ACROSS THE CONTINUUM OF IDD

Several important attributes of people with IDD have direct impact on pain assessment and management: developmental skills and capacities, primary disease effects and comorbid conditions, and challenging behaviors (Bottos & Chambers, 2006; Breau, Stevens, & Grunau, 2006; Kennedy & O'Reilly, 2006; Roane, Fisher, Call, & Kelley, 2006). Family and caregivers are often sources of important and accurate information about the pain, discomfort, and behavior of a nonverbal person. Core pain behaviors common to people with moderate to severe IDD also have been identified.

Verbal communication skills, as well as cognitive and emotional developmental capacities, will have a direct impact on which assessment tool is most appropriate. Assessment and documentation of developmental skills can be found in educational service plans. Colatarci and Nehring (2002) found that direct care providers overestimated the cognitive abilities of people using a numeric rating scale for pain assessment, leading to inadequate pain relief. Some children with mild to moderate IDD may be able to use representative pain tools such as the Faces Pain Scale, Revised (FPS-R; Hicks, von Baeyer, Spafford, van Korlaar, & Goodenough, 2001) to accurately self-report pain (Breau et al., 2006), while people with severe to profound IDD can benefit from use of a pain tool such as the Non-Communicating Children's Pain Checklist (NCCPC-Revised, NCCPC-Postoperative Version; Breau, McGrath, Camfield, & Finley, 2000; Breau, McGrath, Finley, & Camfield, 2004a).

Direct care providers can reasonably predict that certain types of pain will occur with certain primary disease states and comorbid conditions. Pain associated with infection, constipation, GERD, spasticity, accidental injury, surgery, and other procedures can be anticipated, and care can be planned accordingly. Chronic pain may develop from undertreatment of acute pain (WHO, 2006). Types of pain are further discussed in chapter 6. Bottos and Chambers (2006) provide an extensive review of the epidemiology of pain in people with IDD. Direct care providers must anticipate and honor the psychic pain associated with grief, loss, and bereavement. Depression in the population of people with IDD is at least as prevalent as it is in the general population (Pary, El-Defrawi, Khan, Parvin, & Hatch-Warner, 2006).

Challenging behaviors may confound provider assessment of pain, as well as perceptions of a person's capacity to feel pain. Self-injurious behaviors (SIB) occur in 10%–16% of people with IDD (Kennedy & O'Reilly, 2006; Roane et al., 2006;). People who exhibit SIB have been thought to be indifferent to pain or to have qualitatively different pain experiences. Recent work indicates that children with IDD and SIB have pain expression equal to that of children with IDD who do not exhibit SIB (Breau et al., 2003). Physical and/or emotional discomfort may manifest as aggressive or self-injurious behavior (Emmerich, 2006; Kennedy & O'Reilly, 2006). Relief from episodic pain has been associated with decreased incidence of SIB and aggression (Kennedy & O'Reilly, 2006). An analgesic trial is recommended if pain is a possible cause of distress that is not relieved by routine comfort measures (Herr et al., 2006).

Pain Assessment

Identification and measurement of pain is accomplished through the use of reliable and valid pain assessment tools. Reliability refers to a tool's ability to consistently measure a concept, while validity is the tool's ability to measure the concept itself. In the case of pain in people with IDD, this means identifying a given measure of pain (moderate pain, or a treatable threshold of pain) repeatedly and across a population, while also identifying pain itself, rather than another cause for behavioral change, such as depression.

Tools that are designed for the intended population and have been found to be reliable and valid are more likely to identify pain than tools that are designed for other populations. Populations without verbal communication skills may be very different. Tools designed for nonverbal elders with dementia may not capture pain behaviors of a child with severe cognitive and motor disabilities, placing that child at risk for unidentified pain. Validated instruments should be used for pain assessment when available (National Consensus Project for Quality Palliative Care, 2004). The American Society of Pain Management Nursing (ASPMN) clinical practice recommendations emphasize clinician responsibility in choosing reliable, appropriate, clinically feasible, and population-specific assessment tools (Herr et al., 2006).

Pain scales can be verbal, visual, or numeric; observational/behavioral scales are often used for people who are unable to provide self-report, including infants, young children, elders with dementia, and people with IDD. Verbal scales provide language to describe pain, such as mild, moderate, or severe. Numeric scales rate pain severity from 0 to 10, with higher numbers representing more pain. The FPS-R (Hicks, von Baeyer, Spafford, van Korlaar, & Goodenough, 2001) presents sequential pictures of faces depicting pain; the scale can be used with or without a numeric pain rating scale, according to the developmental capacity of the person with pain (von Baeyer, 2001). The FLACC scale (Faces, Legs, Activity, Cry, and Consolabilty), an observational tool developed for infants and young children, has been validated for use in children with severe to profound IDD (Voepel-Lewis, Merkel, Tait, Trzcinka, & Malvia, 2002).

A number of observational/behavioral tools have been developed specifically for use with children and adults with severe to profound levels of IDD. Of these, the Non-Communicating Children's Checklist, in both its revised and postoperative versions (NCCPC-R and NCCPC-PV; Breau, McGrath, Finley, & Camfield, 2004a, 2004b) and the Paediatric Pain Profile (PPP; University College London, 2003) have been validated for use with children with severe to profound IDD. The NCCPC-R and PV were designed for ease of clinical use and do not require a manual. Research is underway to validate the NCCPC with adults in a residential facility (Breau, 2008, personal communication). The Pain and Discomfort Scale (PADS; Bodfish, Harper, Deacon, & Symons, 2001) was developed and validated for use with adults with severe to profound IDD using items similar to the NCCPC (Bodfish et al., 2006). A standardized Pain Examination Procedure (PEP) accompanies the PADS. The PEP was developed to increase tool sensitivity to adult chronic pain and to assist in eliciting and localizing that pain (Bodfish et al., 2006). Table 20.3 lists pain assessment measures that have been developed and/or validated for use with children or adults with IDD.

Ease of use and feasibility of a given tool will depend upon individual and system factors impacting a given clinical situation. The complexity of the 27-item NCCPC-PV may add to decreased ease of use in the acute care setting (Voepel-Lewis et al., 2008). The NCCPC may have clinical feasibility in the home or in settings where caregiver to patient ratios are lower, although this has not yet been evaluated. Tools such as the PPP

Table 20.3
Pain Tools

Pediatric pain

- DESS: Echelle Douleur Enfant San Salvador (Fondacion CNP 1999): Available in French at http://www.CNp.fr/polyhand and embedded in "Validation of a Pain Evaluation Scale for Patients With Severe Cerebral Palsy," by P. Collignon and B. Guisano, 2001, *European Journal of Pain, 5*, pp. 433–442.

- NCCPC-R and NCCPC-PV: Non-Communicating Children's Pain Checklist-Revised and Non-Communicating Children's Checklist-Postoperative Version: Available at http://www.aboutkidshealth.ca/Shared/PDFs/AKH_Breau_post-op.pdf and http://www.aboutkidshealth.ca/Shared/PDFs/AKH_Breau_everyday.pdf

- PPP: Paediatric Pain Profile: Available at http://www.ppprofile.org.uk

- FLACC: Face, Legs, Activity, Cry, Consolabilty Scale: Available at http://painconsortium.nih.gov/pain_scales/

- FACES: The Faces Pain Scale, Revised: Available at http://painsourcebook.ca/pdfs/pps92.pdf

- PICIC: Pain Indicator for Communicatively Impaired Children: Items are available embedded in "Pain in Cognitively Impaired, Non-Communicating Children," by P. Stallard, L. Williams, S. Lenton, and R. Vellman, 2001, *Archives of Disease in Childhood, 85*, pp. 460–462.

- INRS: Individualized Numeric Rating Scale: Tool is embedded in "Pain Assessment in Nonverbal Children With Severe Cognitive Impairments: The Individualized Numeric Rating Scale (INRS)," by J. Solodiuk and M. A. Curley, 2003, *Journal of Pediatric Nursing 18*(4), pp. 295–299.

Adult pain

- PADS: Pain and Discomfort Scale: Available from Western Carolina Research Reports, Western Carolina Center, 300 Enola Rd., Morganton, NC 28655, USA.

- DisDAT: Disability Distress Assessment Tool: Available at http://www.disdat.co.uk

- FACES: The Faces Pain Scale, Revised: Available at http://painsourcebook.ca/pdfs/pps92.pdf

and the Individualized Numeric Rating Scale (INRS; Solodiuk & Curley, 2003) require documentation of pain behavior history and family/caregiver input, providing access to personalized information while fostering alliance with multiple invested caregivers. The Disability Distress Assessment Tool (DisDAT; Northumberland Tyne & Wear National Health Service Trust and St. Oswald's Hospice, 2006) provides an opportunity to record baseline behaviors, from which ease and distress can be identified by multiple caregivers.

Pain Management Interventions

A wide range of therapeutic modalities, medications, and pain management guidelines are available to clinicians managing pain at end of life. Of particular importance is the use of pharmacotherapy for pain and symptom management. In addition to administering and monitoring pharmacotherapy, direct care providers modify environments, provide therapeutic positioning, and modulate sensory experiences for people at end of life. Assessment of patient and provider expectations of a pain management intervention increases communication and collaboration and encourages discussion of realistic expectations. It is unclear if assessment of expectations leads to more positive outcomes (Long & Guite, 2008).

Pharmacotherapy

Children with moderate to severe cerebral palsy receive an average of 3.8 daily medications (Liptak, 2001). Eighty-five percent of children and adults with severe and profound disabilities have seizures, while 65% have severe constipation, 51% have GERD, and 62% have spastic quadriplegic cerebral palsy (Rubin, 2006). Pharmacotherapy for primary and comorbid medical conditions place people with IDD at risk for medication interactions, side effects, and exacerbation of one disease process in the attempt to treat another. The convergence of medication, symptom, and disease is a dynamic phenomenon that requires a nuanced management approach. Pain medication management must be individualized to assure symptom management and relief from pain.

Theoretical frameworks and guidelines exist to guide pain management practices. The World Health Organization Pain Ladder (WHO, 1994, 1990) provides an effective and widely accepted model of pain medication titration, emphasizing a stepwise approach to pain relief. The three-step framework recommends prompt use of nonopioid medications for mild pain, advancing to weak and then strong opioids as quickly as needed to produce relief from moderate or severe pain. Adjuvant medications—those whose primary indication is for conditions other than pain (Taddio & Oberlander, 2006a)—are used at any point to enhance response to primary analgesic therapy. The oral or enteral route of administration is preferred over injection to avoid repeated painful administration.

Components of excellent pain medication guidelines include medication recommendations for given clinical circumstances and conditions, including medication doses, routes, and alternatives. There should be integration of such concepts as opioid titration, equianalgesia, adjuvant pain medication use, and symptom and management. Table 20.4 highlights published pain management guidelines as well as pain guideline sections of comprehensive, evidence-based Web sites committed to excellence in palliative care and pain management. Chapter 6 also provides guidelines for treatment of pain.

Table 20.4
Pain Management Guidelines and Resources

- Pain Treatment Topics Current Pain Treatment Guidelines: Available at http://www.pain-topics.org/guidelines_reports/current_guidelines.php

- National Guidelines Clearinghouse: Available at http://www.guidelines.gov

- American Medical Directors Association. (2003). *Pain management in the long-term care setting: Clinical practice guideline*. Columbia, MD: Author.

- EPERC: End of Life/Palliative Education Resource Center, Fast Facts and Concepts: Pain A Opioids, Pain B Non-Opioids, Pain C Evaluation: Available at http://www.eperc.mcw.edu/ff_index.htm. Also available as a handheld device download at http://www.infingo.com/portal.php

- City of Hope: Pain and symptom management: Pharmacology policies and procedures: Available at http://www.cityofhope.org/prc/pharm.asp

  - Beckman Research Institute Pain and Symptom Management: Available at http://www.cityofhope.org/prc/pain_assessment.asp

  - City of Hope Pain & Palliative Care Resource Center: http://www.cityofhope.org/prc

---

Pharmacotherapy requires careful attention to drug interactions and side effects. Nonsteroidal anti-inflammatory drugs (NSAIDS) may be contraindicated for people with gastritis or congestive heart failure. Opioid medications may have a synergistic effect with other centrally acting medications such as antiepileptics and antispasmodics. Drug induction or inhibition of cytochrome P450 hepatic enzymes may raise or lower serum levels of other medication. Concomitant use of potent P450 3A4 inhibitors such as clarithromycin with long acting opioid preparations such as methadone or the fentanyl patch may result in increased opioid plasma concentrations, leading to risk of respiratory depression (Taketoma, Hodding, & Kraus, 2007). Recently identified genetic differences in hepatic medication metabolism will assist in the identification people of Asian descent at risk for developing Stevens Johnson syndrome with carbamazepine (U.S. Food and Drug Administration, n.d.), an antiepileptic drug sometimes used as a pain adjuvant. Use of routine doses of short-acting benzodiazepines for adjuvant antianxiety pharmacotherapy may not be as effective in people who receive short-acting benzodiazepines routinely for management of spasticity or breakthrough seizures.

People with IDD may require pharmacy compounding of medication for administration via gastrostomy or jejunostomy tube. Certain medications should not be crushed for administration via tube or to be mixed in a vehicle for oral ingestion; direct care providers should consult "do not crush" lists available in drug handbooks (Taketoma, Hodding, & Kraus, 2007).

Patient-controlled analgesia (PCA) may be appropriate at end of life (Prommer, 2008). Clinicians, patients, and families will benefit from protocols to differentiate between people who are able to access PCA, and those who may benefit from the use of an authorized agent, such as a trained family member or health care professional, to administer analgesia on their behalf (Allegreta, 2005; American Society for Pain Management Nursing, 2006).

Historical barriers to the use of opioids at end of life have included concerns for patient addiction and hastening of death from suppression of respiratory effort. People who are actively dying and experiencing pain are not at risk for addiction. Addiction is a disease characterized by compulsive use of a substance, use in the face of harm, use due to craving, and/or poor control over use. In contrast, physical dependence on opioids is a state of adaptation to the medication that will result in withdrawal symptoms in the setting of rapid reduction of the drug dose. Opioid dependence is a normal response to treatment (American Academy of Pain Medicine, American Pain Society, and American Society of Addiction Medicine, 2007; American Society of Interventional Pain Physicians, 2006). Prescribers and caregivers also may be concerned that they will be accused of euthanasia, yet properly titrated morphine at end of life rarely hastens death (Campbell, 2008; von Gunten, 2005). Concerns for hastening death are particularly salient to the care of a vulnerable population whose lives historically have not been valued (Friedman, 2006). To guide care in situations where both pain relief and respiratory suppression are possible with opioid use, providers have turned to the ethical principle of double effect. Double effect holds that an effect that would be morally impermissible if it were caused intentionally is permissible if that harm is unintended, even if that effect can be foreseen (Campbell, 2008; McIntyre, 2008; Schwarz, 2004; von Gunten, 2005).

Table 20.5 provides print, handheld device, and Web-based pharmacology and medication administration resources to assist direct care providers with pain and symptom management. Information about adverse drug events is gathered continuously; it is imperative that the prescribers and professionals responsible for medication administration and education consult the most current medication resources. Several Internet-based applications offer free medication interaction checks: ePocrates.com (http://www.epocrates.com) offers a free online pharmaceutical application with formularies, medication interaction checks, and full drug monographs. Medscape (http://www.medscape.com) offers an online medication interaction application in addition to journal articles and continuing-education offerings. Quinn's (2007) review of online opioid conversion calculators provides an excellent overview of the subject.

COMPLEMENTARY AND ALTERNATIVE THERAPIES

Complementary and alternative medicine (CAM) can be defined as a "group of diverse medical and health care systems, practices, and products that are not generally considered part of conventional medicine" (National Center for Complementary and Alternative Medicine, 2009). Complementary therapies augment standard medical treatment, while alternative therapies replace standard medical treatment. Integrative medicine (IM) "combines mainstream medical therapies and CAM therapies for which there is some high-quality scientific evidence of safety and effectiveness" (National Center for Complementary and Alternative Medicine, 2009). Table 20.6 provides a list of complementary and alternative therapies. Certain CAM therapies may have merit, or may be desired, in end-of-life care and pain management for people with IDD; however, there is little peer-reviewed evidence of safe and effective CAM practice in people with IDD at end of life.

Table 20.5
Medication Administration Resources

- Epocrates Medical PDA Software: Epocrates online includes free access to current concise drug information, mouse-over drug interactions, and a medication interaction feature. *Epocrates Rx*, their basic software, is available for free download; other more comprehensive products are available for purchase: http://www .epocrates.com/

- Hopkins Opioid Program at the Sidney Kimmel Comprehensive Cancer Center at Johns Hopkins: http://www.hopweb.org

- Lacy, C. F., Armstrong, L. L., Goldman, M. P., & Lance, L. L. (Eds.). (2009). *Drug Information Handbook* (18th ed.). Hudson, OH: Lexi-Comp.

- Narcotic Analgesic Converter: http://www.globalrph.com/narcoticonv.htm

- Pujol, L. M., Katz, N. P., & Zacharoff, K. L. (2007). *The PainEdu.org manual: A pocket guide to pain management.* Retrieved March 3, 2008, from http://www .painedu.org

- Quinn, T. E. (2007, February 27). *Pain topics: Converting opioid analgesics, part II: Review of equianalgesic conversion calculators.* Retrieved April 23, 2008, from http:// www.massgeneral.org/PainRelief/Pain%20Topics/Opioid_calculators_V3.07.pdf

- Taketoma, C. K., Hodding, J. H., & Kraus, D. M. (2008). *Pediatric dosage handbook* (15th ed.). Hudson, Ohio: Lexi-Comp. Updated annually, this is a comprehensive medication reference containing extended drug monographs, as well as an extensive appendix, including cyochrome P450 enzyme tables and a list of noncrushable medications. Available in print, PDA, and CD-ROM.

- U.S. Food and Drug Administration. (n.d.). *MedWatch: The FDA safety information and adverse event reporting program.* Retrieved May 3, 2008, from http://www.fda .gov/medwatch/index.htm

Up to 4 in 10 adults and 1 in 9 children in the United States used some form of CAM in 2007 (Barnes, Bloom, & Nahin, 2008). Given such numbers, CAM may already be part of a person's health practices before end-of-life care is sought. Complementary and alternative therapies are most frequently used to address musculoskeletal pain (Barnes et al., 2008; Tsao & Zeltzer, 2005). People turn to CAM because other therapies have not been completely effective, or because a CAM therapy focuses on the health and wellness of the whole person, rather than on illness alone (American Academy of Pediatrics Committee on Children with Disabilities, 2001). Because end-of-life care strives to provide person-centered care that honors individual choices, incorporation of CAM into conventional end-of-life care strategies can be a valuable extension of the continuum of care. Critical evaluation of known risks and benefits of a given CAM modality is crucial as we work with individuals and families to design comprehensive, effective, and individualized plans of care.

The availability of high-quality scientific evidence about CAM therapies is increasing; overall, however, there is a relative dearth of evidence on the use of many CAM

Table 20.6
CAM Modalities

Biologically based practice

Vitamins and minerals	Herbs/botanicals
Functional foods	Probiotics

Energy medicine

Reiki	Therapeutic touch
Magnet therapy	

Manipulative and body-based practices

Massage	Reflexology
Spinal manipulation	

Mind–body medicine

Meditation	Ayurveda
Yoga	Homeopathy
Guided imagery	Naturopathy
Whole medical systems	Traditional Chinese medicine (acupuncture, moxibustion)

Source: National Institute of Health (NIH) Senior Health, 2008, "What Is CAM?"
Retrieved February 22, 2009, from http://www.nihseniorhealth.gov/cam/
whatiscam/01.html

modalities. Much of the research looking at outcomes has been questioned because of methodological issues, such as small sample size. Tsao and Zeltzer (2005) review evidence on CAM approaches for pediatric pain. Aromatherapy, acupuncture, massage, and music therapy have been used at end of life to ameliorate pain, nausea, depression, and anxiety (Dileo & Brandt, 2008; Kutner, 2008; National Cancer Institute, 2008a, 2008b; So, Jiang, & Qin, 2008). Acupuncture, acupressure, and massage therapy have been used for relief of pain associated with the spasticity of cerebral palsy (Liptak, 2005).

It is important to evaluate available evidence on the safety and efficacy of a proposed intervention. Music therapy, guided imagery, aromatherapy, and massage can contribute to increased well-being without a high risk of unintended negative effects. Chiropractic care is contraindicated for people with osteoporosis. Acupuncture may be contraindicated for people who cannot provide feedback on the effect of needling. Many medicinal herbs have known side effects and interactions with prescription medications. Frequent reevaluation of client satisfaction, goals of care, positive therapeutic outcomes, negative side effects, and current research will assure the safety and efficacy of the integrated plan of care.

Discussion of the risks and benefits of individual CAM practices is beyond the scope of this chapter. Important online and print resources exist to assist direct care providers to understand and think critically about CAM and IM, and their role in the care of people with IDD at end of life. National and international professional organizations have established educational and research arms dedicated to the study of CAM. There is a need to investigate the use and effects of these interventions specific to people with IDD so that we may in identify strategies that contribute to high-quality end-of-life care for people with IDD and their families. See Table 20.7 for CAM resources.

PULLING IT ALL TOGETHER

We provide end-of-life care in a broad and interconnected world of professional and personal communities. Professional specialty interest groups provide a nexus of research and clinical practice knowledge. Some professional groups are multidisciplinary, others discipline specific. Family and lay specialty-interest groups articulate human needs and perspectives, allowing us to learn about the relevant issues in providing person-centered care. The Internet increasingly provides a ready access portal to organization-specific content, including extensive online published resources. Content may be free, or may be available for purchase; membership to a given professional organization often includes access to important resources not available to the general public. Selected organizations with resource-rich Internet Web portals are listed in Table 20.8.

Table 20.7
CAM Resources

- The Alternative Medicine Homepage: http://www.pitt.edu/~cbw/altm.html
- Audette, J., & Bailey, A. (Eds.). (2007). *Integrative pain medicine: The science and practice of complementary and alternative medicine in pain management.* Totowa, NJ: Humana Press.
- Bravewell Collaborative: http://www.bravewell.org
- Cochrane Collaboration: http://www.cochrane.org
- Consortium of Academic Health Centers for Integrative Medicine: http://www.imconsortium.org
- Counseling Families Using CAM by the American Academy of Pediatrics: http://pediatrics.aappublications.org/cgi/reprint/107/3/598
- Giese, T., and the Commission on Practice. (2005). Complementary and alternative medicine (CAM) position paper. *American Journal of Occupational Therapy, 59*, 653–655.
- Hospice and Palliative Nurses Association Position Statement: *Complementary Therapies in Palliative Care Nursing Practice*: http://www.hpna.org/DisplayPage.aspx?Title=Position%20Statements
- National Center for Complementary and Alternative Medicine: http://nccam.nih.gov
- Physicians Desk Reference, Inc. (2008). *PDR for nonprescription drugs, dietary supplements, and herbs* (30th ed.). Montvale, NJ: Thomson Reuters.

Table 20.8
Select Professional and Lay Organizations

American Association on Intellectual and Developmental Disabilities (formerly American Association on Mental Retardation): http://www.aamr.org

American Occupational Therapy Association: http://www.aota.org

American Pain Association: http://www.painassociation.org

American Pain Society: http://www.ampainsoc.org

American Physical Therapy Association: http://www.apta.org

American Society for Pain Management Nursing: http://www.aspmn.org

The Arc of the United States: http://www.thearc.org

Association of University Centers on Disabilities: http://www.aucd.org

The Center to Advance Palliative Care: http://www.capc.org

End of Life/Palliative Care Resource Center (EPERC): http://www.eperc.mcw.edu

The Exceptional Parent: http://www.eparent.com

The Family Caregiver Alliance: http://www.caregiver.org

Family Ties of Massachusetts: http://www.massfamilyties.org

Home Health Nurses Association: http://www.hhna.org

Hospice and Palliative Nurses Association: http://www.hpna.org

International Association for the Study of Pain (IASP): http://www.iasp.org

National Hospice and Palliative Care Organization: http://www.nhpco.org

Social Work in Hospice and Palliative Care Network: http://www.swhpn.org

We bring diverse personal and professional experiences to end-of-life care. Different frames of reference also may potentially create barriers to communication and understanding. Diversity of opinion and philosophy enrich and deepen the quality of our care; however, opinion and philosophy must be grounded in knowledge, evidence, and learning from the expertise of others. Direct care providers must seek out education into end-of-life best practices and education that deepens our understanding of the lives of people with IDD and their loved ones. The quality of available curricula for clinicians practicing end-of-life care is striking: University degree programs, palliative and pain management consortia, certification programs, and institutional educational initiatives provide access to creative, excellent, and clinically relevant courses of study. Much current knowledge is directly applicable to the care of people with IDD and their families, yet disability-specific end-of-life needs are only beginning to be articulated.

Current, comprehensive, disability-specific curricula for clinicians are an important priority and are only beginning to emerge (Hahn & Cadogan, 2007; Nehring, 2005). National policy reflects this educational priority and is embodied in University Centers for Excellence in Developmental Disability, located at 67 sites across the United States (http://www.ACUD.org). Continued research into end-of-life pain management for people with IDD and educational curricula reflecting this knowledge are two of many compelling needs. It is necessary to continue to develop discipline-specific educational resources about the complex needs of individuals with IDD approaching end of life. Table 20.9 notes curricula available for direct care providers, including those designed for care of people with IDD.

CONCLUSION

The examples of Aaron and Mrs. Johnson illustrate for direct care providers some of the many complex issues and concerns faced by people with IDD and their families as they cope with life-threatening illness.

Table 20.9
Select Pain and Palliative Care Curricula and Educational Resources

- Hahn, J. E., & Cadogan, M. P. (2007). *A developmental approach to palliative and end of life care—handbook for trainers.* Los Angeles: UCLA School of Nursing.

- Hospice and Palliative Nurses Association. (2007). *Core curriculum for the advanced practice hospice and palliative nurse* (M. J. Perley & C. M. Dahlin, Eds.). Dubuque, IA: Kendall/Hunt.

- Hospice and Palliative Nurses Association. (2005). *Core curriculum for the generalist hospice and palliative care nurse* (2nd ed.). Dubuque, IA: Kendall/Hunt.

- International Association for the Study of Pain (IASP). (2008). *Proposed curricula on pain for Schools of Dentistry (1993), Medicine (1988), Nursing, 2nd ed. (2006), Pharmacy (1992), Psychology (1997), and Occupational/Physical therapy (1994).* Retrieved May 3, 2008, from http://www.iasp-pain.org/AM/Template. cfm?Section=Curricula&Template=/CM/HTMLDisplay.cfm&ContentID=1952

- Initiative for Pediatric Palliative Care (IPPC). (2008, April 27). *IPPC curriculum.* Newton, MA: Center for Applied Ethics at EDC.

- Nehring, W. (Ed.). (2005). *Core curriculum for specializing in intellectual and developmental disabilities: A resource for nurses and other health care professionals.* Boston: Jones and Bartlett.

- University Centers for Excellence in Developmental Disabilities 50 programs in the United States, with links to each found at http://www.aucd.org. Example: Morreim, E. (2005). Ethical challenges in making decisions for, about, and with patients with disabilities. University of Tennessee Boling Center for Developmental Disabilities Interdisciplinary Leadership Training Series: CD-ROMs Fall 2004 through Fall 2006. Memphis: UT Boling Center for Developmental Disabilities. http://www.utmem.edu/bcdd/resources/CD_Roms.htm

- U.S. Veterans Administration; SUMMIT, Stanford University Medical School. (2008). End of life online curriculum. In V. J. Periyakoil (Ed.), *The end-of-life curriculum project.* Retrieved May 3, 2008, from http://endoflife.stanford.edu

In health care, there is often an underappreciation of the importance of discussion, reflection, and sharing perspectives to identifying the needs and concerns of patients, families, and staff. Reflecting together offers staff the opportunity to share and process their responses and feelings to situations that often involve a great deal of suffering for patients and their families. Reflection is itself a resource: careful thought and reflection permit synthesis of the complexities of care.

The authors would like to conclude this chapter by underscoring the critical importance of self-care for all direct care providers who offer caring at end of life. An intentional emphasis on self-care in work settings and in personal lives can provide some counterbalance to the emotional demands that caring during this phase of life entail. Exposure to suffering is an inherent element of caring. Opportunities to share worry, sadness, and other difficult feelings with colleagues at work can provide connection and a way to honor the work and challenges experienced with caring. When providers recognize their unique contributions—easing suffering, mitigating distress, offering healing where cure is not possible—they can recognize the true value and meaning of their work. The meaning and depth of this work are powerful and profound.

REFERENCES

Allegreta, G. (2005). Safety issues in pediatric patient-controlled analgesia. *Pediatric Pain Letter, 7*(2–3). Retrieved February 22, 2009, from http://childpain.org/ppl/issues/v7n2-3_2005/v7n2-3_allegretta.pdf

American Academy of Pain Medicine, American Pain Society, and American Society of Addiction Medicine. (2007). *Definitions related to the use of opioids to relieve pain.* Retrieved May 2, 2008, from http://www.cpmission.com

American Academy of Pediatrics Committee on Children with Disabilities. (2001). Counseling families who choose complementary and alternative medicine for their child with a chronic illness or disability. *Pediatrics, 107*(3), 598–601.

American Association on Intellectual and Developmental Disabilities (AAIDD). (2007, July 5). *AAIDD position statement: Caring at the end of life.* Retrieved February 22, 2009, from http://www.aamr.org/content_170.cfm?navID=31

American Association of Respiratory Care. (2007, December). AARC statement of ethics and professional conduct. Retrieved February 22, 2009, from http://www.aarc.org/resources/position_statements/ethics_detailed.html

American Nurses Association (ANA). (2004). *Intellectual and developmental disabilities nursing: Scope and standards of practice.* Silver Spring, MD: Author.

American Nurses Association (ANA). (2005). *Pain management nursing: Scope and standards of practice.* Silver Spring, MD: Author.

American Nurses Association (ANA). (2007). *Hospice and palliative care scope and standards of practice* (2nd ed.). Silver Spring, MD: Author.

American Nurses Association (ANA). (2008). *Guide to the code of ethics for nurses: Interpretation and application.* Silver Spring, MD: Author.

American Nurses Association (ANA) and Nursing Division of the American Association on Mental Retardation. (2004). *Intellectual and developmental disabilities nursing: Scope and standards of practice.* Silver Spring, MD: Author.

American Occupational Therapy Association Commission on Standards and Ethics (AOTA). (2005). Occupational therapy code of ethics. *American Journal of Occupational Therapy, 59,* 639–642.

American Physical Therapy Association (APTA). (2000, June). *Code of ethics.* Retrieved February 22, 2009, from http://www.apta.org

American Physical Therapy Association (APTA). (2003). *Standards of practice for physical therapy.* Retrieved April 26, 2008, from http://www.apta.org

American Society for Pain Management Nursing. (2006, June). *Authorized and unauthorized ("PCA by proxy") dosing of analgesic infusion pumps*. Retrieved February 22, 2009, from http://www.aspmn.org/Organization/documents/PCAbyProxy-final-EW_004.pdf

American Society of Interventional Pain Physicians. (2006). Opioid guidelines in the management of non-cancer pain. *Pain Physician, 9*, 1–40.

Applebaum, P. (2007). Assessment of patients' competence to consent to treatment. *New England Journal of Medicine, 357*, 1834–1840.

Barnes, P. M., Bloom, B., & Nahin, R. (2008, December 10). Complementary and alternative medicine use among adults and children (CDC National Health Statistics Report No. 12). *National Health Statistics Reports*.

Bodfish, J., Harper, V. N., Deacon, J. M., Deacon, J. R., & Symons, F. J. (2006). Issues in pain assessment for adults with severe to profound mental retardation. In T. Oberlander & F. J. Symons (Eds.), *Pain in children and adults with developmental disabilities* (pp. 173–192). Baltimore, MD: Paul H. Brookes.

Bodfish, J., Harper, V. N., Deacon, J., & Symons, F. (2001). *Identifying and measuring pain in persons with developmental disabilities: A manual for the pain and discomfort scale (PADS)*. Morganton, NC: Western Carolina Center Research Reports.

Bottos, S., & Chambers, C. (2006). The epidemiology of pain in developmental disabilities. In T. F. Oberlander & F. J. Symons (Eds.), *Pain in children and adults with developmental disabilities* (pp. 67–88). Baltimore, MD: Paul H. Brookes.

Breau, L. M., Camfield, C., Symons, F., Bodfish, J., Mackay, A., Finney, G. A., et al. (2003). Relation between pain and self-injurious behavior in nonverbal children with severe cognitive impairments. *Journal of Pediatrics, 142*(5), 498–503.

Breau, L. M., McGrath, P. J., Camfield, C., & Finley, G. A. (2000). Preliminary validation of an observational checklist for persons with cognitive impairments and inability to communicate verbally. *Developmental Medicine & Child Neurology, 42*, 609–619.

Breau, L., McGrath, P., Finley, A., & Camfield, C. (2004a). *Non-communicating children's pain checklist, postoperative version*. Retrieved April 21, 2008, from http://www.aboutkidshealth.ca/Shared/PDFs/AKH_Breau_post-op.pdf

Breau, L., McGrath, P., Finley, A., & Camfield, C. (2004b). *Non-communicating children's pain checklist, revised*. Retrieved April 21, 2008, from http://www.aboutkidshealth.ca/Shared/PDFs/AKH_Breau_everyday.pdf

Breau, L. M., McGrath, P. J., & Zabalia, M. (2006). Assessing pediatric pain and developmental disabilities. In T. F. Oberlander & F. J. Symons (Eds.), *Pain in children and adults with developmental disabilities* (pp. 149–172). Baltimore, MD: Paul H. Brookes.

Breau, L. M., Stevens, B., & Gruneau, R. E. (2006). Developmental issues in acute and chronic pain in developmental disabilities. In T. F. Oberlander & F. J. Symons (Eds.), *Pain in children and adults with developmental disabilities* (pp. 89–108). Baltimore: Paul H. Brookes.

Campbell, M. (2008). Treating distress at the end of life: The principle of double effect. *AACN Advanced Critical Care, 19*(3), 340–344.

Colatarci, S., & Nehring, W. M. (2002). Recognizing and tracking pain in children with developmental disabilities. *The Exceptional Parent, 32*(11), 69–72.

Dileo, C., & Brandt, J. (2008, April 23). Music therapy for end of life care. *Cochrane Database of Systematic Reviews* (2).

Emmerich, M. T. (2006). Community practice for adults. In I. L. Rubin & A. C. Crocker (Eds.), *Medical care of children and adults with developmental disabilities* (2nd ed., pp. 79–88). Baltimore, MD: Paul H. Brookes.

Fishman, L. N., & Bousvaros, A. (2006). Gastrointestinal issues. In I. L. Rubin & A. C. Crocker (Eds.), *Medical care for children and adults with developmental disabilities* (2nd ed., pp. 307–324). Baltimore, MD: Paul H. Brookes.

Friedman, S. L. (2006). End of life care. In L. Rubin & A. Crocker (Eds.), *Medical care of children and adults with developmental disabilities* (pp. 623–631). Baltimore, MD: Paul H. Brookes.

Hahn, J. E., & Cadogan, M. P. (2007). *A developmental approach to palliative and end of life care—handbook for trainers*. Los Angeles: UCLA School of Nursing.

Herr, K., Coyne, P., Key, T., Manworren, R., McCaffery, M., Merkel, S., et al. (2006). Pain assessment in the nonverbal patient: Position statement with clinical practice recommendations. *Pain Management Nursing, 7*(2), 44–52.

Hicks, C., von Baeyer, C., Spafford, P., van Korlaar, I., & Goodenough, B. (2001). The Faces Pain Scale, Revised: Toward a common metric in pediatric pain measurement. *Pain, 93*, 173–183.

Hodgkinson, I. L., Jindrich, M., Duhaut, P., Vadot, J. P., Metton, G., & Bérard, C. (2001). Hip pain in 234 non-ambulatory adolescents and young adults with cerebral palsy: A cross-sectional multicentre study. *Developmental Medicine & Child Neurology, 43*(12), 806–808.

Hospice and Palliative Nurses Association (HPNA). (2005, January). *HPNA position statement: The value of the nursing assistant in end of life care.* Retrieved February 23, 2009, from http://www.hpna.org/filemaintenance_view.aspx?ID=29

Hospice and Palliative Nurses Association (HPNA). (n.d.). *Hospice and Palliative Nurses Association: HPNA Position Statements.* Retrieved February 22, 2009, from http://www.hpna.org/DisplayPage.aspx?Title=Position%20Statements

International Association for the Study of Pain (IASP). (2002, April 20). *Definitions.* Retrieved February 22, 2009, from http://www.iasp-pain.org/AM/Template.cfm?Section=Pain_Definitions&Template=/CM/HTMLDisplay.cfm&ContentID=1728

Kennedy, C. H., & O'Reilly, M. F. (2006). Pain, health conditions, and problem behavior in people with developmental disabilities. In T. F. Oberlander & F. J. Symonds (Eds.), *Pain in children and adults with developmental disabilities* (pp. 121–138). Baltimore, MD: Paul H. Brookes.

King, A., Janicki, M., Kissinger, K., & Lash, S. (2004). *End of life care for people with developmental disabilities: The Last Passages project philosophy and recommendations.* Retrieved February 15, 2009, from http://www.albany.edu/aging/lastpassages

Kutner, J. S. M. (2008). Massage therapy versus simple touch to improve pain and mood in patients with advanced cancer: A randomized trial. *Annals of Internal Medicine, 149*(6), 369–379.

Liptak, G. O. (2001). Health status of children with moderate to severe cerebral palsy. *Developmental Medicine and Child Neurology, 43*(6), 364–370.

Liptak, G. S. (2005). Complementary and alternative therapies for cerebral palsy. *Mental Retardation and Developmental Disabilities Research Reviews, 11*(2), 156–163.

Long, A., & Guite, J. (2008). *Pediatric Pain Letter, 10*(3). Retrieved February 22, 2009, from http://www.childpain.org

Lynn, J., Shuster, J. L., & Kabcenell, A. (2000). *Improving care for the end of life: A sourcebook for health care managers and clinicians.* Santa Monica, CA: Rand Health.

McCaffery, M. (1968). *Nursing practice theories related to cognition, bodily pain, and man-environmental interactions.* Los Angeles: UCLA Students Store.

McIntyre, A. (2008). *Doctrine of double effect* (E. N. Zalta, Ed.). Retrieved February 22, 2009, from http://plato.stanford.edu/archives/fall2008/entries/double-effect/

National Cancer Institute. (2008a, May 29). *Aromatherapy and essential oils PDQ.* Retrieved February 23, 2009, from http://www.cancer.gov/cancertopics/pdq/cam/aromatherapy/HealthProfessional/page8

National Cancer Institute. (2008b, September 26). *Acupuncture PDQ.* Retrieved February 23, 2009, from http://www.cancer.gov/cancertopics/pdq/cam/acupuncture/HealthProfessional/page3

National Center for Complementary and Alternative Medicine. (2009, January 9). *What is complementary and alternative medicine?* Retrieved February 22, 2009, from http://nccam.nih.gov/health/whatiscam

National Consensus Project for Quality Palliative Care. (2004). *Clinical practice guidelines for quality palliative care.* Retrieved February 22, 2009, from http://www.nationalconsensusproject.org/Guideline.pdf

National Institute of Health (NIH) Senior Health. (2008). *What is CAM?* Retrieved February 22, 2009, from http://www.nihseniorhealth.gov/cam/whatiscam/01.html

Nehring, W. (Ed.). (2005). *Core curriculum for specializing in intellectual and developmental disabilities: A resource for nurses and other health care professionals.* Boston: Jones and Bartlett.

Northumberland Tyne & Wear NHS Trust and St. Oswald's Hospice. (2006). *DisDAT.* Retrieved February 22, 2009, from http://www.disdat.co.uk

Oberlander, T. F., & Symonds, F. J. (2006a). An introduction to the problem of pain in developmental disability. In T. F. Oberlander & F. J. Symonds (Eds.), *Pain in children and adults with developmental disabilities* (pp. 1–4). Baltimore, MD: Paul H. Brookes.

Oberlander, T. F., & Symonds, F. J. (Eds.). (2006b). *Pain in children and adults with developmental disabilities.* Baltimore, MD: Paul H Brookes.

Pary, R. J., El-Defrawi, M., Khan, I., Parvin, M., & Hatch-Warner, N. (2006). Depression. In I. L. Rubin & A. C. Crocker (Eds.), *Medical care for children and adults with developmental disabilities* (pp. 489–498). Baltimore: Paul H. Brookes.

Prommer, E. (2008, January). *Fast fact and concept #092: Patient controlled analgesia in palliative care.* Retrieved April 4, 2008, from http://www.eperc.mcw.edu/fastFact/ff_92.htm

Quinn, T. E. (2007, February 27). *Pain topics converting opioid analgesics, part II: Review of equianalgesic conversion calculators.* Retrieved April 23, 2008, from http://www.massgeneral.org/PainRelief/Pain%20Topics/Opioid_calculators_V3.07.pdf

Roane, H., Fisher, W., Call, N., & Kelley, M. (2006). Self-injury, aggression, and pica. In I. L. Rubin & A. C. Crocker (Eds.), *Medical care of children and adults with developmental disabilities* (2nd ed., pp. 498–510). Baltimore, MD: Paul H. Brookes.

Rubin, I. L. (2006). Complex medical problems. In *Medical care for children and adults with developmental disabilities* (2nd ed., pp. 591–602). Baltimore, MD: Paul H. Brookes.

Schwarz, J. K. (2004). The rule of double effect and its role in facilitating good end of life palliative care. *Journal of Hospice and Palliative Nursing, 6*(2), 125–133.

So, P., Jiang, Y., & Qin, Y. (2008, October 8). *Touch therapies for pain relief in adults.* Retrieved February 23, 2009, from http://www.cochrane.org/reviews/en/ab006535.html

Solodiuk, J., & Curley, M. A. (2003). Pain assessment in nonverbal children with severe cognitive impairments: The individualized numeric rating scale (INRS). *Journal of Pediatric Nursing 18*(4), 295–299.

Stallard, P., Williams, L., Lenton, S., & Vellman, R. (2001). Pain in cognitively impaired, noncommunicating children. *Archives of Disease in Childhood, 85,* 460–462.

Symonds, F., Shinde, S., & Gilles, E. (2008). Perspectives on pain and intellectual disability. *Intellectual Disability Research, 52*(4), 275–286.

Taddio, A., & Oberlander, T. F. (2006). Pharmacological management of pain in children and youth with significant neurological impairments. In T. F. Oberlander & F. J. Symons (Eds.), *Pain in children and adults with developmental disabilities* (pp. 193–214). Baltimore, MD: Paul H. Brookes.

Taketoma, C. K., Hodding, J. H., & Kraus, D. M. (Eds.). (2007). *Pediatric dosage handbook* (14th ed.). Hudson, OH: Lexi-Comp.

Texas Administrative Code Title 40 Chapter Rule §95.128. (2008). Retrieved May 2, 2008, from http://www.sos.state.tx.us/tac/

Tsao, J. C., & Zeltzer, L. (2005). Complementary and alternative medicine approaches for pediatric pain: A review of the state-of-the-science. *Evidence Based Complimentary and Alternative Medicine, 2*(2), 149–159.

University College London. (2003). *Paediatric pain profile.* Retrieved February 22, 2009, from http://www.pppprofile.org.uk

U.S. Food and Drug Administration. (n.d.). *MedWatch: The FDA safety information and adverse event reporting program.* Retrieved May 3, 2008, from http://www.fda.gov/medwatch/index.html

Voepel-Lewis, T., Malviya, S., Tait, A. R., Merkel, S., Foster, R., Krane, E., et al. (2008). A comparison of the clinical utility of pain assessment tools for children with cognitive impairment. *Pediatric Anesthesiology, 106*(1), 72–78.

Voepel-Lewis, T., Merkel, S., Tait, A., Trzcinka, A., & Malvia, S. (2002). Reliability of the Faces, Legs, Arms, Cry, Consolability Observational Tool as a measure of pain in children with cognitive impairment. *Pediatric Anesthesia, 95*(5), 1224–1229.

von Baeyer, C. (2001). *Pediatric pain sourcebook: The Faces Pain Scale, Revised (in English and French).* Retrieved February 22, 2009, from http://painsourcebook.ca/pdfs/pps92.pdf

von Gunten, C. (2005, August). *Fast fact and concept #008; morphine and hastened death.* Retrieved March 22, 2008, from http://www.eperc.mcw.edu/fastFact/ff_008.htm

Winter, S., & Kiely, M. (2006). Cerebral palsy. In I. Rubin & A. Crocker (Eds.), *Medical care for children and adults with developmental disabilities* (2nd ed., pp. 233–248). Baltimore, MD: Paul H. Brookes.

World Health Organization (WHO). (1990). *WHO's pain ladder*. Retrieved February 22, 2009, from http://www.who.int/cancer/palliative/painladder/en/index.html

World Health Organization (WHO). (1994). *Cancer pain relief* (2nd ed.). Geneva: Authors

World Health Organization (WHO). (2006). Pain associated with neurological disorders. In *Neurological disorders: Public health challenges* (pp. 127–140). Geneva: Author.

World Health Organization (WHO). (2009). *WHO palliative care*. Retrieved February 22, 2009, from http://www.who.int/cancer/palliative/en/

FURTHER READING

Abbatiello, G. (2005). End of life planning: Parenting a child with an intellectual disability. *The Exceptional Parent, 35*(11) 33–34.

Cavanaugh, P. E. (2004). At home: Care options at the end of life. *The Exceptional Parent, 34*(12), 46–48.

Cavanaugh, P. E. (2005). History of end-of-life care for people with disabilities. *The Exceptional Parent, 35*(3), 61–64.

Center for Excellence in Aging Services. (2004, December). *End of life care for people with developmental disabiilties bibliograhy*. Retrieved February 22, 2009, from http://www.albany.edu/aging/lastpassages/lp-bibliography.htm#

Faulkner, L. R. (2007). *End of life care for persons with intellectual disabilities: The New York policies*. Retrieved February 22, 2009, from http://kennedyinstitute.georgetown.edu/inteldisabres/EID2007v10n2.pdf

Friedman, S. L., Choueri, R., & Gilmore, D. (2008). Staff carers' understanding of end of life care. *Journal of Policy and Practice in Intellectual Disabilities, 5*(1), 56–64.

Friedman, S. L., & Gilmore, D. (2007). Factors that impact resuscitation preferences for young people with severe developmental disabilities. *Intellectual and Developmental Disabilities, 45*(2), 90–97.

Hadden, K. L., & vonBaeyer, C. L. (2002). Pain in children with cerebral palsy: Common triggers and expressive behaviors. *Pain, 99*, 281–288.

Hospice Foundation of America. (2006). *Pain management at the end of life: Bridging the gap between knowledge and practice* (K. J. Doka, Ed.). Washington, DC: Hospice Foundation of America.

Kingsbury, L. A. (2004). Person centered planning in the communication of end of life wishes. *The Exceptional Parent, 34*(11), 44–47.

Lohiya, G.-S., Tan-Figueroa, L., & Crinella, F. (2003). End of life care for a man with developmental disabilities. *Journal of the American Board of Family Practice Medicine, 16* (1), 58–62.

McKearnan, K. A., Kieckhefer, G. M., Engel, J. M., Jensen, M. P., & Labyak, S. (2004). Pain in children with cerebral palsy: A review. *Journal of Neuroscience Nursing, 36*(5), 252–259.

Rader, R. (2003). Last passages. *The Exceptional Parent, 33*(6), 6–7.

Rosello, A. H. (2007, June). *Understanding chronic pain and disability in young people: A study with Catalan school children*. Retrieved May 15, 2008, from http://www.tesisenxarxa.net/TESIS_URV/AVAILABLE/TDX-1207107-174513//TESIS_AHR1.pdf

Solomon, M. Z. (2005). New and lingering controversies in pediatric end-of-life care. *Pediatrics, 116*(4), 872–883.

Tuffrey-Wijne, I. (2003). The palliative care needs of people with intellectual disabilities: A literature review. *Palliative Medicine, 17*(1), 55–62.

Tuffrey-Wijne, I., Bernal, J., Butler, G., Hollins, S., & Curfs, L. (2007). Using nominal group technique to investigate the views of people with intellectual disabilities on end of life care provision. *Journal of Advanced Nursing, 58*(1), 80–89.

Postscript

SANDRA L. FRIEDMAN AND DAVID T. HELM

Each of the chapters in this book provides insight into the current state of care and support at the end of life for people with intellectual and developmental disabilities (IDD). Here we hope to pull together some of these ideas to help generate additional discussions on how to better the end-of-life process. As with all social phenomena, patterns evolve at variable rates with unexpected occurrences shaping societies' views and practices. Underlying the expected and unexpected social landscape is the push to champion the rights, needs, and dignity of all people in every aspect of the life cycle, including death.

This book has informed us that despite the social progress that has been made over the years, people with disabilities continue to face situations in which they are not accepted as being equal. At times they are stigmatized to the extent that they are considered second-class citizens and, as such, they are not entitled to the same benefits as the rest of society. These negative images are often unconsciously integrated into the thoughts and words of even those who consider themselves rather progressive. Negative images in the media, jokes, slips of the tongue, and teasing continue to occur, usually without intent or even realization of their offensive connotations or effects. Language serves as a reflection of our ideas and beliefs—hence the importance of "person-first" language that is more than just politically correct verbiage.

As we have become more sensitized to the issues faced by people with disabilities, there have been many positive changes to laws and policies that affect their lives, including end-of-life practices. However, this publication has underscored the need for review of a number of national, state, and local policies as they relate to people with IDD at the end of life. For example, the Home and Community Based (HCBS) Medicaid waiver programs, which affect issues related to health and end-of-life care, would benefit from more national uniformity. Medicaid and Medicare policies should be reviewed in all states in order to better meet the needs of patients at the end of life. Inadequate policies and regulations have been cause for additional burdens to some people with disabilities at the end of life, at times forcing relocation just when consistency of care is crucial. Bureaucratic oversight of death may also result in treating the end of life as a sentinel event rather than a natural process, adding extra stress to those who were involved in the care of the person who died.

While we were reminded of the importance of actively involving people with disabilities in decisions that affect them, the scope of this book did not lend itself to fully discussing the crucial role of the self-advocate movement. In this struggle for social change, self-advocates can and do make a difference in how society treats people with disabilities. They play an essential part in heightening our awareness of the issues, speaking up regarding these individuals' civil rights, and articulating issues that are important to them. A number of authors have provided guidance about how to determine what is essential for each individual. We must be wary of thinking that all people with disabilities or self-advocates have the same wishes and needs, as individual differences and desires are relevant to all people.

We also cannot assume that just because people may have significant disabilities and/or are dependent on medical technology, that they necessarily have a poor quality of life or are suffering. Assumptions of suffering and futility have been revealed as being subjective words that are widely misinterpreted. Simple comments, such as referring to someone as "suffering from cerebral palsy" or "wheelchair bound," help perpetuate these misperceptions. New technologies and innovative procedures and protocols will continue to emerge, and they will likely have a continued effect on life span and the way in which people live and engage with their communities. This increase in life span among people with disabilities has been another recurring theme. People are receiving better medical care, with advances in treatments and medical management. These potential improvements in care pose new options for them. Within the changes that confront us in our professional work, we must protect and acknowledge the importance of the autonomy of individuals to make choices. However, autonomy does not mean that we are free to make decisions that threaten respect for the value of human life. Conversely, in making autonomous decisions, one also runs the risk of wanting to do everything to fight the inevitability of imminent death. There does come a time when respect for an individual may mean knowing when to stop intensive and intrusive treatments.

It is important that access to care be readily available in a way that is responsive to the needs of people with IDD. While most medical issues for people with IDD are similar to those of the general population, people with disabilities may require extra time and support to process information and express themselves. They also may require additional social supports for medical appointments and procedures. Access may refer to having medical care providers available who will take a person's health care coverage, often in the form of public assistance. Access may refer to physically being able to get to an appointment, as well as having adequate and appropriate space to be comfortable within the office itself for the necessary examinations and testing. Access may also refer to having physicians available within patients' geographical locations who are knowledgeable and well versed in the needs of people with disabilities.

Unfortunately, too many medical providers—including medical students, residents, fellows, primary care providers, medical specialists, nurses, physician assistants, and nurse practitioners—have limited formal training or even exposure to the needs of people with IDD. With more people with IDD residing in the community, it is important for primary care providers to be able to address the needs of people with disabilities. However, of great concern is the fact that there is a critical shortage of primary care providers in the United States, with the prospect that things will likely worsen, particularly for adults seeking medical care (Bodenheimer, 2006; American College of Physicians, 2008). More graduating medical students plan to pursue medical specialty careers, resulting in a critical shortage of primary care providers and no apparent solution to this problem is in sight. In addition, physicians who do provide primary care are often uncomfortable discussing potential life-threatening situations and death with their patients in nonacute situations. Waiting until a critical episode is not the best time to initially broach these discussions with a person who has chronic medical conditions, including those with IDD.

The Medical Home—as endorsed by the American Academy of Pediatrics (AAP), American Academy of Family Physicians (AAFP), American College of Physicians (ACP), and the American Osteopathic Association (AOA)—seems to provide a natural fit to meet the many medical needs of people with IDD, including end-of-life care (AAFP, AAP, ACP, and AOA, 2007). It is a model of care that is concerned with the whole person, emphasizing community-based care, quality, and safety. The Medical Home provides coordinated, physician-directed care that is comprehensive and integrated with other agencies and health systems. A patient is cared for within the context of his or her family, community, and culture, with emphasis on safety, quality, and accessibility (Homer et al., 2008). This model of care has been lauded as being particularly appropriate for individuals with special health care needs, which are usually complex and ongoing. However, medical and nonmedical care providers need to be reimbursed fairly with adequate and appropriate available resources. It is important for providers to be versed in how to make sound decisions from medical, legal, and ethical standpoints, as well as when to obtain outside assistance from experts in ethics and law. One size does not fit all—no matter the level of cognitive functioning; thus cultural differences and beliefs are critical factors to consider in the care of all people, including people with disabilities.

Consideration of these differences is also relevant after someone dies. When we think about grief and bereavement in the context of people with IDD, we often think about how families cope with the loss of their loved one. In this book, we have been informed about the real and varied emotional responses, as well as the spiritual needs, of people with disabilities when faced with their own life-threatening illness or condition. Similarly, people with IDD experience losses of their parents, roommates, caregivers, companions, and friends. While grief and bereavement may be articulated and manifested differently at times, it should be identified and addressed expeditiously and with sensitivity. People with IDD should be able to feel safe in their surroundings and comfortable in expressing their emotions. Most important is understanding that people with IDD go through a grief process like anyone else who has lost someone close to them.

Just as funding for support of comprehensive and relevant end-of-life care for people with IDD is needed, so is access to educational materials, training, and support for caregivers. There are many resources and curricula available, both hard copy and electronic. However, it is unclear how often they are accessed and used by providers and agencies. The unique needs of people with IDD call for, at times, modification of some of the resources available for the general population. In addition to the multiple resources for direct-care providers regarding palliative care and pain management provided in this book, the National Center for the Medical Home Initiative for Children (American Academy of Pediatrics, 2008) also provides resources for the practitioner regarding palliative care and end-of-life issues. It is important for practitioners to avail themselves of resources to assist them to engage in timely discussions with their patients and their patients' families regarding their preferences and goals for interventions in the event of an acute, serious, or potentially life-threatening episode. Similarly, we must be cognizant of those who suggest that structured curricula alone do not necessarily result in significant improvement in care (Himelstein, 2006). Certainly, improvements can be made toward educating providers about IDD and end-of-life care in general, as well as improvements of similar resources for people with IDD. Ongoing experiential support and education relating to particular situations provides an added element to the process of learning how to care for people at the end of life. Caregivers also benefit from programs that provide emotional support. Caring for a dying family member or patient can be rewarding yet difficult. Nonfamily providers also have emotional responses to the stress of the care and the death of a patient, which should be addressed and supported with adequate resources.

All in all, we need a more compassionate society that treats people equally, including those with IDD. Appropriate policies and legislation need to be enacted that support end-of-life care that is just, equitable, humane, and sensible. In so doing, more people will have access to care within their home community. Readily available medical and social services also may help patients and their families avoid higher cost hospital or nursing home care. It has been said that a society can be judged by how it treats it most vulnerable members. Our society has made many gains over the years, but it still has a way to go.

References

American Academy of Family Practice, American Academy of Pediatrics, American College of Physicians, and American Osteopathic Association. (2007). *Joint principles of the patient-centered medical home*. Retrieved March 27, 2009, from http://www.medicalhomeinfor.org/

American Academy of Pediatrics. (2008). National Center for the Medical Home Initiative. *Palliative care tools for providers*. Retrieved August 26, 2009, from http://www.medicalhomeinfo.org/tools/palliative%20care.html

American College of Physicians. (2008). Achieving a high-performance health care system with universal access: What the United States can learn from other countries. *Annals of Internal Medicine, 148*, 55–75.

Bodenheimer, T. (2006). Primary care—will it survive? *New England Journal of Medicine, 355*, 861–864.

Himelstein, B. P. (2006). Palliative care for infants, children, adolescents, and their families. *Journal of Palliative Medicine, 9*, 163–181.

Homer, C. J., Klatka, K., Romm, D., Kuhlthau, K., Bloom, K., Newcheck, P., et al. (2008). A review of the evidence for the medical home for children with special health care needs. *Pediatrics, 122*, e922–e937.

About the Editors

Sandra L. Friedman, MD, MPH, MS. Sandra Friedman is section head of Neurodevelopmental and Behavioral Pediatrics at the Children's Hospital (TCH) in Denver, Colorado, and associate professor of Pediatrics at the University of Colorado Denver School of Medicine. She is a developmental pediatrician who has been involved in developmental assessment and management of children with a wide range of developmental problems and special health care needs, formerly at the Developmental Medicine Center at Children's Hospital Boston (CHB) and currently at the Child Development Unit at TCH. She functioned as director of the Neurodevelopmental Disabilities residency program at CHB and Harvard Medical School. She also was director of pediatric training for the Leadership Education in Neurodevelopmental Disabilities (LEND) program and a member of the Ethics Advisory Committee. Dr. Friedman has served as medical director of Seven Hills Pediatric Center, caring for children and youth with severe intellectual and developmental disabilities and complex medical problems. She was president of the Medicine Division of the American Association on Intellectual and Developmental Disabilities (AAIDD) and currently is a member of their board of directors.

David T. Helm, PhD. David Helm is director of the Leadership Education in Neurodevelopmental Disabilities, or LEND program, at the Institute for Community Inclusion, a University Center of Excellence in Developmental Disabilities (ICI/UCEDD), dually situated at the University of Massachusetts Boston and at CHB. He is also an adjunct lecturer at Harvard School of Public Health and Bentley University and affiliated with Boston College and Boston University. Dr. Helm is a medical sociologist and has worked in the field of developmental disabilities for over 35 years. He has partnered with families in developing programs in their homes, directed a center for youth transitioning from school to employment, and trained graduate students and professionals across disciplines who are entering the field. Dr. Helm has been director of training, program coordinator, and now director for the LEND program at CHB since 1990. He continues to serve on various boards and advisory committees in the community and has been an AAIDD member for many years.

The editors have in part been supported by funds from the U.S. Department of Health and Human Services, Maternal and Child Health Bureau (Grant No. T73MC00020), and the Administration on Developmental Disabilities (Grant No. 90DD0575).

Contributors

Katherine Ast, LCSW · Assistant Director, Clinical Services, Residential Administration, Anixter Center, Chicago, Illinois

Anne-Marie Barron, PhD, PMHCNS-BC · Associate Professor and Associate Chair for Undergraduate Nursing, Simmons College; Psychiatric Clinical Nurse Specialist, Inpatient Oncology & Bone Marrow Transplant Unit, Massachusetts General Hospital, Boston, Massachusetts

Lauren C. Berman, MSW, LICSW · Director of Social Work, Institute for Community Inclusion/Leadership Education in Neurodevelopmental Disabilities Program, Children's Hospital Boston; Adjunct Faculty, Boston University School of Social Work and Simmons College School of Social Work, Boston, Massachusetts

Reva Bess · Manager, Roscoe CILA, Anixter Center, Chicago, Illinois

Anne L. Botsford, LMSW, PhD · Professor, Marist College, School of Social and Behavioral Sciences, Poughkeepsie, New York

Jeffrey P. Burns, MD, MPH · Chief, Division of Critical Care Medicine, and Co-Chair, Ethics Committee, Children's Hospital Boston; Associate Professor of Anesthesia and Pediatrics, Harvard Medical School, Boston, Massachusetts

Marykay Castrogiovanni · Assistant Director, Residential Administration, Anixter Center, Chicago, Illinois

Patricia Conway, RN, BA, CDDN · Medical Services Coordinator, Residential Administration, Anixter Center, Chicago, Illinois

David Coulter, MD · Associate Professor of Neurology, Harvard Medical School, Department of Neurology, Children's Hospital Boston, Massachusetts

Kenneth J. Doka, PhD · Professor of Gerontology, the College of New Rochelle; Senior Consultant, the Hospice Foundation of America, New Rochelle, New York

Sari Edelstein, PhD, RD · Associate Professor of Nutrition, Simmons College, Boston, Massachusetts

Marc Emmerich, MD · Developmental Disabilities Internal Medicine, Boston's Community Medical Group, Boston Medical Center, Boston, Massachusetts

Bill Gaventa, MDiv · Associate Professor and Director, Community and Congregational Supports, the Elizabeth M. Boggs Center on Developmental Disabilities, UMDNJ–Robert Wood Johnson Medical School, New Brunswick, New Jersey

Tawara Goode, MA · Assistant Professor and Director, National Center for Cultural Competence, University Center for Excellence in Developmental Disabilities, Center for Child and Human Development, Georgetown University Medical Center, Washington, DC

John J. Hardt, PhD · Assistant Professor, Neiswanger Institute for Bioethics and Health Policy, Loyola University Chicago Stritch School of Medicine, Chicago, Illinois

Julie Hauer, MD · Assistant Professor of Pediatrics, Director, Pediatric Palliative Care, University of Minnesota, Children's Hospital Gillette/Children's Specialty Healthcare, St. Paul, Minnesota

Betsy Bradford Johnson, MA, MEd · Consultant in Health Care Ethics; Affiliated with the Commonwealth of Massachusetts Department of Developmental Services, Central-West Region, Palmer, Massachusetts; Affiliated with the Renal Transplant Program of Baystate Medical Center, Springfield, Massachusetts

Angela King, MSSW · Vice President of Aging Services, Volunteers of America, Alexandria, VA

Leigh Ann C. Kingsbury, MPA · Gerontologist, InLeadS Consulting and Training, New Bern, North Carolina

So Yun Kwan, MSW, LICSW · Medical/Surgical Intensive Care Unit, Children's Hospital Boston, Boston, Massachusetts

Judith M. Levy, MSW, MA · Acting Director, Maryland Center for Developmental Disabilities; Director, Department of Social Work; Chair, Ethics Committee, Kennedy Krieger Institute, Baltimore, Maryland

Vanessa Ludlow, RD, LDN · Education Coordinator, Clinical Nutrition Service, and Clinical Nutrition Specialist, Children's Hospital Boston, Boston, Massachusetts

Zana Marie Lutfiyya, PhD · Professor and Associate Dean, Graduate Programs, Faculty of Education, University of Manitoba, Winnipeg, Manitoba

Patricia Maloof, PhD · Medical Anthropologist and Senior Consultant, National Center for Cultural Competence, Center for Child and Human Development, Georgetown University, Washington, DC

Christine Mitchell, RN, MS, MTS · Director, Office of Ethics, and Co-Chair, Ethics Committee, Children's Hospital Boston; Associate Director of Clinical Ethics, Division of Medical Ethics, Harvard Medical School, Boston, Massachusetts

Patricia N. Rissmiller, RN, DNSc, C-PNP · Associate Professor and Coordinator, Pediatric Nurse Practitioner Program, Simmons College · Boston, Massachusetts

Teresa A. Savage, PhD, RN · Assistant Professor of Research, Maternal-Child Nursing, College of Nursing, University of Illinois at Chicago; Consultant, Donnelley Family Disability Ethics Program, Rehabilitation Institute of Chicago, Chicago, Illinois

Karen D. Schwartz · Doctoral Candidate · Faculty of Education, University of Manitoba, Winnipeg, Canada

Peter J. Smith, MD, MA · Assistant Professor, Section of Developmental and Behavioral Pediatrics, MacLean Center for Clinical Medical Ethics, University of Chicago Medical Center, Chicago, Illinois

Amy Stevens, MSN, CPNP · Pediatric Nurse Practitioner, Seven Hills Pediatric Center, Groton, Massachusetts

Maureen van Stone, Esq, MS · Director, Project HEAL, Kennedy Krieger Institute, Baltimore, Maryland

Robert M. Veatch, PhD · Professor, Medical Ethics, Kennedy Institute of Ethics, Georgetown University, Washington, DC

Sharon Weston, MS, RD, LDN · Clinical Dietitian Specialist, Children's Hospital Boston, Boston, Massachusetts

Index

Note: The *italicized f* and *t* following page numbers refer to figures and tables, respectively.